Statistical Methods for Survival Trial Design

With Applications to Cancer Clinical Trials Using R

Chapman & Hall/CRC Biostatistics Series

Shein-Chung Chow, Duke University of Medicine
Byron Jones, Novartis Pharma AG
Jen-pei Liu, National Taiwan University
Karl E. Peace, Georgia Southern University
Bruce W. Turnbull, Cornell University

Recently Published Titles

Repeated Measures Design with Generalized Linear Mixed Models for Randomized Controlled Trials
Toshiro Tango

Clinical Trial Data Analysis Using R and SAS, Second Edition
Ding-Geng (Din) Chen, Karl E. Peace, Pinggao Zhang

Clinical Trial Optimization Using R
Alex Dmitrienko, Erik Pulkstenis

Cluster Randomised Trials, Second Edition
Richard J. Hayes, Lawrence H. Moulton

Quantitative Methods for HIV/AIDS Research
Cliburn Chan, Michael G. Hudgens, Shein-Chung Chow

Sample Size Calculations in Clinical Research, Third Edition
Shein-Chung Chow, Jun Shao, Hansheng Wang, Yuliya Lokhnygina

Randomization, Masking, and Allocation Concealment
Vance Berger

Statistical Topics in Health Economics and Outcomes Research
Demissie Alemayehu, Joseph C. Cappelleri, Birol Emir, Kelly H. Zou

Applied Surrogate Endpoint Evaluation Methods with SAS and R
Ariel Alonso, Theophile Bigirumurame, Tomasz Burzykowski, Marc Buyse, Geert Molenberghs, Leacky Muchene, Nolen Joy Perualila, Ziv Shkedy, Wim Van der Elst

Medical Biostatistics, Fourth Edition
Abhaya Indrayan, Rajeev Kumar Malhotra

Self-Controlled Case Series Studies: A Modelling Guide with R
Paddy Farrington, Heather Whitaker, Yonas Ghebremichael Weldeselassie

Bayesian Methods for Repeated Measures
Lyle D. Broemeling

Modern Adaptive Randomized Clinical Trials: Statistical and Practical Aspects
Oleksandr Sverdlov

Medical Product Safety Evaluation: Biological Models and Statistical Methods
Jie Chen, Joseph Heyse, Tze Leung Lai

Statistical Methods for Survival Trial Design: With Applications to Cancer Clinical Trials Using R
Jianrong Wu

For more information about this series, please visit: https://www.crcpress.com/go/biostats

Statistical Methods for Survival Trial Design

With Applications to Cancer Clinical Trials Using R

Jianrong Wu

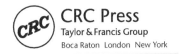

CRC Press
Taylor & Francis Group
Boca Raton London New York

CRC Press is an imprint of the
Taylor & Francis Group, an **informa** business

A CHAPMAN & HALL BOOK

CRC Press
Taylor & Francis Group
6000 Broken Sound Parkway NW, Suite 300
Boca Raton, FL 33487-2742

First issued in paperback 2020

© 2018 by Taylor & Francis Group, LLC
CRC Press is an imprint of Taylor & Francis Group, an Informa business

No claim to original U.S. Government works

Version Date: 20180509

ISBN-13: 978-0-367-73432-9 (pbk)
ISBN-13: 978-1-138-03322-1 (hbk)

Library of Congress Cataloging-in-Publication Data

Names: Wu, Jianrong, author.
Title: Statistical methods for survival trial design : with applications to cancer clinical trials using R / Jianrong Wu.
Description: Boca Raton : Taylor & Francis, 2018. | Includes bibliographical references and index.
Identifiers: LCCN 2018008225 | ISBN 9781138033221 (hardback)
Subjects: LCSH: Clinical trials--Statistical methods. |
Cancer--Research--Methodology. | Medicine--Research--Methodology. | R
(Computer program language)
Classification: LCC R853.C55 W8 2018 | DDC 610.72/4--dc23
LC record available at https://lccn.loc.gov/2018008225

**Visit the Taylor & Francis Web site at
http://www.taylorandfrancis.com**

**and the CRC Press Web site at
http://www.crcpress.com**

Contents

Preface

The clinical trial has become a major research tool for developing advanced cancer treatments. In recent years, the pharmaceutical industry, hospitals, and other research centers have been increasingly active in conducting cancer clinical trials with time-to-event endpoints. Statistical methods for designing and monitoring such trials have been available for many years, and a number of books have addressed this topic, including those by Chow et al. (2003), Julious (2010), Cook and DeMets (2008), Jennison and Turnbull (2000), and Proschan et al. (2006). However, as none of these books was written specifically to address the design and monitoring of survival clinical trials, they contain only limited material on that topic. For example, in the book by Julious, only one chapter discusses sample size calculation under the exponential model and proportional hazards model, and some of the presented approaches to sample size calculation and adjusting for loss to follow-up are inappropriate. The book by Chow et al. is also limited with regard to its discussion of the exponential model, and its presentation of the method of Lakatos for complex survival trial design not only lacks sufficient detail but also contains errors. The book by Jennison and Turnbull is an excellent reference for group sequential trial design, but its coverage of survival trial design is limited to a single chapter.

Cancer treatment has progressed dramatically in recent decades, such that it is now common to see a cure or long-term survival in a significant proportion of patients with various types of cancer, e.g., breast cancer, non-Hodgkin lymphoma, leukemia, prostate cancer, melanoma, or head and neck cancer (Ewell and Ibrahim, 1997). Until now, however, the principles of designing survival trials in which a proportion of the participants are expected to be cured have not been published in any book or implemented in any commercially available software.

This book is intended to provide a comprehensive introduction to the most commonly used methods for survival trial design and monitoring and to highlight some recent developments in the area. I hope this book will serve as a reference book for researchers conducting clinical trials with survival endpoints and for statisticians designing survival clinical trials for the pharmaceutical industry, hospitals, or other cancer research centers. It may also serve as a textbook for graduate students in the biostatistics field who wish to learn survival analysis and/or acquire basic knowledge of clinical trial design and sample size calculation.

The main focus of this book is on the methodology of sample size calculation, and clinical trial design and monitoring are illustrated using data from real cancer clinical trials. The book has 12 chapters. Chapter 1 introduces the general and statistical aspects of cancer survival trial design. Chapter 2 introduces several parametric survival distributions that are commonly used for trial design, along with basic methods for survival data analysis, including parametric maximum likelihood estimation, nonparametric Kaplan-Meier estimation, the log-rank test, and the semiparametric Cox regression model. Chapter 3 presents basic convergence concepts, counting processes, martingales, and the martingale central limit theorem (without giving the proof). Those readers who are interested only in applications can bypass this chapter. In Chapter 4, we first introduce the sample size calculation under the Weibull model, considering the exponential model as a special case. In Chapter 5, three widely used sample size formulae, namely those of Schoenfeld, Rubenstein, and Freedman, are derived under the proportional hazards model. A precise formula and an exact formula are also derived in this chapter as extensions of the Schoenfeld formula. Chapter 6 discusses sample size calculation under the Cox regression model for adjusting covariates. Complex survival trial designs are discussed in detail in Chapter 7, which includes the Lakatos Markov chain model, along with an R code for sample size calculation. Sample size calculations under the proportional hazards cure model are discussed in Chapter 8. Chapter 9 presents a general group sequential procedure based on the sequential conditional probability ratio test developed by Xiong (1995) and Xiong et al. (2003). Group sequential trial design under the Weibull model and the proportional hazards model is discussed in Chapter 10. Chapter 11 introduces group sequential trial design using historical control data. The final chapter discusses some practical aspects of survival trial design, including sample size calculation under the competing risk model.

Each chapter is essentially self-contained. Thus, a reader interested in a particular topic need not read the entire book but can turn straight to the chapter of interest and use the formula and R code therein for the sample size calculation without knowing the details of how the formula is derived.

I have greatly benefited from many discussions with colleague Dr. Xiaoping Xiong regarding his sequential conditional probability ratio test. I give special thanks to Drs. Hua Liang, Lili Zhao, Liang Zhu, and Shengping Yang for their enthusiastic support in providing critical reviews and comments. I also thank Dr. Keith A. Laycock for providing scientific editing of the entire book. In addition, I thank St. Jude Children's Research Hospital and University of Kentucky for their support in this undertaking.

List of Figures

List of Tables

1

Introduction to Cancer Clinical Trials

A cancer clinical trial is a planned experiment involving cancer patients. Each trial is based on a limited number of patients who satisfy certain study inclusion/exclusion criteria. The goal is to make a decision about how a new treatment should be conducted in a general patient population who require the treatment in the future. Because cancer clinical trials involve human subjects, they must be conducted in a manner that meets current ethical standards. Before participating in a trial, patients or their legal guardian must sign an informed consent form. In the consent form, patients must be fully informed about the nature of the studies to be conducted, the research goals, the potential benefits, and possible risks.

Cancer clinical trials study the toxicity and efficacy of experimental cancer therapies through four phases of clinical trials, designated phase I to IV. A phase I trial is often a drug safety study. Usually, for an anticancer chemotherapy, both the toxicity and the efficacy increase as the drug dose level increases. Thus, a phase I trial is intended to define a dose with a maximum tolerable toxicity level through drug dose-escalation. The defined dose is called the maximum tolerated dose (MTD) and is further investigated in a phase II trial for safety and efficacy. Common designs of a phase I trial include the traditional 3+3 design (Kelly and Halabi, 2010), the rolling 6 design (Skolnik et al., 2008), or model-based dose-escalation designs, such as the continual reassessment method (CRM) (O'Quigley, et al., 1990) and escalation with overdose control (EWOC) (Babb et al., 1998). A phase II trial is usually a small-scale, single-arm study in which patients are treated with the experimental therapy only. The primary objectives of phase II trials are to determine the safety and primary efficacy of the experimental therapy and to see whether the new treatment has sufficient antitumor activity to warrant a further large-scale, randomized phase III study. The primary endpoint of a phase II trial is usually the tumor response to a frontline therapy. Disease relapse-free survival (RFS) or event-free survival (EFS) could also be the primary endpoint for a phase II trial, where RFS is defined as the time interval from date on study (or date of diagnosis) to disease relapse or last follow-up, and EFS is defined as the time interval from date on study (or date of diagnosis) to an event (relapse, progression, a second malignant neoplasm, or death) or last follow-up. If an experimental therapy is shown to have anticancer activity through a phase II trial, we proceed to a phase III trial. A phase III trial is usually a large-scale, randomized study to compare the efficacy of a new treatment (the experimental arm) to that of the best current standard therapy (the control arm). Patients are allocated to a treatment arm by a randomization procedure. The primary endpoint of a phase III trial is usually overall survival (OS) or EFS, where OS is defined as the time interval from the date of randomization to the date of death or last follow-up; and EFS is defined as the time interval from the date of randomization to the date of an event (relapse, progression, a second malignant neoplasm or death) or last follow-up; Phase IV trials further evaluate the effectiveness and long-term safety of a drug or treatment. They usually take place after the drug or treatment has been approved by the Food and Drug Administration (FDA) for standard use. Several hundred to several thousand subjects may participate in a phase III or phase IV trial.

1.1   General Aspects of Cancer Clinical Trial Design

Many aspects must be considered when designing a clinical trial. These include the idea for improving treatment, the study objectives, specific hypotheses, the treatment plan, patient eligibility criteria, the method of randomization and blinding, the sample size calculation and statistical analysis plan (ASP), protocol development, database issues, and trial monitoring for safety and ethics considerations (Piantadosi, 1997). To develop a clinical trial, we first need to define the study objectives, including one or more primary objectives and several secondary and exploratory objectives; to specify the eligibility criteria and treatment plan; to determine the magnitude of treatment difference (effect size) to be detected; to specify how treatment assignment will be accomplished via stratification and randomization; and to examine the historical data to identify the statistical model or distribution assumptions to be used for the sample size calculation. A well-designed clinical trial minimizes the variability of the evaluation and provides an unbiased estimation of the treatment effect by avoiding confounding factors. Randomization insures that each patient has an equal chance of receiving any of the treatments under study and generates comparable treatment groups that are alike in all important aspects except for the treatment each group receives.

1.1.1   Study Objectives

The research questions to be addressed in a clinical trial are summarized in the study objectives, which are classified as primary objectives, secondary objectives, and exploratory objectives according to the importance of the research questions. The primary endpoint in a phase III cancer clinical trial with a time-to-event endpoint is often OS or EFS. Feasibility and quality of life (QoL) could be the secondary objectives, and supportive care and pharmacokinetic (PK) studies may be the exploratory objectives.

1.1.2   Treatment Plan

A detailed plan that describes the patient's treatment is needed, and the treatment schedule and duration are prescribed in the study protocol. Different types of cancer trial have different treatment plans. In a phase III cancer clinical trial, there are two types of treatments; one is the standard treatment and the other is the experimental treatment. The standard treatment is the best treatment known for a specific type of cancer. As the clinical trials are completed, more knowledge is accumulated and standard treatments evolve. Experimental treatments are medical therapies intended to treat cancer by improving on standard treatments. A cancer treatment plan usually begins with induction chemotherapy, which is followed by local control with surgery and radiation and maintenance therapy.

1.1.3   Eligibility Criteria

In a cancer clinical trial, the investigators must specify the inclusion and exclusion criteria for the study. The inclusion criteria are characteristics that the prospective patients must have if they are to be included in the study, whereas the exclusion criteria are those characteristics that disqualify prospective patients from inclusion in the study. The inclusion and exclusion criteria may include factors such as age, sex, race, ethnicity, type and stage of disease, previous treatment history, and the presence or absence of other medical, psychosocial, or emotional conditions.

1.1.4   Statistical Considerations

The study protocol must specify clearly the statistical considerations relating to the trial design and analysis plan. The protocol often specifies the study objectives and the patient groups for each objective; defines the outcome variables; provides the sample size calculation or accrual and follow-up duration for the primary objectives; provides the interim analysis plan or stopping rules for futility and/or efficacy; and specifies the randomization and stratification procedure. Finally, the data management and data safety monitoring plans should also be included in the protocol.

1.2   Statistical Aspects of Cancer Survival Trial Design

1.2.1   Randomization

In general, a randomized trial is an essential tool for testing the efficacy of a treatment because randomization tends to produce comparable treatment groups with regard to known or unknown risk factors. A simple (complete) randomization (e.g., tossing a coin or using tables of random numbers) is completely unpredictable; however, it is not quite sufficient by itself to guarantee comparable treatment arms unless the sample size is large. In small or moderate-size studies, major imbalances in important patient characteristics can occur by chance, even with a randomization procedure. Thus, it is necessary to incorporate a stratification procedure for the randomization, particularly for a small and moderate-size study.

1.2.2   Stratification

Patient characteristics or risk factors incorporated into the randomization scheme to achieve balance are called stratification factors. Stratification factors should be those strongly associated with outcome (e.g., tumor response or survival). In general, we recommend using no more than three stratification factors in cancer clinical trials because too many strata will result in too few patients within each stratum and hence reduce the power of the trials. Stratified randomization is achieved by performing a separate randomization procedure within each stratum. For example, suppose that in a study, age and gender are the two most important stratification factors. To ensure a balance of age and gender between the two treatment groups, the study will be stratified on age (e.g., age < 10 vs. ≥ 10 years old) and (male vs. female) (two stratification factors, each with two levels), and a simple (or blocked) randomization will be performed within each of the four defined patient strata: age < 10 and male; age < 10 and female; age ≥ 10 and male; age ≥ 10 and female. Stratified randomization ensures not only that the numbers in the treatment groups are closely balanced within each stratum but also that the treatment groups are similar with respect to the important prognostic factors. The basic benefits of randomization include eliminating selection bias; balancing the study arms with respect to prognostic variables (known and unknown); and forming a basis for statistical tests. The ethics and feasibility of randomization must also be considered before designing a randomized trial.

1.2.3   Blinding

Human behavior is influenced by what we know or believe. In research, there is a particular risk of expectations influencing findings and leading to biased results. Blinding is usually used to try to eliminate such bias. For example, medical staff caring for patients in a randomized trial should be blinded to treatment allocation to minimize possible bias in patient management and in assessing disease status. A trial in which only the patient is blinded is called single-blinded trial. If neither the patient nor the clinician is aware of the treatment assignment, the trial is called a double-blinded trial. Sometimes, to avoid bias in the data analysis, the statistician is blinded to the outcome too.

TABLE 1.1: Hypothesis decision process

	Null Hypothesis	
Decision	True	False
Reject H_0	Type I error α	Correct $1 - \beta$
Accept H_0	Correct $1 - \alpha$	Type II error β

1.2.4 Sample Size Calculation

Clinical trials can be designed in many ways, but the type most frequently encountered is the comparative trial, in which two or more treatments are compared. The primary objective is usually represented by a hypothesis being tested for the primary endpoint. For the sample size calculation, the hypothesis is formulated as a null hypothesis and an alternative hypothesis. The null hypothesis, H_0, is that the effect of the experimental therapy on the outcome is no different from that of the control, whereas the alternative hypothesis, H_1, is that the effect of the experimental therapy on the outcome differs from that of the control. The determination of the sample size of a survival trial depends on the following factors: an estimate of the primary endpoint of interest in the control group (based on historical data, e.g., the 5-year survival probability); a clinically meaningful minimal effect size; the accrual period or accrual rate and duration of follow-up; the type I error or significance level α (the probability of rejecting the null hypothesis when the null is true, i.e., the false positive rate); and the type II error β (the probability of accepting the null hypothesis when the null is false, i.e., the false negative rate); where $1 - \beta$ is the power, which is the probability of rejecting the null hypothesis when the null is false. The two-way decision process is shown in Table 1.1 with the corresponding probabilities associated with each decision. Although it would be desirable to simultaneously minimize both the type I and type II errors, this is not possible. Thus, in a trial, the experimenter specifies a tolerable probability for a type I error α, which is usually chosen to be 0.01, 0.05, or 0.1, and a power $1 - \beta$, which is usually chosen to be 80%, 85%, or 90%, to determine the required sample size n that achieves the desired power $1 - \beta$.

The appropriate sample size for a clinical trial is a major component of the study design. Many other aspects of the clinical trial depend on the sample size, including how the trial will be organized and how many treatment centers are required, etc. Furthermore, selecting an appropriate sample size is crucial to the outcome of the clinical trial. If the sample size is too small to yield meaningful results, it puts patients at risk for no potential benefit. If the sample size is too large, it wastes resources, thereby jeopardizing the completion of the trial. Thus, it is necessary to calculate the sample size required for the study to detect a prespecified minimal clinically meaningful effect size with constrained type I error and power. The sample size calculation procedure consists of two important elements: the hypothesis of interest and the test statistic. First, the null and alternative hypotheses need to be specified. Second, a proper test statistic must be determined, and the asymptotic or exact distribution of the test statistic under the null and alternative must be derived. The sample size can then be evaluated with the pre-specified type I error α, power of $1 - \beta$, effect size, and other design parameters, such as the variance of the test statistic.

Suppose that, using a typical frequentist hypothesis-testing procedure, we wish to test the following one-sided hypothesis for the mean of a continuous outcome variable:

$$H_0 : \mu \leq \mu_0 \quad \text{vs.} \quad H_1 : \mu > \mu_0 \tag{1.1}$$

and the study is powered at an alternative $\mu = \mu_1 (> \mu_0)$.

Now, given the type I error α and power of $1 - \beta$ under the alternative $H_1 : \mu = \mu_1$ with an effect size $\omega = \mu_1 - \mu_0 > 0$, the sample size can be calculated based on the following assumptions. Assume that statistic U under the H_0 is asymptotically normal distributed with mean μ_0 and variance σ_0^2/n. Let $\hat{\sigma}^2$ be a consistent estimate of σ_0^2 under the null; then, a test statistic for testing the hypothesis (1.1) is given by

$$Z = \frac{\sqrt{n}(U - \mu_0)}{\hat{\sigma}} \xrightarrow{\mathcal{D}} N(0, 1),$$

where the symbol $\xrightarrow{\mathcal{D}}$ represents "convergence in distribution" and $N(0, 1)$ represents the standard normal distribution function with zero mean and unit variance, which is given by

$$\Phi(x) = \int_{-\infty}^{x} \frac{1}{\sqrt{2\pi}} e^{-\frac{u^2}{2}} du.$$

Thus, for a one-sided test, we reject H_0 if $Z > z_{1-\alpha}$, where $z_{1-\alpha}$ is the $1 - \alpha$ percentile of the standard normal distribution, that is, $z_{1-\alpha} = \Phi^{-1}(1 - \alpha)$.

Assume that under alternative $\mu = \mu_1$, $\hat{\sigma}^2$ converges in probability to σ^2; then, Z is asymptotically normal distributed with mean $\sqrt{n}\omega/\sigma$ and unit variance. Thus, the power $1 - \beta$ to detect an alternative $\mu = \mu_1$ satisfies the following equations:

$$
\begin{aligned}
1 - \beta &= P(Z > z_{1-\alpha}|H_1) \\
&= P\left(\frac{\sqrt{n}(U - \mu_0)}{\hat{\sigma}} > z_{1-\alpha}|H_1\right) \\
&\simeq P\left(\frac{\sqrt{n}(U - \mu_1)}{\hat{\sigma}} > z_{1-\alpha} - \frac{\sqrt{n}\omega}{\sigma}|H_1\right) \\
&\simeq \Phi\left(-z_{1-\alpha} + \frac{\sqrt{n}\omega}{\sigma}\right).
\end{aligned}
$$

It follows that

$$
(z_{1-\alpha} + z_{1-\beta})\sigma = \sqrt{n}\omega.
$$

Therefore, we obtain the sample size by solving n from the above equation as

$$
n = \frac{(z_{1-\alpha} + z_{1-\beta})^2\sigma^2}{\omega^2},
$$

where the (asymptotic) variance σ^2 can be estimated from historical data.

If we are interested in a two-sided hypothesis

$$
H_0 : \mu = \mu_0 \quad \text{vs.} \quad H_1 : \mu \neq \mu_0,
$$

we reject H_0 if $|Z| > z_{1-\alpha/2}$.

Then, the power to detect an alternative $\mu = \mu_1(\neq \mu_0)$ is

$$
\begin{aligned}
1 - \beta &= P(|Z| > z_{1-\alpha/2}|H_1) \\
&= P(Z > z_{1-\alpha/2}|H_1) + P(Z < -z_{1-\alpha/2}|H_1).
\end{aligned}
$$

If the study is expected to increase the mean so that $\omega = \mu_1 - \mu_0 > 0$, the probability of Z having a value less than $-z_{1-\alpha/2}$ will be small. That is, $P(Z < -z_{1-\alpha/2}|H_1) \simeq 0$. Therefore, the power of the study satisfies the following equations:

$$
\begin{aligned}
1 - \beta &= P(|Z| > z_{1-\alpha/2}|H_1) \\
&\simeq P\left(\frac{\sqrt{n}(U - \mu_1)}{\sigma} > z_{1-\alpha/2} - \frac{\sqrt{n}\omega}{\sigma}|H_1\right) \\
&\simeq \Phi\left(-z_{1-\alpha/2} + \frac{\sqrt{n}\omega}{\sigma}\right),
\end{aligned}
$$

which is equivalent to

$$
(z_{1-\alpha/2} + z_{1-\beta})\sigma = \sqrt{n}\omega.
$$

Thus, the required sample size n for a two-sided test can be solved from this equation as

$$
n = \frac{(z_{1-\alpha/2} + z_{1-\beta})^2\sigma^2}{\omega^2}.
$$

Hence, to calculate the sample size for a two-sided test, we can still use the sample size formula for a one-sided test if we replace α by $\alpha/2$.

There are several important steps in the sample size calculation. The key step is choosing an appropriate hypothesis of interest and a test statistic. The sample size calculation is related to a number of factors, such as the type I error, power, effect size, and design parameters. To make a connection among these factors, we need to derive the (asymptotic) distributions of the test statistic under the null and alternative hypotheses. Specifically, the sample size calculation procedure can be summarized as follows:

- Specify the null and alternative hypotheses of interest.

- Specify the minimal clinically meaningful effect size.

- Choose a test statistic

- Derive the asymptotic or exact distributions of the test statistic under the null and alternative hypotheses.

- Link the sample size to the type I error, power, effect size, and design parameters (e.g., variance) by using the distribution of the test statistic.

The type I error, power, sample size, effect size, and design parameters are related by the sample size formula. If only one of these elements is unknown, it can be determined from the others. In a sample size calculation, the hypothesis and test statistic are two key components to consider. If a different hypothesis of interest is considered or a different test statistic is chosen, the sample size formula may be different. A fundamental rule of sample size determination is that the method of calculation should be based on the planned method of analysis.

The sample size is often derived under the fixed alternative hypothesis. However, when the asymptotic distribution of the test statistic is difficult to derive under the fixed alternative, a local or contiguous alternative (the terms "local alternative" and "contiguous alternative" are used interchangeably) hypothesis can also be considered by assuming that the alternative value of the testing parameter is located at the local of the null value, that is, $H_1 : \mu_1 = \mu_{1n} = \mu_0 + n^{-1/2}b$, where $b < \infty$. When a local alternative is considered in the sample size calculation, the asymptotic distribution of the test statistic needs to be derived under the local alternative.

2

Survival Analysis

2.1 Survival Distribution

A cancer clinical trial is usually a planned experiment to study the survival of a group of cancer patients and make inferences regarding the general patient population. Each patient has a failure time after the patient is enrolled in the study. In general, the failure time of an individual is a nonnegative random variable T, which follows the survival distribution of the population. The survival distribution is defined by the probability that T exceeds a value of time t, that is,

$$S(t) = P(T > t), \quad 0 < t < \infty,$$

which is a right-continuous function and satisfies the following (Figure 2.1)

- $S(t) = 0$ if $t < 0$ and $S(0) = 1$

- $\lim_{t \to \infty} S(t) = 0$

- $S(t)$ is a monotonically decreasing function

The hazard function $\lambda(t)$ is defined as

$$\lambda(t) = \lim_{h \to 0+} P(t \le T < t + h | T \ge t)/h,$$

which specifies the instantaneous rate (risk or hazard) at which failures occur for subjects that are surviving at time t. $\lambda(t)h$ is the approximate probability that an individual will die in the interval $[t, t+h)$, conditional on that patient having survived to time t. The cumulative hazard function is given by

$$\Lambda(t) = \int_0^t \lambda(u)du.$$

The relationship between the survival distribution function and the cumulative hazard function is as follows:

$$S(t) = e^{-\Lambda(t)} = e^{-\int_0^t \lambda(u)du},$$

or equivalently,

$$\Lambda(t) = -\log S(t).$$

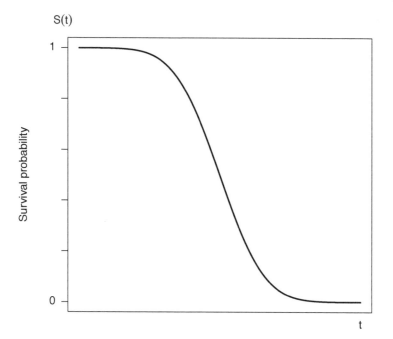

FIGURE 2.1: Graphic representation of the survival distribution function.

For a continuous failure time, the density function of T is given by

$$f(t) = -\frac{dS(t)}{dt}$$

and the hazard function

$$\lambda(t) = \frac{f(t)}{S(t)},$$

or equivalently,

$$f(t) = \lambda(t)S(t).$$

The mean and variance of the survival time T can be calculated by

$$
\begin{aligned}
\mathrm{E}(T) &= \int_0^\infty t f(t)dt, \\
\mathrm{Var}(T) &= E(T^2) - \{E(T)\}^2 \\
&= \int_0^\infty t^2 f(t)dt - \{E(T)\}^2.
\end{aligned}
$$

Because the survival distribution is usually skewed, the median survival time is used as a center measurement instead of the mean. The median survival time T is defined as

$$m(T) = S^{-1}(0.5),$$

where the inverse survival function $S^{-1}(\cdot)$ is defined as

$$S^{-1}(p) = \min\{t; S(t) < p\},$$

where $0 < p \leq 1$ (Figure 2.2).

The survival data obtained from clinical trials are usually modeled by parametric survival distributions. In the following subsections, several widely used parametric survival distributions are introduced and their characteristics are summarized.

2.1.1 Exponential Distribution

The failure time T follows an exponential distribution with a scale parameter $\lambda > 0$ if its probability density function is defined by

$$f(t) = \lambda e^{-\lambda t}, \quad t > 0,$$

and 0 otherwise. The survival distribution is given by

$$S(t) = e^{-\lambda t}, \quad t > 0,$$

the hazard function by

$$\lambda(t) = \lambda,$$

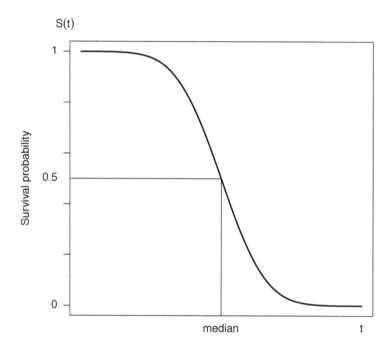

FIGURE 2.2: Graphic representation of the median survival time.

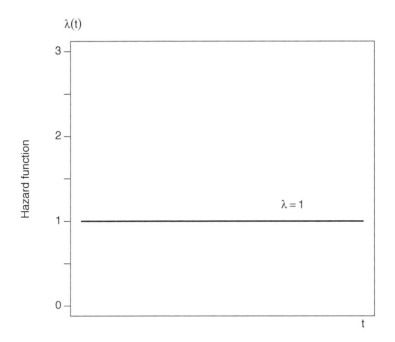

FIGURE 2.3: Hazard function of exponential distribution with hazard parameter λ.

and the cumulative hazard function by (Figure 2.3)

$$\Lambda(t) = \lambda t.$$

The mean and variance of the exponential distribution are

$$E(T) = \frac{1}{\lambda}, \quad \text{Var(T)} = \frac{1}{\lambda^2},$$

and the median survival time is given by $m = \lambda^{-1} \log(2)$.

The exponential distribution is the simplest and most important distribution in survival studies. Its hazard function is constant over time, that is, the hazard of failure at any time after the time origin is then the same, irrespective of the time elapsed.

2.1.2   Weibull Distribution

The failure time T follows the Weibull distribution, with a shape parameter $\kappa > 0$ and a scale parameter $\rho > 0$, if its probability density function is defined by

$$f(t) = \kappa \rho^\kappa t^{\kappa-1} e^{-(\rho t)^\kappa}, \quad t > 0,$$

and 0 otherwise. The survival distribution is given by

$$S(t) = e^{-(\rho t)^\kappa}, \quad t > 0,$$

and the hazard function by

$$\lambda(t) = \kappa \rho^\kappa t^{\kappa-1},$$

the cumulative hazard function by

$$\Lambda(t) = \rho^\kappa t^\kappa.$$

The mean, variance, and median of the Weibull distribution are as follows:

$$
\begin{aligned}
E(T) &= \rho^{-1} \Gamma(1 + \frac{1}{\kappa}), \\
\mathrm{Var(T)} &= \rho^{-2} \left[\Gamma(1 + \frac{2}{\kappa}) - \{\Gamma(1 + \frac{1}{\kappa})\}^2 \right], \\
m &= \rho^{-1} \{\log(2)\}^{1/\kappa},
\end{aligned}
$$

where $\Gamma(\cdot)$ is known as the function given by

$$\Gamma(x) = \int_0^\infty u^{x-1} e^{-u} du.$$

The hazard function of the Weibull distribution depends on the scale parameter ρ and the shape parameter κ. When the shape parameter $\kappa = 1$, the Weibull distribution reduces to the exponential distribution, and $\kappa < 1$ and $\kappa > 1$ correspond to the decreasing and increasing hazard functions, respectively (Figure 2.4).

2.1.3   Gamma Distribution

A random variable T is said to have a Gamma distribution, with a shape parameter k and a scale parameter λ, if its probability density function is given by

$$f(t) = \frac{\lambda^k t^{k-1} e^{-\lambda t}}{\Gamma(k)}, \quad t > 0,$$

where $k, \lambda > 0$. The gamma survival distribution is given by

$$S(t) = 1 - I_k(\lambda t), \quad t > 0,$$

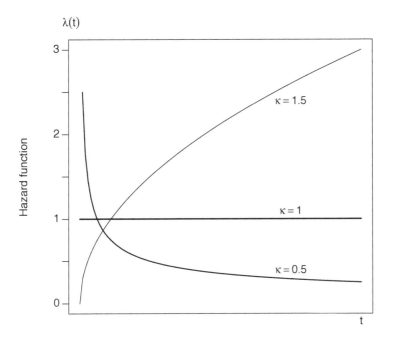

FIGURE 2.4: Hazard functions of the Weibull distribution with shape parameter $\kappa = 0.5, 1, 1.5$ and scale parameter $\rho = 1$.

where $I_k(\cdot)$ is known as the incomplete gamma function, given by

$$I_k(x) = \frac{1}{\Gamma(k)} \int_0^x u^{k-1} e^{-u} du,$$

the cumulative hazard function is given by

$$\Lambda(t) = -\log S(t),$$

and the hazard function by

$$\lambda(t) = \frac{f(t)}{S(t)}.$$

The hazard function $\lambda(t)$ increases monotonically if $k > 1$, decreases if $k < 1$, and is constant if $k = 1$ (exponential model) (Figure 2.5). The mean and variance of the gamma distribution are

$$E(T) = \frac{k}{\lambda} \quad \text{and} \quad \text{Var}(T) = \frac{k}{\lambda^2},$$

respectively.

2.1.4 Gompertz Distribution

The probability density function of a Gompertz distribution with parameters θ and γ is such that

$$f(t) = \theta e^{\gamma t} e^{-\frac{\theta}{\gamma}(e^{\gamma t} - 1)}, \quad t > 0,$$

where $\theta > 0$. The survival distribution is given by

$$S(t) = e^{-\frac{\theta}{\gamma}(e^{\gamma t} - 1)}, \quad t > 0,$$

the cumulative hazard function by

$$\Lambda(t) = \frac{\theta}{\gamma}(e^{\gamma t} - 1),$$

and the hazard function by

$$\lambda(t) = \theta e^{\gamma t}.$$

The median survival time of the Gompertz distribution is

$$m = \gamma^{-1} \log \left\{ 1 - \frac{\log(1+\pi)/2}{\log(\pi)} \right\},$$

where $\pi = e^{\theta/\gamma}$. For positive values of γ, the hazard increases and $S(\infty) = 0$. If $\gamma < 0$, then $S(\infty) = e^{\theta/\gamma} = \pi$. Thus, the Gompertz distribution with $\gamma < 0$ describes a population with a non-zero portion of cure (long-term survivors). The survival distribution $S(t)$ is discontinuous at $\gamma = 0$; that discontinuity is removable by defining $S(t) = \exp(-\theta t)$ when $\gamma = 0$. The Gompertz hazard function increases and decreases monotonically, according to whether $\gamma > 0$ or $\gamma < 0$, respectively (Figure 2.6).

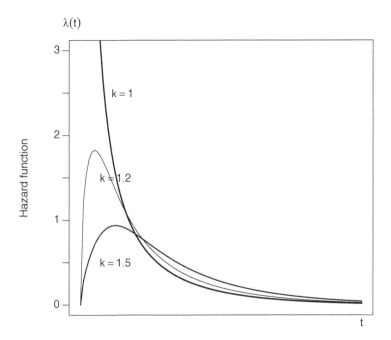

FIGURE 2.5: Hazard functions of the gamma distribution with shape parameter $k = 1, 1.2, 1.5$ and scale parameter $\lambda = 1$.

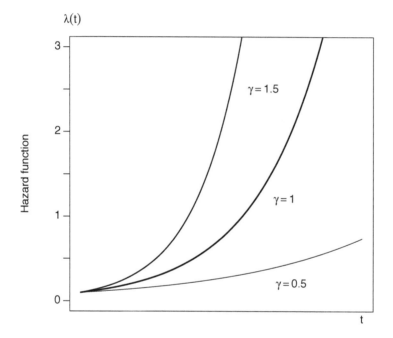

FIGURE 2.6: Hazard functions of the Gompertz distribution with shape parameter $\gamma = 0.5, 1, 1.5$ and scale parameter $\theta = 0.1$.

2.1.5 Log-Normal Distribution

A random variable T is said to have a log-normal distribution if $\log T$ has a normal distribution with mean μ and variance σ^2. The probability density function of T is given by

$$f(t) = \frac{1}{\sqrt{2\pi}\sigma t} e^{-\frac{(\log t - \mu)^2}{2\sigma^2}}, \quad t > 0,$$

where $\sigma > 0$. The log-normal survival distribution is given by

$$S(t) = 1 - \Phi\left(\frac{\log t - \mu}{\sigma}\right), \quad t > 0,$$

where $\Phi(\cdot)$ is the standard normal distribution function. The cumulative hazard function is given by

$$\Lambda(t) = -\log S(t),$$

and the hazard function by

$$\lambda(t) = \frac{f(t)}{S(t)}.$$

The hazard function $\lambda(t)$ increases to the maximum and then decreases to zero as t goes to infinity (Figure 2.7). The mean and variance of the log-normal distribution are

$$E(T) = e^{\mu + \sigma^2/2}$$

and

$$\text{Var}(T) = e^{2\mu + \sigma^2}(e^{\sigma^2} - 1),$$

respectively, and the median survival time is $m = e^\mu$.

2.1.6 Log-Logistic Distribution

A random variable T is said to have a log-logistic distribution, with shape parameter p and scale parameter λ, if its probability density function is given by

$$f(t) = \frac{p\lambda t^{p-1}}{(1 + \lambda t^p)^2}, \quad t > 0,$$

where p and $\lambda > 0$. The survival function is given by

$$S(t) = \frac{1}{1 + \lambda t^p},$$

the cumulative hazard function by

$$\Lambda(t) = \log(1 + \lambda t^p),$$

and the hazard function by

$$\lambda(t) = \frac{p\lambda t^{p-1}}{1 + \lambda t^p}.$$

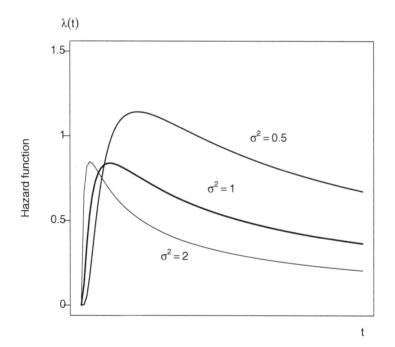

FIGURE 2.7: Hazard functions of the log-normal distribution with location parameter $\mu = 0$ and $\sigma^2 = 0.5, 1, 2$.

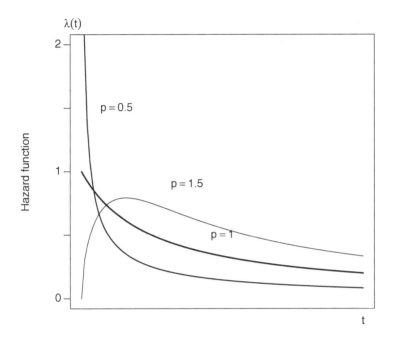

FIGURE 2.8: Hazard functions of the log-logistic distribution with shape parameter $p = 0.5, 1, 1.5$ and scale parameter $\lambda = 1$.

This hazard function decreases monotonically if $p \leq 1$, but if $p > 1$, the hazard function has a single mode (Figure 2.8). The median survival time of the log-logistic distribution is $m = \lambda^{-1/p}$.

2.2 Survival Data

In a typical cancer clinical trial, patients are not all recruited at exactly the same time but accrue over a period of months or years. After recruitment, the patients are followed up until they die or until the end of the study. Such recruitment is often referred to as "staggered entry." For each patient, we define the survival or failure time as the interval from the date of randomization to the date of death or the date of last follow-up. The actual survival times or failure times (the terms "survival time" and "failure time" are used interchangeably) will be observed for a number of patients, but some patients may be lost to follow-up and others will still be alive at the end of the study. Thus, the survival data from a clinical trial are usually subjected to right censoring, in which the trial ends before the event of interest (e.g., death) is observed in the study (terms "event," "death," and "failure" are also used interchangeably); for example, if patients who are still alive at the end of study, are lost to follow-up, or withdraw from the study are censored, this is known as right censoring. Patients who are still alive at the time the trial is terminated are administratively censored. Therefore, what can be observed is not the true failure time T but the minimum of the true failure time and the censoring time C, as well as an indication of whether the observed time was a true failure time (T) or a censored observation (C). Thus, the observed failure time is $X = T \wedge C$, and the failure indicator is $\Delta = I(T < C)$, where $x \wedge y = \min\{x, y\}$, and $I(A)$ is an indicator function of a set A. The right censored survival time for five patients in a clinical trial is illustrated in Figure 2.9, in which the time of entry to the trial is represented by a "$\bullet$", subjects 1, 2, and 4 died ("$\times$") during the course of study, subject 3 was lost to follow-up ("$\circ$") and subject 5 was still alive ("$\diamond$") at the end of study. Thus, the observed survival data $\{(X_i, \Delta_i), i = 1, \ldots, 5\}$ for the five patients are $(6, 1), (7, 1), (4, 0), (2.5, 1)$, and $(6, 0)$, respectively.

Survival time is nonnegative, and its distribution is generally not symmetrical. Thus, it is not reasonable to assume that the survival time follows a normal distribution. However, we can adopt an alternative distribution, as discussed in the previous section, for the survival data analysis.

Example 2.1 *Prostatic cancer trial*

A randomized controlled trial for prostatic cancer was begun in 1967 by the Veteran's Administration Cooperative Urological Research Group. The trial was double blind and two of the treatments in the trial were a placebo and 1.0 mg of diethylstilbestrol (DES), which were administered daily by mouth. The time origin of the study was the date on which a patient was randomized to a treatment, and the endpoint was the death from prostatic cancer. The primary objective of the trial is to determine if patients treated with DES survived longer than those treated with the placebo.

The full data set is given by Andrews and Herzberg (1985). A subset of 38 patients presenting with Stage III cancer is presented in Table 2.1, where the survival times are given in months (Collett, 2003). The observed survival time T, the censoring indicator Δ (status: 0-censored, 1-died from prostatic cancer) and treatment group (1-placebo, 2-DES), and prognostic factors, such as age at study entry, serum hemoglobin level, size of tumor, and Gleason index, are also recorded in Table 2.1. It was also of interest to determine if any of these covariates were associated with survival time. If so, the effect of these variables would need to be adjusted for the comparison of survival between two treatment groups. However, since this was a randomized trial,

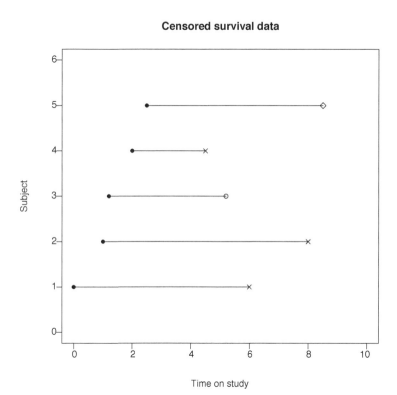

FIGURE 2.9: Graphic representation of accrual, follow-up, and censoring of survival data.

one should expect that the distributions of the prognostic factors would be balanced between the two treatment groups. Thus, comparing the difference in survival distributions between two treatment groups may still be valid without considering the known or unknown prognostic factors in the comparison.

TABLE 2.1: Survival times of patients with prostatic cancer in a randomized clinical trial to compare two treatments (placebo vs. DES)

Patient ID	Treatment group	Time	Status	Age	Serum level	Tumor size	Gleason index
1	1	65	0	67	13.4	34	8
2	2	61	0	60	14.6	4	10
3	2	60	0	77	15.6	3	8
4	1	58	0	64	16.2	6	9
5	2	51	0	65	14.1	21	9
6	1	51	0	61	13.5	8	8
7	1	14	1	73	12.4	18	11
8	1	43	0	60	13.6	7	9
9	2	16	0	73	13.8	8	9
10	1	52	0	73	11.7	5	9
11	1	59	0	77	12	7	10
12	2	55	0	74	14.3	7	10
13	2	68	0	71	14.5	19	9
14	2	51	0	65	14.4	10	9
15	1	2	0	76	10.7	8	9
16	1	67	0	70	14.7	7	9
17	2	66	0	70	16	8	9
18	2	66	0	70	14.5	15	11
19	2	28	0	75	13.7	19	10
20	2	50	1	68	12	20	11
21	1	69	1	60	16.1	26	9
22	1	67	0	71	15.6	8	8
23	2	65	0	51	11.8	2	6
24	1	24	0	71	13.7	10	9
25	2	45	0	72	11	4	8
26	2	64	0	74	14.2	4	6
27	1	61	0	75	13.7	10	12
28	1	26	1	72	15.3	37	11
29	1	42	1	57	13.9	24	12
30	2	57	0	72	14.6	8	10
31	2	70	0	72	13.8	3	9
32	2	5	0	74	15.1	3	9
33	2	54	0	51	15.8	7	8
34	1	36	1	72	16.4	4	9
35	2	70	0	71	13.6	2	10
36	2	67	0	73	13.8	7	8
37	1	23	0	68	12.5	2	8
38	1	62	0	63	13.2	3	8

Note: Treatment group: 1, placebo; 2, DES. Status: 0, censored; 1, died from prostatic cancer.

2.3 Fitting the Parametric Survival Distribution

When designing a clinical trial, one needs to explore the survival distribution of the control group. It is often the case that a parametric model is tried to see if it fits the data from historical control trials well, because if the assumption of a particular parametric model is valid, inferences based on such an assumption will be more precise and efficient. The Weibull distribution plays a central role in the analysis of survival data. Clinical trial designs based on the Weibull distribution will also be discussed in this book. Thus, how to fit the Weibull distribution by using maximum likelihood methods will be discussed in this section. Other parametric survival distributions can be fitted similarly by using maximum likelihood methods but are not discussed in this book.

For notation convenience, we convert the scale parameter ρ of the Weibull distribution to $\lambda = \rho^\kappa$. Thus, the failure time T has the density function

$$f(t) = \kappa \lambda t^{\kappa-1} e^{-\lambda t^\kappa}$$

and the survival distribution function is given by

$$S(t) = e^{-\lambda t^\kappa}.$$

Assume that during the accrual phase of a trial, n subjects are enrolled in the study in a staggered fashion, and let T_j and C_j denote, respectively, the failure time and censoring time of the jth subject, with both being measured from the time of study entry. We assume that the failure time T_j is independent of the censoring time C_j and that $(T_1, C_1), \ldots, (T_n, C_n)$ are independent and identically distributed pairs, where T_j has a distribution $S(t)$. Then, the observed survival data are $\{X_i = T_i \wedge C_i, \Delta_i = I(T_i < C_i), i = 1, \cdots, n\}$, which is a random sample from the Weibull distribution with unknown hazard parameter λ and shape parameter κ. The observed likelihood function of (κ, λ) is proportional to

$$L(\kappa, \lambda) = \prod_{i=1}^{n} f(X_i)^{\Delta_i} S(X_i)^{1-\Delta_i} = \prod_{i=1}^{n} \left\{ \lambda \kappa X_i^{\kappa-1} \right\}^{\Delta_i} e^{-\lambda X_i^\kappa}$$

(see Appendix 1) and the log-likelihood function becomes

$$\ell(\kappa, \lambda) = \log(\kappa\lambda) \sum_{i=1}^{n} \Delta_i + (\kappa - 1) \sum_{i=1}^{n} \Delta_i \log X_i - \lambda \sum_{i=1}^{n} X_i^\kappa.$$

Therefore, the maximum likelihood estimates (MLEs) of κ and λ can be obtained by solving the score equations:

$$\frac{d}{\hat{\lambda}} - \sum_{i=1}^{n} X_i^{\hat{\kappa}} = 0$$

and

$$\frac{d}{\hat{\kappa}} + \sum_{i=1}^{n} \Delta_i \log(X_i) - \hat{\lambda} \sum_{i=1}^{n} X_i^{\hat{\kappa}} \log(X_i) = 0, \tag{2.1}$$

where $d = \sum_{i=1}^{n} \Delta_i$ is the total number of failures. Thus, the MLE of λ is given by

$$\hat{\lambda} = \frac{d}{\sum_{i=1}^{n} X_i^{\hat{\kappa}}}, \tag{2.2}$$

and substituting for $\hat{\lambda}$ in equation (2.1) we have

$$\frac{d}{\hat{\kappa}} + \sum_{i=1}^{n} \Delta_i \log(X_i) - \frac{d}{\sum_{i=1}^{n} X_i^{\hat{\kappa}}} \sum_{i=1}^{n} X_i^{\hat{\kappa}} \log(X_i) = 0.$$

This is a nonlinear equation in $\hat{\kappa}$, which can only be solved by using an iterative numerical procedure. Once the estimate $\hat{\kappa}$ has been obtained, equation (2.2) can be solved to obtain $\hat{\lambda}$. Thus, the Weibull distribution is estimated by $\hat{S}(t) = e^{-\hat{\lambda} t^{\hat{\kappa}}}$.

2.4 Kaplan-Meier Estimates

In this section, we will discuss nonparametric methods of estimating the survival distribution for censored survival data. The parametric survival distributions discussed in the previous section can be estimated using maximum likelihood methods. However, all parametric models have restricted assumptions and it may not be possible to fit them to the observed data. Nonparametric methods are more flexible, with no assumptions regarding the form of the underlying distribution. They are less efficient than parametric methods when the survival times follow a theoretical distribution but more efficient when no suitable theoretical distributions are known.

The survival distribution can be estimated nonparametrically from observed survival data by using the method of Kaplan and Meier (1958). Suppose that patients have failures in the follow-up period at distinct times $t_1 < t_2 < \cdots < t_k$ in a sample of size n with an unknown survival function S. Suppose that there are d_j failures at t_j and c_j patients are censored in the interval $[t_j, t_{j+1})$ at times $t_{j1}, \ldots, t_{jc_j}, j = 0, \ldots, k$, where $t_0 = 0$ and $t_{k+1} = \infty$. Let $n_j = (c_j + d_j) + \cdots + (c_k + d_k)$ be the number of individuals at risk at a time just prior to t_j. Then, the probability of failure at t_j is

$$P(T = t_j) = S(t_j^-) - S(t_j),$$

where $S(t^-) = \lim_{u \to t^-} S(u)$ (the superscript "t^-" indicates that the limit is a left-handed limit), and the contribution to the likelihood of a censored survival time at t_{jl} is

$$P(T > t_{jl}) = S(t_{jl}).$$

Therefore, the likelihood of the data is given by

$$L = \prod_{j=0}^{k} \left\{ [S(t_j^-) - S(t_j)]^{d_j} \prod_{l=1}^{c_j} S(t_{jl}) \right\}$$

(Kalbfleisch and Prentice, 2002). The maximum likelihood estimate (MLE) is defined as

$$\hat{S} = \arg \max_S L.$$

Clearly, $\hat{S}(t)$ is a discrete survival function with hazard rate $\hat{\lambda}_1, \ldots, \hat{\lambda}_k$ at failure time $t_1, \ldots, t_k$. Thus,

$$\hat{S}(t_j) = \prod_{l=1}^{j}(1 - \hat{\lambda}_l)$$

and

$$\hat{S}(t_j^-) = \prod_{l=1}^{j-1}(1 - \hat{\lambda}_l).$$

Because $t_{jl} \geq t_j$, $S(t_{jl})$ is maximized by taking $S(t_{jl}) = S(t_j)$; thus, $\hat{\lambda}_1, \ldots, \hat{\lambda}_k$ are chosen to maximize the likelihood function L, which can be expressed as

$$L = \prod_{j=1}^{k} \lambda_j^{d_j}(1 - \lambda_j)^{n_j - d_j},$$

which in turn gives

$$\hat{\lambda}_j = \frac{d_j}{n_j}, \quad j = 1, \ldots, k.$$

This MLE is given as the Kaplan-Meier estimator of the survival function of T in the form

$$\hat{S}(t) = \prod_{t_j \leq t} \left(\frac{n_j - d_j}{n_j} \right).$$

The following recursive formula is useful for calculating the probability of a patient being alive at time t_j:

$$\hat{S}(t_j) = \hat{S}(t_{j-1})\left(1 - \frac{d_j}{n_j}\right),$$

where $t_0 = 0$ and $\hat{S}(0) = 1$. The value of $\hat{S}(t)$ is constant between the times of failure, and, therefore, it is a step function that changes its value only at the time of each failure. Note: If the largest observation is a censored survival time, say, t^*, then $\hat{S}(t)$ is undefined for $t > t^*$. If the largest observed survival time t_k is a failure, then $\hat{S}(t)$ is zero for $t > t_k$. The Kaplan-Meier estimate is a step function which may be inconvenient for some applications. A smoothed estimate of the survival distribution can be obtained using **logspline** methods (Kooperberg and Stone, 1992).

Efron (1967) has shown that $\hat{S}(t)$ is a consistent estimator of $S(t)$ and that

$$n^{1/2}[\hat{S}(t) - S(t)] \xrightarrow{D} N(0, \sigma_t^2),$$

where

$$\sigma_t^2 = [S(t)]^2 \int_0^t \frac{\lambda(t)}{S(t)G(t)} dt,$$

in which $\lambda(t)$ is the hazard function and $G(t) = P(C > t)$ is the censoring distribution. Thus, the asymptotic variance of $\hat{S}(t)$ can be estimated by

$$\widehat{\text{Var}}(\hat{S}(t)) = [\hat{S}(t)]^2 \sum_{t_j \le t} \frac{d_j}{n_j(n_j - d_j)}, \tag{2.3}$$

which is known as Greenwood's formula (Greenwood, 1926). Therefore, a $100(1 - \alpha)\%$ confidence interval for $S(t)$ is given by

$$\hat{S}(t) \pm z_{1-\alpha/2} \sqrt{\widehat{\text{Var}}(\hat{S}(t))}.$$

A better confidence interval can be obtained by using a log-log transformation, which is given by

$$\hat{S}(t)^{\exp(\pm z_{1-\alpha/2}\hat{v}_t)},$$

where $\hat{v}_t^2 = \widehat{\text{Var}}(\hat{S}(t))/[\hat{S}(t) \log \hat{S}(t)]^2$.

The hazard function $\lambda(t)$ in the interval $t_j \le t < t_{j+1}$ can be roughly estimated by

$$\hat{\lambda}(t) = \frac{d_j}{n_j \tau_j}, \quad t_j \le t < t_{j+1},$$

where $\tau_j = t_{j+1} - t_j$.

Example 2.2 *Continuation from Example 2.1*

There were 18 patients in the placebo group, and five patients died at times $t_1 = 14, t_2 = 26, t_3 = 36, t_4 = 42$, and $t_5 = 69$ months, respectively. Thus, the time interval $[0, \infty)$ can be divided into six sub-intervals as $[0, 14), [14, 26), [26, 36), [36, 42), [42, 69)$ and $[69, \infty)$. The number of patients at risk before each failure time point is $n_0 = 18, n_1 = 17, n_2 = 14, n_3 = 13, n_4 = 12$, and $n_5 = 1$; the number of deaths at each failure time point is $d_0 = 0, d_1 = 1, d_2 = 1, d_3 = 1, d_4 = 1$, and $d_5 = 1$; and the number of censorings in each failure time interval is $c_0 = 1, c_1 = 2, c_2 = 0, c_3 = 0, c_4 = 10$,

TABLE 2.2: Calculation of the Kaplan-Meier estimate for the data from Example 2.1

Interval	t_j	n_j	d_j	c_j	$(n_j - d_j)/n_j$	$\hat{S}(t_{j-1}) \times \frac{n_j - d_j}{n_j} = \hat{S}(t_j)$
$[0, 14)$	0	18	0	1	(18-0)/18=1.000	1.000
$[14, 26)$	14	17	1	2	(17-1)/17=0.941	$1.000 \times 0.941 = 0.941$
$[26, 36)$	26	14	1	0	(14-1)/14=0.929	$0.941 \times 0.929 = 0.874$
$[36, 42)$	36	13	1	0	(13-1)/13=0.923	$0.874 \times 0.923 = 0.807$
$[42, 69)$	42	12	1	10	(12-1)/12=0.917	$0.807 \times 0.917 = 0.740$
$[69, \infty)$	69	1	1	0	(1-1)/1=0.000	$0.000 \times 0.740 = 0.000$

and $c_5 = 0$. Thus, the Kaplan-Meier survival distribution estimate can be calculated using the recursive formula

$$\hat{S}(t_j) = \frac{n_j - d_j}{n_j} \hat{S}(t_{j-1}),$$

(see Table 2.2 for the calculations); the Kaplan-Meier survival curve and 95% confidence limits are shown in Figure 2.10.

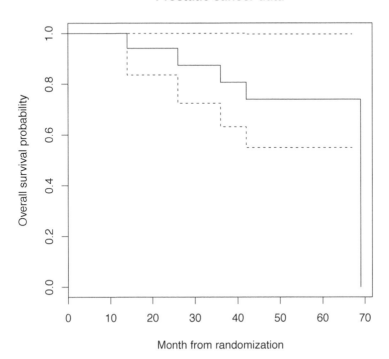

Prostatic cancer data

FIGURE 2.10: The solid line step function is the Kaplan-Meier curve and the dotted lines are the 95% confidence limits.

2.5   Median Survival Time

Since the distribution of survival times tends to be positively skewed, the median survival time is the preferred summary measure of the central location of the survival distribution. The median survival time m is the time beyond which 50% of the subjects in the population are expected to survive, that is, m satisfies the condition $S(m) = 0.5$. If the survival distribution $S(t)$ is estimated by a Kaplan-Meier survival function $\hat{S}(t)$, the median survival time can be estimated as

$$\hat{m} = \min\{t_j, \hat{S}(t_j) < 0.5\},$$

where t_j is the jth ordered failure time, $j = 1, 2, \ldots, k$. In the particular case where the survival function $\hat{S}(t)$ is exactly equal to 0.5 at an interval $[t_j, t_{j+1})$, the median estimate is not unique but is often taken to be $\hat{m} = (t_j + t_{j+1})/2$. The asymptotic distribution of the median estimate $\hat{m}$ is

$$\sqrt{n}(\hat{m} - m) \xrightarrow{D} N(0, \sigma^2),$$

where n is the sample size (e.g., Reid, 1981). The asymptotic variance σ^2 is given by

$$\sigma^2 = \{f(m)\}^{-2} S^2(m) \int_0^m \frac{\lambda(t)dt}{S(t)G(t)} \simeq \frac{n\text{Var}\{\hat{S}(m)\}}{f^2(m)},$$

where $f(t)$ and $\lambda(t)$ are the density and hazard function, respectively, and $G(t) = P(C > t)$ is the censoring survival distribution. Thus, the asymptotic variance of $\hat{m}$ can be estimated by

$$\hat{\text{Var}}(\hat{m}) = \frac{1}{\hat{f}^2(\hat{m})} \widehat{\text{Var}}\{\hat{S}(\hat{m})\},$$

where $\hat{f}$ is an estimate of the density function f, and $\widehat{\text{Var}}\{\hat{S}(\hat{m})\}$ is given by Greenwood's formula (2.3) at $t = \hat{m}$. To use this asymptotic variance formula, we have to estimate the density function f. A common type of density estimation is a window estimate obtained by using a kernel function. For example, Kosorok (1999) proposed an optimal window estimate based on the kernel function

$$\hat{f}(\hat{m}) = \int n^{1/5} \hat{Q}^{-1} K \left(\frac{\hat{m} - x}{n^{-1/5} \hat{Q}} \right) d\hat{F}(x),$$

where $\hat{F} = 1 - \hat{S}$, $\hat{Q}$ is twice the estimated interquartile range of $F = 1 - S$, and the kernel function $K(\cdot)$ is a triangular function on $[-1, 1]$,

$$K(x) = \begin{cases} x + 1 & -1 \leq x \leq 0 \\ 1 - x & 0 < x \leq 1 \\ 0 & |x| > 1. \end{cases}$$

In a cancer survival trial, there may be interest in comparing the median survival times of two treatment groups. Assume a survival function S_i, a density f_i and a median m_i for two treatment groups $i = 1, 2$, and let $\hat{S}_i(t)$ be the Kaplan-Meier survival function estimate and $\hat{m}_i$ be the median estimate. We are interested in the difference in the medians $m_d = m_2 - m_1$ (the treatment effect is quantified by the difference in the medians). An estimate of m_d is $\hat{m}_d = \hat{m}_2 - \hat{m}_1$, and a $100(1 - \alpha)\%$ large-sample asymptotic confidence interval of m_d can be obtained as

$$\hat{m}_d \pm z_{1-\alpha/2}\hat{se}(\hat{m}_d),$$

where

$$\hat{se}(\hat{m}_d) = \{\widehat{\mathrm{Var}}(\hat{m}_1) + \widehat{\mathrm{Var}}(\hat{m}_2)\}^{1/2}.$$

Here, the variances $\widehat{\mathrm{Var}}(\hat{m}_1)$ and $\widehat{\mathrm{Var}}(\hat{m}_2)$ can be estimated by a kernel density estimation, as discussed above. To avoid density estimation for a small sample study, an alternative way to estimate the variance of the median is to use the bootstrap method (Wu, 2011).

If there is interest in testing the hypothesis of equality of the medians,

$$H_0 : m_1 = m_2 \quad vs. \quad H_1 : m_1 \neq m_2,$$

then the following test statistic can be used:

$$Z = \frac{\hat{m}_d}{\hat{se}(\hat{m}_d)},$$

which is asymptotically standard normal distributed. Thus, the test rejects the null hypothesis if $|Z| > z_{1-\alpha/2}$. Rahbar et al. (2012) proposed an alternative test statistic to test the hypothesis of equality of several medians.

2.6 Log-Rank Test

The treatment effect of a trial with survival endpoints is often detected by the log-rank test, which is a nonparametric procedure for testing the hypothesis of equality of two or more survival distribution functions. For example, the hypothesis of interest in a two-arm trial is

$$H_0 : S_1(t) = S_2(t) \quad vs. \quad H_1 : S_1(t) \neq S_2(t), \tag{2.4}$$

where $S_1(t)$ and $S_2(t)$ represent the survival distribution of two groups with indexes 1 and 2. Trials based on hypothesis (2.4) are often referred to as superiority trials. There are other types of hypothesis that may be of interest in cancer survival trial designs, such as a noninferiority trial or an equivalence trial. In this book, however, we will only discuss superiority trial design.

TABLE 2.3: Number of failures at the jth failure time in each of two groups

Group	Number of failures at t_j	Number of survivors beyond t_j	Number at risk just before t_j
I	d_{1j}	$n_{1j} - d_{1j}$	n_{1j}
II	d_{2j}	$n_{2j} - d_{2j}$	n_{2j}
Total	d_j	$n_j - d_j$	n_j

Assume that the unique and ordered failure times for two groups are denoted by $t_1 < t_2 < \cdots < t_k$. Let d_{1j} be the number of failures and n_{1j} be the number at risk in group 1 at time t_j. Let d_{2j} and n_{2j} be the corresponding number in group 2. Then, $d_j = d_{1j} + d_{2j}$ represents the number of failures in both groups at time t_j, and $n_j = n_{1j} + n_{2j}$ is the number at risk in both groups at time t_j. The situation is summarized in Table 2.3.

We can consider this table as tabulating failures occurring within the interval $[t_j, t_j + \Delta t)$, where Δt is defined as a small increment of time t, then we have, conditional on n_{ij}, that d_{ij} has, approximately, a binomial distribution with mean $E d_{ij} = n_{ij} \lambda_{ij} \Delta t$, where $\lambda_{ij} = \lambda_i(t_j)$ is the hazard rate for group i at time t_j. Following Cook and DeMets (2005), the joint distribution of d_{1j} and d_{2j} conditional on n_{1j} and n_{2j} is

$$
\begin{aligned}
p(d_{1j}, d_{2j}) &= \binom{n_{1j}}{d_{1j}} \binom{n_{2j}}{d_{2j}} (\lambda_{1j} \Delta t)^{d_{1j}} (1 - \lambda_{1j} \Delta t)^{n_{1j} - d_{1j}} \\
&\quad \times (\lambda_{2j} \Delta t)^{d_{2j}} (1 - \lambda_{2j} \Delta t)^{n_{2j} - d_{2j}} \\
&\simeq \binom{n_{1j}}{d_{1j}} \binom{n_{2j}}{d_{2j}} \lambda_{1j}^{d_{1j}} \lambda_{2j}^{d_{2j}} \Delta t^{d_j}.
\end{aligned}
$$

The conditional distribution for (d_{1j}, d_{2j}), given d_j, is

$$
\begin{aligned}
p(d_{1j}, d_{2j} | d_j) &= \frac{p(d_{1j}, d_{2j})}{\sum_{s=0}^{d_j} p(s, d_j - s)} \\
&\simeq \frac{\binom{n_{1j}}{d_{1j}} \binom{n_{2j}}{d_{2j}} \lambda_{1j}^{d_{1j}} \lambda_{2j}^{d_{2j}}}{\sum_{s=0}^{d_j} \binom{n_{1j}}{s} \binom{n_{2j}}{d_j - s} \lambda_{1j}^{s} \lambda_{2j}^{d_j - s}}.
\end{aligned}
\qquad (2.5)
$$

Let the hazard ratio $\delta = \lambda_{2j} / \lambda_{1j}$ be a constant (independent of j); then

$$
p(d_{1j}, d_{2j} | d_j) = \frac{\binom{n_{1j}}{d_{1j}} \binom{n_{2j}}{d_{2j}} \delta^{d_{2j}}}{\sum_{s=0}^{d_j} \binom{n_{1j}}{s} \binom{n_{2j}}{d_j - s} \delta^{d_j - s}}.
$$

This conditional distribution is known as the non-central hypergeometric distribution and depends on the hazard ratio δ only. The null hypothesis

$H_0 : \lambda_1(t) = \lambda_2(t)$ for all t is equivalent to $H_0 : \delta = 1$. Thus, under the null hypothesis, the conditional distribution simplifies as

$$p(d_{1j}, d_{2j}|d_j) = \frac{\binom{n_{1j}}{d_{1j}}\binom{n_{2j}}{d_{2j}}}{\sum_{s=0}^{d_j}\binom{n_{1j}}{s}\binom{n_{2j}}{d_j-s}},$$

which is known as the central hypergeometric distribution. Therefore, under H_0, the conditional mean of d_{1j} is

$$e_{1j} = E[d_{1j}|n_{1j}, n_{2j}, d_j] = \frac{n_{1j}d_j}{n_j},$$

and its variance is

$$v_{1j} = \text{Var}[d_{1j}|n_{1j}, n_{2j}, d_j] = \frac{n_{1j}n_{2j}d_j(n_j - d_j)}{n_j^2(n_j - 1)}.$$

If the true underlying hazard is uniformly larger (or smaller) in group 1 than in group 2, then we expect that d_{1j} will be systematically larger (or smaller) than its expected value under the null in group 1. This suggests that the following test statistic,

$$U = \sum_{j=1}^{k}(d_{1j} - e_{1j}), \qquad (2.6)$$

which is the overall sum of the observed number of failures minus its conditional expectation under the null, is a measure of the degree of departure from the null suggested by the data. Notice that $d_{1j} - e_{1j}$ are not independent over the observed failure times; however, it can be shown that they are uncorrelated (Proschan et al., 2006, page 41). The variance of U can then be estimated by

$$V = \sum_{j=1}^{k}\frac{n_{1j}n_{2j}d_j(n_j - d_j)}{n_j^2(n_j - 1)}. \qquad (2.7)$$

Furthermore, by the martingale central limiting theorem (see Chapter 4), we have the following test statistic:

$$L = \frac{U}{\sqrt{V}} \xrightarrow{\mathcal{D}} Z \sim N(0, 1). \qquad (2.8)$$

This test is usually known as the log-rank test or Mantel-Haenszel test (Mantel, 1966). The log-rank test is valid for any alternative hypothesis including those for which the proportional hazards assumption does not hold. It can be shown, however, that the log-rank test is optimal for the proportional hazards alternatives (see Chapter 4), but its power is lower than that of other tests

TABLE 2.4: Test statistics and weight function

Statistic	Weight
Log-rank	$w_j = 1$
Gehan-Wilcoxon	$w_j = n_j$
Prentice-Wilcoxon	$w_j = S(t_j^-)$
Harrington-Fleming	$w_j = \hat{S}^\rho(t_j^-)$
Tarone-Ware	$w_j = \sqrt{n_j}$

against nonproportional hazards alternatives. If we desire higher power for particular nonproportional hazards alternatives, the test can be modified to improve its power by replacing the sum in test statistic U by a weighted sum, with weights chosen to optimize the test for the alternative of interest (Cook and DeMets, 2008). In general, the weighted log-rank test is any test in the form

$$L_w = \frac{U_w}{\sqrt{V_w}} = \frac{\sum_{j=1}^k w_j(d_{1j} - e_{1j})}{\sqrt{\sum_{j=1}^k w_j^2 v_{1j}}},$$

where $\{w_j, j = 1, \ldots, k\}$ are the nonnegative weights. The case where $w_j = 1$ gives the ordinary log-rank test L. The case where $w_j = n_j$ is known as the Gehan-Wilcoxon test. By using this test, early failures receive higher weight than do later failures, and this test will be more sensitive to differences between the two groups that occur early. Harrington and Fleming (1982) proposed a general family of weight functions, the $\mathcal{G}^\rho$ family, that uses weight $w_j = \hat{S}^\rho(t_j^-)$, where $\hat{S}(t^-)$ is the left-continuous version of the Kaplan-Meier estimate computed from the pooled sample of two groups. This class contains as special cases the ordinary log-rank test ($\rho = 0$), which assigns equal weights throughout the study, and the Prentice-Wilcoxon test ($\rho = 1$), which assigns more weight on early survival differences (see Table 2.4). Greater flexibility can be provided by choosing values of ρ between 0 and 1. The relative efficiency of various members of these families of tests have been explored by Tarone and Ware (1997) and Harrington and Fleming (1982).

Remark 1: Notice that the log-rank score $U = \sum_{j=1}^k d_{1j} - \sum_{j=1}^k e_{1j} = O_1 - E_1$ is the difference between the total observed (O_1) and expected (E_1) number of deaths in group 1. Similarly, if we define the total observed $O_2 = \sum_{j=1}^k d_{2j}$ and expected $E_2 = \sum_{j=1}^k e_{2j}$ number of deaths in group 2, where $e_{2j} = n_{2j}d_j/n_j$, as $n_{1j} + n_{2j} = n_j$ and $d_{1j} + d_{2j} = d_j$, respectively, then, we have $O_1 - E_1 + O_2 - E_2 = 0$, that is $U = O_1 - E_1 = -(O_2 - E_2)$. Thus, using the difference between the total observed and expected number of deaths in group 1 or group 2 will result in the same statistic (except for the sign of the test statistic).

Remark 2: The log-rank score $U = \sum_{j=1}^{k}(d_{1j} - e_{1j})$ can be rewritten as

$$U = \sum_{j=1}^{k} \frac{n_{1j}n_{2j}}{n_j}(\hat{\lambda}_{1j} - \hat{\lambda}_{2j}),$$

where $\hat{\lambda}_{ij} = d_{ij}/n_{ij}$ is the estimated hazard rate at the jth failure of group $i = 1, 2$. Thus, it is a type of weighted difference of the estimated hazard rates between two groups.

Example 2.3 *Melanoma patient data*

Thirty melanoma patients were studied to compare the ability of Bacillus Calmette Guerin (BCG) and Corynebacterium parvum (C. parvum) immunotherapies to prolong survival time (Table 2.5, also see Lee and Wang, 2013). The age, sex, disease stage, treatment and survival time are given in Table 2.5. All the patients' tumors were resected before treatment began and thus had no evidence of melanoma at the time of first treatment. The study objective is to compare the survival distributions between treatment groups. To visualize the difference in the survival distributions of the two groups, Kaplan-Meier estimates are plotted in Figure 2.11. The survival curves clearly show that patients treated with C. parvum had a slightly better survival experience than did patients treated with BCG. Let $S_1(t)$ and $S_2(t)$ be the survival distributions of the BCG and C. parvum groups, respectively. The hypothesis

$$H_0 : S_1(t) = S_2(t) \quad vs. \quad H_0 : S_1(t) \neq S_2(t)$$

will be tested by using the log-rank test. The required calculations are laid out in Table 2.6. We begin by ordering the observed death times (t_j) across the two groups (shown in column 1 of Table 2.6. The numbers of death times (d_{1j} and d_{2j}) and the numbers at risk (n_{1j} and n_{2j}) at each death time are calculated and shown in columns 2 to 5 of Table 2.6. The final three columns give the values of e_{1j}, e_{2j} and v_{1j}. The total values in the last row of Table 2.6 are $O_1 = O_2 = 5$, $E_1 = 3.68$ and $E_2 = 6.32$. Then $U = O_1 - E_1 = 5 - 3.68 = 1.32$ and $O_2 - E_2 = 5 - 6.32 = -1.32$; thus, we verify the equation $U = O_1 - E_1 = -(O_2 - E_2)$. The observed value of the log-rank test statistic is $L^0 = (5 - 3.68)/\sqrt{2.31} = 0.8685$, with a two-sided p-value=$2\{1 - \Phi(0.8685)\} = 0.385$. Thus, the difference in the survival distribution of the two treatment groups is not significant. Therefore, we do not reject the null hypothesis that the two survival distributions are equal. However, this study had a limited number of failures in each group and thus had a limited power to detect difference.

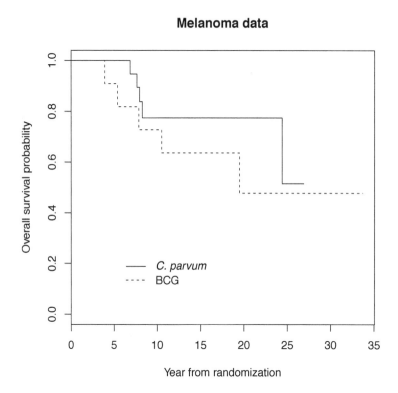

FIGURE 2.11: Kaplan-Meier Survival Curves of patients receiving BCG and C. parvum.

TABLE 2.5: Data for 30 resected melanoma patients in a clinical trial

Patient ID	Age	Sex	Initial stage	Treatment group	Survival time	Censoring indicator
1	59	2	3B	1	33.7	0
2	50	2	3B	1	3.9	1
3	76	1	3B	1	10.5	1
4	66	2	3B	1	5.4	1
5	33	1	3B	1	19.5	1
6	23	2	3B	1	23.8	0
7	40	2	3B	1	7.9	1
8	34	1	3B	1	16.9	0
9	34	1	3B	1	16.6	0
10	38	2	2	1	33.7	0
11	54	2	2	1	17.1	0
12	49	1	3B	2	8	1
13	35	1	3B	2	26.9	0
14	22	1	3B	2	21.4	0
15	30	1	3B	2	18.1	0
16	26	2	3B	2	16	0
17	27	1	3B	2	6.9	1
18	45	2	3B	2	11	0
19	76	2	3A	2	24.8	0
20	48	1	3A	2	23	0
21	91	1	4A	2	8.3	1
22	82	2	4A	2	10.8	0
23	50	2	4A	2	12.2	0
24	40	1	4A	2	12.5	0
25	34	1	3A	2	24.4	1
26	38	1	4A	2	7.7	1
27	50	1	2	2	14.8	0
28	53	2	2	2	8.2	0
29	48	2	2	2	8.2	0
30	40	2	2	2	7.8	0

Note: Sex: 1, male; 2, female. Treatment group: 1, BCG; 2, *C. parvum*. Censoring indicator: 1, dead; 0, alive. Survival times are in months.

TABLE 2.6: Calculation of the log-rank test statistic for the data from Example 2.3

t_j	d_{1j}	d_{2j}	n_{1j}	n_{2j}	$e_{1j} = \frac{n_{1j}d_j}{n_j}$	$e_{2j} = \frac{n_{2j}d_j}{n_j}$	$v_{1j} = \frac{n_{1j}n_{2j}d_j(n_j-d_j)}{n_j^2(n_j-1)}$
3.9	1	0	11	19	11/30	19/30	$11 \times 19 \times (30-1)/(30^2 \times (30-1))$
5.4	1	0	10	19	10/29	19/29	$10 \times 19 \times (29-1)/(29^2 \times (29-1))$
6.9	0	1	9	19	9/28	19/28	$9 \times 19 \times (28-1)/(28^2 \times (28-1))$
7.7	0	1	9	18	9/27	18/27	$9 \times 18 \times (27-1)/(27^2 \times (27-1))$
7.9	1	0	9	16	9/25	16/25	$9 \times 16 \times (25-1)/(25^2 \times (25-1))$
8.0	0	1	8	16	8/24	16/24	$8 \times 16 \times (24-1)/(24^2 \times (24-1))$
8.3	0	1	8	13	8/21	13/21	$8 \times 13 \times (21-1)/(21^2 \times (21-1))$
10.5	1	0	8	12	8/20	12/20	$8 \times 12 \times (20-1)/(20^2 \times (20-1))$
19.5	1	0	4	5	4/9	5/9	$4 \times 5 \times (9-1)/(9^2 \times (9-1))$
24.4	0	1	2	3	2/5	3/5	$2 \times 3 \times (5-1)/(5^2 \times (5-1))$
Total	5	5			3.68	6.32	2.31

2.7   Cox Regression Model

When analyzing survival data, there is usually interest in the association between the survival time and one or more explanatory variables, such as age, gender, or treatment group. The Cox regression model (Cox, 1972) enables such an analysis of survival data.

The Cox regression model assumes that the conditional hazard function of T, given Z, has the form

$$\lambda(t|Z) = \lambda_0(t)e^{\theta' Z},$$

where $\lambda_0(t)$ is the baseline hazard function, $Z = (Z_1, \ldots, Z_p)'$ is a $p \times 1$ column vector of covariates, $\theta = (\theta_1, \ldots, \theta_p)'$ is a $p \times 1$ is a vector of unknown regression coefficients, and x' indicates a vector transpose. The Cox regression model states that the ratio of the hazard functions for two subjects with different covariates is constant. Under this model, the conditional density and survival functions of T, given Z, have the forms

$$f(t|Z) = \lambda_0(t)e^{\theta' Z}e^{-\Lambda_0(t)e^{\theta' Z}}$$

and

$$S(t|Z) = [S_0(t)]^{e^{\theta' Z}},$$

where $\Lambda_0(t)$ and $S_0(t)$ are the baseline cumulative hazard function and baseline survival function, respectively. The conditional cumulative hazard function of T, given Z, has the form

$$\Lambda(t|Z) = \Lambda_0(t)e^{\theta' Z}.$$

Now suppose that the data consist of n observed survival times, denoted by $X_1, \ldots, X_n$ subject to right censoring and let $\Delta_1, \ldots, \Delta_n$ be the failure indicators. Furthermore we assume that there are no tied failure times. Then the partial likelihood function can be expressed in the form

$$L(\theta) = \prod_{i=1}^{n} \left\{ \frac{e^{\theta' Z_i}}{\sum_{j \in \mathcal{R}(X_i)} e^{\theta' Z_j}} \right\}^{\Delta_i},$$

where $Z_j = (Z_{1j}, \ldots, Z_{pj})'$, and $\mathcal{R}(X_i) = \{j : X_j \geq X_i\}$ is the indicator set for subjects at risk just prior to X_i. The partial log-likelihood function is given by

$$\ell(\theta) = \sum_{i=1}^{n} \Delta_i \left\{ \theta' Z_i - \log \sum_{j \in \mathcal{R}(X_i)} e^{\theta' Z_j} \right\},$$

and the score function, first derivative of the partial log-likelihood, is given by

$$U(\theta) = \sum_{i=1}^{n} \Delta_i \left\{ Z_i - \frac{\sum_{j \in \mathcal{R}(X_i)} e^{\theta' Z_j} Z_j Y_j(t)}{\sum_{j \in \mathcal{R}(X_i)} e^{\theta' Z_j} Y_j(t)} \right\}.$$

The maximum partial likelihood estimate $\hat{\theta}$ of θ can be obtained by solving the score equation $U(\hat{\theta}) = 0$ numerically using the Newton-Raphson iterative procedure

$$\theta_{s+1} = \theta_s + \{V(\theta_s)\}^{-1} U(\theta_s),$$

for $s = 0, 1, 2 \ldots$, where $V(\theta)$ is the observed Fisher information matrix, negative second derivatives of the partial log-likelihood, which is given by

$$V(\theta) = \sum_{i=1}^{n} \Delta_i \left\{ \frac{\sum_{j \in \mathcal{R}(X_i)} e^{\theta' Z_j} Z_j Z_j' Y_j(t)}{\sum_{j \in \mathcal{R}(X_i)} e^{\theta' Z_j} Y_j(t)} \right.$$
$$\left. - \frac{\sum_{j \in \mathcal{R}(X_i)} e^{\theta' Z_j} Z_j Y_j(t) \sum_{j \in \mathcal{R}(X_i)} e^{\theta' Z_j} Z_j' Y_j(t)}{\left(\sum_{j \in \mathcal{R}(X_i)} e^{\theta' Z_j} Y_j(t) \right)^2} \right\}.$$

The variance of $\hat{\theta}$ can be estimated by the inverse Fisher information matrix $\text{Var}(\hat{\theta}) = \{V(\hat{\theta})\}^{-1}$.

3

Counting Process and Martingale

In this chapter, we review some basic convergence concepts and notations that are often used in the development of statistics theory (DasGupta, 2008). We will also introduce the counting process and martingale theories, which are the fundamental tools for deriving the asymptotic distribution of the test statistics in a survival analysis (Fleming and Harrington, 1991).

3.1   Basic Convergence Concepts

Definition 3.1 *Let $\{X_n, X\}$ be random variables defined on a common probability space. We say X_n converges to X in probability if $\forall \epsilon > 0$, $P(|X_n - X| > \epsilon) \to 0$ as $n \to \infty$. If X_n converges in probability to zero, then we write $X_n \xrightarrow{P} 0$ and also $X_n = o_p(1)$ and if $a_n X_n \xrightarrow{P} 0$ for some constant sequence a_n, then we write $X_n = o_p(\frac{1}{a_n})$.*

Definition 3.2 *A sequence of random variables X_n is said to be bounded in probability if $\forall \epsilon > 0$, and one can find a constant c and an integer n_0 such that $P(|X_n| > c) \le \epsilon$ for all $n \ge n_0$. If X_n is bounded in probability, then we write $X_n = O_p(1)$. If $a_n X_n = O_p(1)$ for a constant sequence a_n, then we write $X_n = O_p(\frac{1}{a_n})$.*

Definition 3.3 *Let $\{X_n, X\}$ be random variables defined on a common probability space. We say X_n converges almost surely to X if $P(X_n \to X) = 1$. We write $X_n \xrightarrow{a.s} X$.*

Definition 3.4 *Let $\{X_n, X\}$ be random variables defined on a common probability space. We say X_n converges in distribution to X if $P(X_n \le x) \to P(X \le x)$ as $n \to \infty$ at every point x that is a continuity point of the distribution of X. We write $X_n \xrightarrow{D} X$.*

We next state two fundamental theorems known as the laws of large numbers.

Theorem 3.1 (Khintchine) *Suppose $X_n, n \ge 1$ are independent and identically distributed with a finite mean μ. Let $\bar{X}_n = \sum_{j=1}^{n} X_j / n$. Then $\bar{X}_n \xrightarrow{P} \mu$.*

This is known as the weak law of large numbers. The next theorem is known as the strong law of large numbers.

Theorem 3.2 (Kolmogorov) *Suppose $X_n, n \geq 1$ are independent and identically distributed, then $\bar{X}_n$ has an a.s. limit iff $E|X_1| < \infty$, in which case, $\bar{X}_n \xrightarrow{a.s.} \mu = E(X_1)$.*

The following theorem of Slutsky is simple but very useful for deriving the asymptotic distribution of test statistics.

Theorem 3.3 (Slutsky)
(i) If $X_n \xrightarrow{D} X$ and $Y_n \xrightarrow{P} c$ where c is a constant, then $X_n + Y_n \xrightarrow{D} X + c$.
(ii) If $X_n \xrightarrow{D} X$ and $Y_n \xrightarrow{P} c$ where c is a constant, then $X_n Y_n \xrightarrow{D} cX$.
(iii) If $X_n \xrightarrow{D} X$ and $Y_n \xrightarrow{P} c \neq 0$, then $X_n / Y_n \xrightarrow{D} X/c$.

The most fundamental result on the convergence in law is the central limit theorem (CLT). We state the finite variance case below.

Theorem 3.4 Central Limit Theorem
Let $X_n, n \geq 1$ be independent and identically distributed random variables with $E(X_n) = \mu$ and $Var(X_n) = \sigma^2 < \infty$. Then

$$\frac{\sqrt{n}(\bar{X} - \mu)}{\sigma} \xrightarrow{D} Z \sim N(0, 1).$$

3.2 Counting Process Definition

The counting process theory for censored survival data was developed by Aalen (1975). It plays an important role in the development of asymptotic distributions of test statistics for censored survival data, such as log-rank tests. References for the counting process theory include *Counting Processes and Survival Analysis* (Fleming and Harrington, 1991), *Statistical Models Based Counting Processes* (Anderson, et al., 1993), and *The Statistical Analysis of Failure Time Data* (Kalbfleisch and Prentice, 2002). For the convenience of the reader, we will briefly introduce the counting process and martingale theory in the remainder of this chapter.

Definition 3.5 *A stochastic process is a family of random variables $X = \{X(t), t \in \Gamma\}$ indexed by a set Γ.*
From this definition, $X(t)$ is a random variable for each t, and set Γ indexes time, which is either $\{0, 1, 2, \dots\}$ for a discrete-time process or $[0, \infty)$ for a continuous-time process.
A stochastic process $N = \{N(t), t \geq 0\}$ is a counting process if

- $N(0) = 0$

- $N(t) < \infty$

- *Sample paths are right-continuous and piecewise constant and have only jump discontinuities, with a jump size of 1.*

For a counting process N, we denote $dN(t) = N((t + dt)^-) - N(t^-)$ to be the number of failures that occur in the interval $[t, t + dt)$, where $N(t^-) = \lim_{\Delta t \to 0} N(t - \Delta t)$ is the value of the process at the instant before t. For a continuous failure time random variable, where it is assumed that no subject experiences multiple failures at any instant and that no two subjects experience a failure at the same instant, the jump size $dN(t) = 1$ when a failure occurred at time t and 0 otherwise. If N is a counting process, H is a function of time, then $\int_s^t H(u)dN(u)$ is the Stieltjes integral representation of the sum of the values of H at the jump times of N over the interval $(s, t]$.

Example 3.1 *Counting process*

Suppose T is a continuous nonnegative failure time variable subject to right censoring by an independent censoring time C. Let $X = T \wedge C$; and $\Delta = I(T < C)$, then $N(t) = \Delta I(X \leq t)$ is a continuous-time counting process (see Figure 3.1) that records a failure up to time t when $\Delta = 1$. Two useful integration expressions with respect to the counting process $N = \{N(t), t \geq 0\}$ are as follows:

$$\int_0^\infty H(u)dN(u) = \Delta H(X),$$

$$\int_0^t H(u)dN(u) = \Delta I(X \leq t)H(X),$$

where $H(t)$ is a bounded function of time.

3.3 Filtration and Martingale

An increasing family of σ-algebras $\{\mathcal{F}_t, t \geq 0\}$ is called a filtration. Thus, for a filtration $\{\mathcal{F}_t, t \geq 0\}$,

- $\mathcal{F}_s \subset \mathcal{F}_t$ if $s \leq t$

- $\mathcal{F}_t$ is usually generated by some stochastic processes $X = \{X(t), t \geq 0\}$, that is, $\mathcal{F}_t = \sigma\{X(s) : 0 \leq s \leq t\}$.

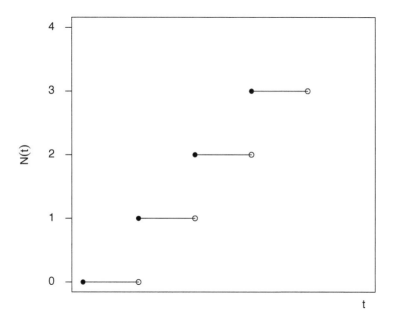

FIGURE 3.1: Graphic representation of a counting process.

- $\mathcal{F}_t$ represents the past history up to time t.

- $\mathcal{F}_{t-} = \sigma\{\bigcup_{h>0} \mathcal{F}_{t-h}\}$ represents the history up to just before t.

A stochastic process $X = \{X(t), t \geq 0\}$ is adapted to $\{\mathcal{F}_t, t \geq 0\}$ if $X(t)$ is measurable with respect to $\mathcal{F}_t$ for any t. A right-continuous stochastic process $\{X(t), t \geq 0\}$ is a martingale with respect to the filtration $\{\mathcal{F}_t, t \geq 0\}$ if

- X is adapted to $\{\mathcal{F}_t, t \geq 0\}$.

- $E|X(t)| < \infty$ for any $t < \infty$.

- $E(X(t)|\mathcal{F}_s) = X(s)$ for any $t > s$.

A stochastic process $X = \{X(t), t \geq 0\}$ is called a sub-martingale if $E(X(t)|\mathcal{F}_s) \geq X(s)$ for any $t > s$. Note that the martingale condition $E(X(t)|\mathcal{F}_s) = X(s)$ for any $t > s$ is equivalent to $E(dX(t)|\mathcal{F}_{t-}) = 0$ for all t, where $dX(t) = X((t+dt)^-) - X(t^-)$ is the increment of X over the interval $[t, t+dt)$.

3.4   Martingale Central Limit Theorem

A is predictable with respect to filtration $\{\mathcal{F}_{t-}, t \geq 0\}$ if it is measurable with respect to the smallest σ-algebra generated by the adapted left-continuous processes.

Theorem 3.5 *(Doob-Meyer Decomposition)*
Let X be a right-continuous nonnegative sub-martingale with respect to the filtration $\{\mathcal{F}_t, t \geq 0\}$. Then there is a unique right continuous predictable process A such that $A(0) = 0$, $EA(t) < \infty$ for any t, and $X - A$ is an $\mathcal{F}_t$-martingale. A is called the compensator of X.

Corollary *For a counting process $N = \{N(t), t \geq 0\}$ with $EN(t) < \infty$, for any t, there is a unique compensator A such that $A(0) = 0$ and $N - A$ is an $\mathcal{F}_t$-martingale.*

Example 3.2 *Independent censoring model*

Consider an independent censoring model, in which the failure time T and censoring time C are independent, and $X = T \wedge C$ and $\Delta = I(T < C)$. Let $Y(t) = I(X \geq t)$ and $N(t) = \Delta I(X \leq t)$, and define the filtration $\mathcal{F}_t = \sigma\{N(s), Y(s+) : 0 \leq s \leq t\}$. Let $\lambda(t)$ be the hazard function of T. Under the independent censoring model, it can be shown approximately that

$$P(t \leq T < t + dt | X \geq t) = \lambda(t)dt,$$

that is, $\lambda(t)dt = E\{dN(t)|X \geq t\}$. Then it follows that

$$E\{dN(t)|\mathcal{F}_{t-}\} = I(X \geq t)\lambda(t) = dA(t).$$

Let $M(t) = N(t) - A(t)$, then $E\{dM(t)|\mathcal{F}_{t-}\} = E\{dN(t) - dA(t)|\mathcal{F}_{t-}\} = 0$; thus, $M(t) = N(t) - A(t)$ is an $\mathcal{F}_t$ martingale, where $A(t) = \int_0^t Y(u)\lambda(u)du$.

A multivariate process $\{N_1(t), \ldots, N_n(t), t \geq 0\}$ is called a multivariate counting process if each $N_i(t)$ is a counting process and no two component processes jump at the same time.

Theorem 3.6 *Let $\{N_1(t), \ldots, N_n(t), t \geq 0\}$ be a multivariate counting process, with $A_j(t)$ being the compensator of $N_j(t)$, and $M_j(t) = N_j(t) - A_j(t)$, and let $U_{n,l}(t) = \sum_{j=1}^n \int_0^t H_{j,l}(u)dM_j(u)(l = 1, \ldots r)$, where $H_{j,l}(t)$ are bounded $\mathcal{F}_t$ predictable processes. Then*
(i) $U_{n,l}$ is a martingale,
(ii) $EU_{n,l}(t) = 0$,
(iii) $Cov\{U_{n,l}(s), U_{n,k}(t)\} = \sum_{j=1}^n \int_0^{t \wedge s} E\{H_{j,l}(u)H_{j,k}(u)dA_j(u)\}$.

Theorem 3.7 *(Martingale Central Limit Theorem)*
Let $\{N_1(t), \ldots, N_n(t), t \geq 0\}$ be a multivariate counting process, with $A_j(t)$ being the compensator of $N_j(t)$, and $M_j(t) = N_j(t) - A_i(t)$, and let $U_n(t) = \sum_{j=1}^n \int_0^t H_j(u)dM_j(u)$, where $H_i(t)$ are bounded $\mathcal{F}_t$ predictable processes. If for all $t > 0$,
(C1) $\sum_{j=1}^n \int_0^t H_j^2(u)dA_j(u) \xrightarrow{P} \sigma^2(t) < \infty$, as $n \to \infty$,
(C2) $\sum_{j=1}^n \int_0^t H_j^2(u)I\{|H_j(u)| > \epsilon\}dA_j(u) \xrightarrow{P} 0$, as $n \to \infty$, $\forall \epsilon > 0$,
then $n^{-1/2}U_n(t) \xrightarrow{D} W(t)$, where $W(t)$ is a continuous Gaussian process with
(i) $W(0) = 0$,
(ii) $EW(t) = 0$,
(iii) $E\{W(s)W(t)\} = \sigma^2(s \wedge t)$.

3.5   Counting Process Formulation of Censored Survival Data

Assume that $\{(T_j, C_j), j = 1, \ldots, n\}$ are independent and identical distributed failure times and censoring times and that T_j is a continuous random variable independent of C_j. Let $X_j = T_j \wedge C_j$, $\Delta_j = I(T_j < C_j)$, $Y_j(t) = I(X_j \geq t)$, and $N_j(t) = \Delta_j I(X_j \leq t)$. If we define the filtration as $\mathcal{F}_t = \sigma\{N(s), Y(s+) : 0 \leq s \leq t\}$, then $M_j(t) = N_j(t) - \int_0^t Y_j(u)\lambda_j(u)du$ is an $\mathcal{F}_t$ martingale, where $\lambda_j(t)$ is the hazard function of T_j. Applying the martingale central limit theorem to the independent random censorship model, we have the following results:

Properties *Let $U_n(t) = \sum_{j=1}^{n} \int_0^t H_j(u)dM_j(u)$, where $H_j(t)$ is a bounded left-continuous $\mathcal{F}_t$-predictable process, then*

(i) $U_n(t)$ is a martingale with $EU_n(t) = 0$,

(ii) $Var\{U_n(t)\} = \sum_{j=1}^{n} \int_0^t E\{H_j^2(u)Y_j(u)\lambda_j(u)\}du$.

Furthermore, if the following conditions are satisfied as $n \to \infty$,

(C1) $\sum_{j=1}^{n} \int_0^t H_j^2(u)Y_j(u)\lambda_j(u)du \overset{P}{\to} \sigma^2(t) < \infty$,

(C2) $\sum_{j=1}^{n} \int_0^t H_j^2(u)I\{|H_j(u)| > \epsilon\}Y_j(u)\lambda_j(u)du \overset{P}{\to} 0$, for any $\epsilon > 0$,

then, by the martingale central limit theorem, $n^{-1/2}U_n(t) \overset{D}{\to} W(t)$, where $W(t)$ is a Gaussian process with properties of (i) to (iii) of theorem 3.4.4.

Properties *Let $U_{n,l}(t) = \sum_{j=1}^{n} \int_0^t H_{j,l}(u)dM_j(u), l = 1, 2$ such that $H_{j,l}(t)$ is a bounded left-continuous $\mathcal{F}_t$-predictable process, then for any $l, k \in \{1, 2\}$*

(i) $U_{n,l}(t)$ is a martingale with $EU_{n,l}(t) = 0$,

(ii) $Var\{U_{n,l}(t)\} = \sum_{j=1}^{n} \int_0^t E\{H_{j,l}^2(u)Y_j(u)\lambda_j(u)du\}$,

(ii) $Cov\{U_{n,l}(t), U_{n,k}(t)\} = \sum_{j=1}^{n} \int_0^t E\{H_{j,l}(u)H_{j,k}(u)Y_j(u)\lambda_j(u)du\}$.

4

Survival Trial Design under the Parametric Model

4.1 Introduction

A phase III cancer clinical trial typically compares an experimental therapy to a standard (control) therapy. The primary objective is usually to study if the experimental therapy results in better survival. It is widely acknowledged that the most appropriate way to compare treatments is through a randomized clinical trial. The randomization guarantees that there is no systematic selection bias in the treatment allocation. Therefore, phase III trials are usually conducted as confirmatory and multicenter studies.

In a cancer survival trial with an overall survival endpoint, patients enter the study in a staggered fashion. They are randomized to one of two (or more) groups for treatment and followed to the end of the study. At the final analysis, some patients may have died. For those patients who remain alive, the total time of observation will vary, depending upon when in the accrual period they were randomized to a treatment group. The actual survival time for these patients is unknown. The survival time of a patient is defined as the time interval between the time origin (e.g., date of randomization) and the date of death or date of last follow-up. A patient who is still alive at the date of last follow-up is censored. The power of the study to detect the difference in survival between treatment groups is determined by the number of deaths observed rather than the number of patients enrolled in the study.

The methods for sample size calculation under the exponential model have been discussed extensively in the literature by George and Desu (1974), Lachin (1981), Rubinstein et al. (1981), Makuch and Simon (1982), Schoenfeld and Richter (1982), Lachin and Foulkes (1986), and many others. The exponential model has a constant hazard rate during the entire study period, and this is usually invalid in a long-period survival trial. In this chapter, we will extend the sample size calculation to the Weibull model.

TABLE 4.1: Lengths of remission of leukemia patients

Treatment	Length of remission (weeks)										
6-MP	6*	6	6	6	7	9*	10*	10	11*	12	16
	17*	19*	20*	22	23	25*	32*	32*	34*	35*	
Placebo	1	1	2	2	3	4	4	5	5	8	8
	8	8	11	11	12	12	15	17	22	23	

Note: *: censored observation.

4.2 Weibull Model

We first illustrate the motivation to use the Weibull model for survival trial design with an example given by Cox and Oakes (1984). In that trial, 6-mercaptopurine (6-MP) was compared to a placebo for the maintenance of complete remission in patients with acute leukemia who had undergone steroid therapy (Freireich et al., 1963). The sequential phase of the trial was stopped after 21 pairs of subjects had been enrolled and followed until at least one member of each pair experienced relapse. The lengths of complete remission (in weeks) of these 42 subjects are presented in Table 4.1, where censored values are denoted with asterisks.

Figure 4.1 shows the Kaplan-Meier curves and fitted Weibull distributions with a common shape parameter $\hat{\kappa} = 1.366$ and scale parameters $\hat{\rho}_1 = 0.1056$ and $\hat{\rho}_2 = 0.0297$ for placebo and 6-MP treatment, respectively. The Weibull distributions fit the Kaplan-Meier curves well. From the fitted curves for 6-MP and placebo, there is strong evidence that patients receiving 6-MP have longer remissions than do those receiving placebo. Thus, the Weibull distribution is the potential model for such clinical trial designs.

We start with a parametric MLE test under the Weibull model because it is simple and its asymptotic distribution is easy to derive and hence the sample size can be calculated. Assume that failure time variable T_i of a subject from the ith group follows the Weibull distribution with a common shape parameter κ and a scale parameter ρ_i, where $i = 1, 2$. That is, T_i has a survival distribution function

$$S_i(t) = e^{-(\rho_i t)^\kappa}$$

and a hazard function

$$h_i(t) = \kappa \rho_i^\kappa t^{\kappa-1}.$$

The shape parameter κ indicates the cases of increasing ($\kappa > 1$), constant ($\kappa = 1$) or decreasing ($\kappa < 1$) hazard functions. In a cancer trial, the median survival time is an intuitive endpoint for clinicians. The median survival time of the ith

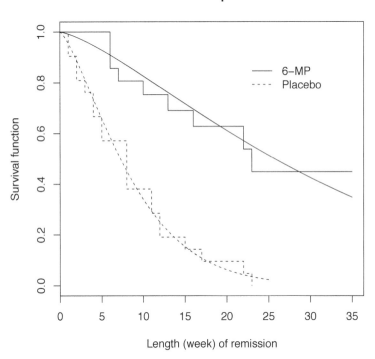

FIGURE 4.1: Kaplan-Meier curves (step functions) and fitted Weibull distributions (smooth curves) for 6-MP arm and placebo arm, respectively.

group for the Weibull distribution can be calculated as $m_i = \rho_i^{-1}\{\log(2)\}^{1/\kappa}$. Therefore, the Weibull survival distribution can be expressed as

$$S_i(t) = e^{-\log(2)(\frac{t}{m_i})^\kappa}, \quad i = 1, 2.$$

A one-sided hypothesis of a randomized two-arm trial defined by median survival times can be expressed as

$$H_0 : m_2 \le m_1 \quad vs. \quad H_1 : m_2 > m_1. \tag{4.1}$$

To derive the test statistics, we assume that the shape parameter κ is known or can be estimated from historical data. Good-quality historical data from a standard treatment group can provide estimates of the Weibull parameters that are reliable for study design. For notational convenience, we convert the scale parameter ρ_i to a hazard parameter $\lambda_i = \rho_i^\kappa = \log(2)/m_i^\kappa$, and the corresponding survival distribution is $S_i(t) = e^{-\lambda_i t^\kappa}$. Then the hypothesis (4.1) on median survival times is equivalent to the following hypothesis:

$$H_0 : \delta \ge 1 \quad vs. \quad H_1 : \delta < 1,$$

where $\delta = \lambda_2/\lambda_1 = (m_1/m_2)^\kappa$ is the hazard ratio.

4.3   Test Statistic

Suppose that during the accrual phase of the trial, n_i subjects of the ith group are enrolled in the study in a staggered fashion, and let T_{ij} and C_{ij} denote, respectively, the failure time and censoring time of the jth subject in the ith group, with both being measured from the time of study entry. We assume that the failure time T_{ij} is independent of the censoring time C_{ij} (independent censorship model), and that $\{(T_{ij}, C_{ij}); j = 1, \cdots, n_i\}$ are independent and identically distributed for $i = 1, 2$, respectively. The observed failure time and failure indicator are $X_{ij} = T_{ij} \wedge C_{ij}$ and $\Delta_{ij} = I(T_{ij} \le C_{ij})$, respectively, for $j = 1, \cdots, n_i$, $i = 1, 2$. Further assume that T_{ij} follows the Weibull distribution with shape parameter κ and hazard parameter λ_i. On the basis of the observed data $\{(X_{ij}, \Delta_{ij}), \quad j = 1, \cdots, n_i, \ i = 1, 2\}$, the likelihood function for (λ_1, λ_2) is given by

$$L(\lambda_1, \lambda_2) = \lambda_1^{d_1} \lambda_2^{d_2} e^{-\lambda_1 U_1 - \lambda_2 U_2},$$

where $d_i = \sum_{j=1}^{n_i} \Delta_{ij}$ is the total number of failures observed in the ith group and $U_i = \sum_{j=1}^{n_i} X_{ij}^\kappa$ is the cumulative follow-up time penalized by the Weibull shape parameter κ (see Appendix A).

To drive the test statistics, we convert (λ_1, λ_2) to (ψ, χ), where $\psi = \log(\lambda_1/\lambda_2)$ and $\chi = \lambda_2$. Then, the log-likelihood for (ψ, χ) is given by

$$\ell(\psi, \chi) = d_1 \log(\chi) + \psi d_1 + d_2 \log(\chi) - \chi e^\psi U_1 - \chi U_2.$$

By solving the following score equations:

$$\ell_\psi(\psi, \chi) = d_1 - \chi e^\psi U_1,$$
$$\ell_\chi(\psi, \chi) = \frac{d_1}{\chi} + \frac{d_2}{\chi} - e^\psi U_1 - U_2,$$

where ℓ_ψ and ℓ_χ represent the first derivatives of $\ell(\psi, \chi)$ with respect to ψ and χ, the maximum likelihood estimates of ψ and χ are

$$\hat{\psi} = \log\left(\frac{U_2 d_1}{U_1 d_2}\right) \quad \text{and} \quad \hat{\chi} = \frac{d_2}{U_2}.$$

The observed Fisher information matrix, a negative second derivatives matrix of $\ell(\psi, \chi)$ with respect to ψ and χ, evaluated at $(\psi, \chi) = (\hat{\psi}, \hat{\chi})$, is given by

$$J(\hat{\psi}, \hat{\chi}) = \begin{pmatrix} d_1 & U_2 d_1 d_2^{-1} \\ U_2 d_1 d_2^{-1} & U_2^2 d_2^{-2}(d_1 + d_2) \end{pmatrix},$$

and the variance of $\hat{\psi}$ can then be estimated by $J^{\psi\psi} = (d_1^{-1} + d_2^{-1})$, which is the (1,1) entry in the inverse of the Fisher information matrix $J^{-1}(\hat{\psi}, \hat{\chi})$. Therefore, the MLE test statistic of $\hat{\psi}$ is given by

$$Z = (\hat{\psi} - \psi)(J^{\psi\psi})^{-1/2}.$$

4.4 Distribution of the MLE test

Under the null hypothesis $H_0 : \delta = 1$, or $\psi = -\log(\delta) = 0$, the test statistic Z reduces to

$$Z = \log(U_2 d_1/U_1 d_2)(d_1^{-1} + d_2^{-1})^{-1/2}.$$

Under the alternative hypothesis $H_1 : \delta \neq 1$, we have $d_i/n_i \to p_i = E_{\lambda_i}(\Delta)$ and $\hat{\psi} \to \psi = -\log(\delta)$; then, $n_1^{-1/2} \log(U_2 d_1/U_1 d_2)(d_1^{-1} + d_2^{-1})^{-1/2} \to -\log(\delta)(p_1^{-1} + \omega^{-1} p_2^{-1})^{-1/2}$, where $\omega = n_2/n_1$. Therefore, based on the asymptotic theory for parametric survival models (Borgan, 1984), we have the following results: under the null hypothesis $H_0 : \delta = 1$, the test statistic $Z = \log(U_2 d_1/U_1 d_2)(d_1^{-1} + d_2^{-1})^{-1/2} \xrightarrow{D} N(0, 1)$ and under the alternative hypothesis $H_1 : \delta \neq 1$, $Z = \log(U_2 d_1/U_1 d_2)(d_1^{-1} + d_2^{-1})^{-1/2} \xrightarrow{D} N(\mu_1, 1)$, where $\mu_1 = -n_1^{1/2} \log(\delta)(p_1^{-1} + \omega^{-1} p_2^{-1})^{-1/2}$. Thus, the one-sided p-value for testing hypothesis (4.1) can be calculated by

$$p = P(Z > Z^0) = 1 - \Phi(Z^0),$$

where Z^0 is the observed value of the test statistic Z. If the hypothesis is a two-sided

$$H_0 : \delta = 1 \quad vs. \quad H_1 : \delta \neq 1,$$

then a two-sided p-value for testing the hypothesis can be calculated by

$$p = P(|Z| > |Z^0|) = 2\{1 - \Phi(|Z^0|)\}.$$

Example 4.1 *Acute Leukemia Trial*

If we fit the Weibull model to the acute leukemia trial data given in Table 4.1, the MLE of the common shape parameter is $\hat{\kappa} = 1.366$ and the MLEs of the scale parameters are $\hat{\rho}_1 = 0.1056$ and $\hat{\rho}_2 = 0.0297$ for the placebo and 6-MP groups, respectively. Hence, the estimated median survival times are $m_1 = \hat{\rho}_1^{-1} \log(2)^{1/\hat{\kappa}} = 7.24$ (weeks) and $m_2 = \hat{\rho}_2^{-1} \log(2)^{1/\hat{\kappa}} = 25.75$ (weeks) for the placebo and 6-MP groups, respectively. The observed numbers of failures are $d_1 = 21$ and $d_2 = 9$, and the penalized cumulative follow-up times are $U_1 = 452.979$ and $U_2 = 1096.141$ for placebo and 6-MP, respectively. Thus, the MLE of ψ is $\hat{\psi} = \log(1096.141 \times 21/452.979 \times 9) = 1.731$, and its variance estimate is $J^{\psi\psi} = (1/21 + 1/9) = 0.1587$. Then, the observed MLE test becomes $Z^0 = 1.731/\sqrt{0.1587} = 4.345$, and a two-sided p-value of the MLE test Z is $p = 2\{1 - \Phi(4.345)\} = 0.000014$. If the nonparametric log-rank test is applied to this data, the observed log-rank test $L^0 = 4.09878$ and a two-sided p-value for the log-rank test is $p = 2\{1 - \Phi(4.09878)\} = 0.000042$. Therefore, based on either the parametric MLE test or the nonparametric log-rank test, the observed difference in the survival distributions for those patients receiving 6-MP and those receiving the placebo is statistically significant, and we can then conclude that treatment with 6-MP reduces the disease recurrence rate.

4.5 Sample Size Formula

The asymptotic distribution of the test statistic Z derived in the previous section allows us to calculate the required sample size for the trial design. Under the null hypothesis, Z is approximately standard normal distributed. Thus, given a one-sided type I error α, we reject the null hypothesis H_0 if $Z > z_{1-\alpha}$. Under the alternative hypothesis $H_1 : \delta < 1$, Z is approximately normal distributed with mean $\mu_1 = -n_1^{1/2} \log(\delta)(p_1^{-1} + \omega^{-1}p_2^{-1})^{-1/2}$ and unit variance. Therefore, the power $(1 - \beta)$ of the Z test under the alternative hypothesis can be calculated as follows:

$$\begin{aligned}
1 - \beta &= P(Z > z_{1-\alpha}|H_1) \\
&= P(Z - \mu_1 > z_{1-\alpha} - \mu_1|H_1) \\
&\simeq \Phi\{-n_1^{1/2} \log(\delta)(p_1^{-1} + \omega^{-1}p_2^{-1})^{-1/2} - z_{1-\alpha}\}.
\end{aligned}$$

Thus, based on the Z test, the sample size of the first group can be calculated as

$$n_1 = \frac{(z_{1-\alpha} + z_{1-\beta})^2 (p_1^{-1} + \omega^{-1} p_2^{-1})}{[\log(\delta)]^2}. \tag{4.2}$$

The total sample size for the two groups is $n = (\omega + 1)n_1$.

For a two-sided test hypothesis

$$H_0 : \delta = 1 \quad vs. \quad H_1 : \delta \neq 1,$$

by the argument presented in Chapter 1, replace α by $\alpha/2$, then the sample size of the first group is given by

$$n_1 = \frac{(z_{1-\alpha/2} + z_{1-\beta})^2 (p_1^{-1} + \omega^{-1} p_2^{-1})}{[\log(\delta)]^2},$$

and the total sample size for the two groups is

$$n = \frac{(\omega + 1)(z_{1-\alpha/2} + z_{1-\beta})^2 (p_1^{-1} + \omega^{-1} p_2^{-1})}{[\log(\delta)]^2}. \tag{4.3}$$

4.6   Sample Size Calculation

To calculate the number of subjects required for the study, we need to calculate p_i, the probability of a subject in the ith group having an event during the study, that is $p_i = E_{\lambda_i}(\Delta)$, where $i = 1, 2$. Let $f_i(t)$, $S_i(t)$, and $\lambda_i(t)$ be the density, survival distribution, and hazard function of the control group ($i = 1$) and treatment group ($i = 2$). Under the independent censorship assumption, that is, where T and C are independent, we have

$$
\begin{aligned}
p_i = E_{\lambda_i}(\Delta) &= P_{\lambda_i}(T < C) \\
&= \int_0^\infty P_{\lambda_i}(T < C | T = t) f_i(t) dt \\
&= \int_0^\infty P(C > t) f_i(t) dt \\
&= \int_0^\infty G(t) S_i(t) \lambda_i(t) dt, \quad i = 1, 2, \tag{4.4}
\end{aligned}
$$

where $G(t) = P(C > t)$ is the common survival distribution function of the censoring time for the two groups, which is a common assumption for the randomized trial. Otherwise, the censoring process may be informative which inflates the estimate of the treatment effect and biases the results. To calculate this probability, we have to specify the censoring distribution $G(t)$, which is usually difficult during the design stage. However, it is typically assumed that subjects are accrued uniformly over an accrual period of length t_a and followed for a period of length t_f, and that no subject is lost to follow-up during the study; then, the censoring distribution $G(t)$ is a uniform distribution over $[t_f, t_a + t_f]$, which is usually called administrative censoring. The density function $a(t)$ of the entry times and the corresponding survival distribution $G(t) = A(\tau - t)$ of the administrative censoring times are given as follows, where $A(\cdot)$ is the distribution function of entry time:

$$a(t) = \begin{cases} \frac{1}{t_a} & \text{if } 0 < t \leq t_a \\ 0 & \text{otherwise} \end{cases} \qquad G(t) = \begin{cases} 1 & \text{if } 0 < t \leq t_f \\ \frac{t_a + t_f - t}{t_a} & \text{if } t_f < t \leq \tau \\ 0 & \text{if } t > \tau \end{cases}$$

and $\tau = t_a + t_f$ is the study duration. Thus, the probability of a subject having an event during the study given by (4.4) can be simplified as

$$p_i = 1 - \frac{1}{t_a} \int_{t_f}^{t_a + t_f} S_i(t) dt, \quad i = 1, 2, \tag{4.5}$$

where $S_i(t) = e^{-\log(2)\left(\frac{t}{m_i}\right)^\kappa}$ for the Weibull model (see Appendix B). This integration can be calculated numerically. Therefore, by using the relationship $\lambda_i = \log(2)/m_i^\kappa$, $\delta = \lambda_2/\lambda_1$, and $\lambda_i = -\log S_i(x)/x^\kappa$, where x is a landmark time point, given any one set of the following design parameters:

1. $\kappa, m_1, m_2, \alpha, \beta, \omega, t_f, t_a$;
2. $\kappa, m_1, \delta, \alpha, \beta, \omega, t_f, t_a$;
3. $\kappa, \lambda_1, \delta, \alpha, \beta, \omega, t_f, t_a$;
4. $\kappa, S_1(x), \delta, \alpha, \beta, \omega, t_f, t_a, x$;
5. $\kappa, S_1(x), S_2(x), \alpha, \beta, \omega, t_f, t_a, x$,

the number of subjects n required for the study can be calculated using formulae (4.3) and (4.5).

Remark 1: When $\kappa = 1$, the sample size formula (4.3) reduces to the formula developed by Schoenfeld and Richter (1982) for the exponential model.

Remark 2: Two Weibull distributions with shape parameters κ_1 and κ_2 satisfy the proportional hazards model if and only if $\kappa_1 = \kappa_2$.

Remark 3: Formula 4.3 was first derived by Heo et al. (1998) under the Weibull model, but their formula for calculating the failure probability, $p_i = 1 - P_i(t_a) S_i(t_f)$, where

$$S_i(t_f) = e^{-\log(2)\frac{t_f^\kappa}{m_i^\kappa}}$$

$$P_i(t_a) = \frac{1}{t_a} \int_0^{t_a} S_i(t_a - u) du.$$

was in error. This calculation holds for the exponential model ($\kappa = 1$), but it is incorrect for the Weibull distribution when $\kappa \neq 1$. Furthermore, they did not specify the test statistics for the sample size calculation. It is dangerous to calculate the sample size without specifying the test statistic, because different test statistics may use different methods to determine the sample size and may have different powers for the study.

Remark 4: Wu (2015) derived an alternative sample size formula under the Weibull model by using the test statistic

$$Z = \frac{\hat{\phi}_1 - \hat{\phi}_2}{\{\hat{\phi}_1^2/(9d_1) + \hat{\phi}_2^2/(9d_2)\}^{1/2}},$$

where $\hat{\phi}_j = (d_j/U_j)^{1/3}$, which has better small sample property (Sprott, 1973).

Remark 5: We can write the sample size formula (4.3) in terms of the number of failures $d_i = n_i p_i$ as follows:

$$d_1^{-1} + d_2^{-1} = \frac{[\log(\delta)]^2}{(z_{1-\alpha/2} + z_{1-\beta})^2}.$$

This formula was first derived by Rubinstein et al. (1981) under the exponential model. In Chapter 5 we will show that it holds for the log-rank test as well. This formula is very useful for designing unbalanced randomized clinical trials.

Remark 6. In an actual trial design, if there are historical data for the standard treatment group showing that the Weibull distribution provides a satisfactory model and gives reliable estimates for the median survival time (m_1) and the shape parameter κ, and if the investigators can also provide an estimate of the median survival time m_2 or hazard ratio δ based on a literature review or data from a pilot study on the experimental treatment or from the investigators' expectation for the experimental treatment (the minimal clinically meaningful effect size), then the trial can be designed as discussed above.

Remark 7. The most common entry method is uniform accrual, which assumes that patients enter the study at a constant rate over the accrual period. However, in practice, the accrual rate is rarely constant throughout the accrual period. For example, Barthel et al. (2006) gave examples of trials dealing with small populations or rare diseases, in which the limited number of cases can be exhausted quickly and further enrollment may slow down. Therefore, an increasing or decreasing accrual distribution may be used in the sample size calculation. Specifically, the censoring distribution considered in the trial design can then represent increasing or decreasing accruals (Maki, 2006). Then, the integrations in formula (4.4) can be calculated by numeric integrations, for example, by using the R function 'integrate.'

Remark 8. Clinical trials with time-to-event endpoints have an accrual period, t_a, the period during which patients enter the study, and a follow-up period,

t_f, the period from the end of accrual until the end of study or analysis of the data. The follow-up period substantially reduces the number of patients required in a clinical trial, because without it, little information would be provided by patients who entered the trial near the end of the accrual period.

4.7 Accrual Duration Calculation

When designing an actual trial with accrual time t_a, calculating the sample size is usually impractical because we may not be able to enroll the planned number of patients within the given accrual duration. It is more practical to design the study by starting with the given accrual rate r, which can usually be estimated from historical enrollment data, and then calculating the required accrual time t_a. This can be accomplished under the Weibull model assumption by defining a root function of the accrual time t_a,

$$\text{root}(t_a) = rt_a - \frac{(\omega + 1)(z_{1-\alpha} + z_{1-\beta})^2(p_1^{-1} + \omega^{-1}p_2^{-1})}{[\log(\delta)]^2}, \qquad (4.6)$$

where the failure probabilities p_1 and p_2 can be calculated by (4.5). The accrual time t_a can now be obtained by solving the root equation $\text{root}(t_a) = 0$ numerically in Splus/R using the 'uniroot' function. The total sample size required for the study is approximately $n = [rt_a]^+$, where $[x]^+$ denotes the smallest integer greater than x.

4.8 Example and R code

Example 4.2 *The PBC Trial*

Between January 1974 and May 1984, the Mayo Clinic conducted a double-blind randomized trial on treating primary biliary cirrhosis of the liver (PBC), comparing the drug D-penicillamine (DPCA) with a placebo (Fleming and Harrington, 1991). PBC is a rare but fatal chronic liver disease of unknown cause, with a prevalence of approximately 50 cases per million in the population. The primary pathologic event appears to be the destruction of the interlobular bile ducts, which may be mediated by immunologic mechanisms. Of 158 patients treated with DPCA, 65 died. The median survival time was 9 years (the full dataset is given in Appendix D of the report by Fleming and Harrington, 1991). Suppose investigators want to design a randomized two-arm phase III trial using DPCA treatment as the standard treatment. The primary endpoint of the study is overall survival. The survival distribution of

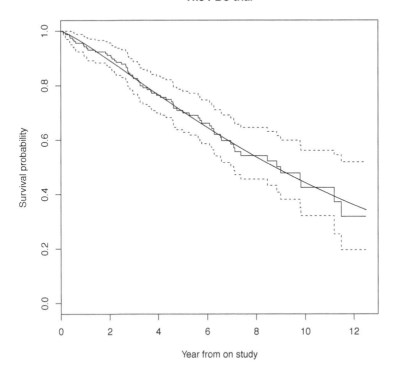

FIGURE 4.2: The step function is the Kaplan-Meier survival curve and the dotted lines are the 95% confidence limits. The solid curve is the fitted Weibull survival distribution function.

the Mayo Clinic DPCA arm was estimated by the Kaplan-Meier method and the Weibull model (Figure 4.2).

The Weibull distribution fitted the Kaplan-Meier curve well with shape parameter $\hat{\kappa} = 1.22$ and median survival time $\hat{m}_1 = 9$ (years). We assume that the failure time of patients on the experimental treatment follows the Weibull distribution with shape parameter $\kappa = 1.22$ and median survival time m_2. The study aim is to test the following hypothesis:

$$H_0 : m_2 \leq m_1 \quad vs. \quad H_1 : m_2 > m_1,$$

with a one-sided significance level of $\alpha = 0.05$ and power of $1 - \beta = 90\%$ to detect a 5-year increase in the median survival times with the standard treatment. To calculate the sample size, we assume a uniform accrual with accrual period $t_a = 6$ years and follow-up $t_f = 3$ years, no patient loss to follow-up, and equal allocation. We calculate the sample size by using formula

(4.2):

$$n_1 = \frac{(z_{1-\alpha} + z_{1-\beta})^2 (p_1^{-1} + \omega^{-1} p_2^{-1})}{[\log(\delta)]^2},$$

where $z_{1-\alpha} = 1.645$, $z_{1-\beta} = 1.282$, $\delta = (m_1/m_2)^\kappa = (9/14)^{1.22} = 0.583$, and $\omega = 1$. The probability of death is calculated by

$$p_i = 1 - \frac{1}{t_a} \int_{t_f}^{t_a+t_f} e^{-\log(2)(\frac{t}{m_i})^\kappa} dt, \quad i = 1, 2,$$

through numerical integration using the R function 'integrate,' as $p_1 = 0.341$ and $p_2 = 0.218$. Thus, the required sample size of the control group is $n_1 = (1.645+1.282)^2 \times (0.341^{-1}+0.218^{-1})/[\log(0.583)]^2 \simeq 222$, and the total sample size for the two groups is $n = (\omega+1)n_1 = 444$ patients. As indicated previously, in the clinical trial design, it is more practical to design the study by starting with the given accrual rate r and then calculating the required accrual time t_a. For example, assume the accrual rate is $r = 74$ patients per year. Then, the accrual period t_a can be calculated using formula (4.6). By numerical iteration using the R function 'uniroot,' we obtain the accrual period $t_a = 6$ years and the total sample size $n = 6 \times 74 = 444$ patients, which is the same as the sample size obtained above. If the accrual is faster than expected, e.g., the accrual rate is $r = 100$ patients per year, then a shorter accrual period $t_a = 4.9$ years and more patients $n = 490$ are needed for the study. The R function 'Duration' is given below for the duration and sample size calculations.

```
############################ Input parameters ############################
### kappa is the Weibull shape parameter; m1 is median survival for control;###
### alpha and beta are the type I and type II errors and power=1-beta;     ###
### delta is the hazard ratio; r is the accrual rate; tf is follow-up time; ###
### omega is the allocation ratio of treatment to control (n2/n1).          ###
############################################################################
Duration=function(kappa, m1, delta, alpha, beta, r, tf, omega)
{
 root=function(ta)
 {lambda1=log(2)/m1^kappa; lambda2=delta*lambda1; tau=ta+tf
  S1=function(t){exp(-lambda1*t^kappa)}
  S2=function(t){exp(-lambda2*t^kappa)}
  p1=1-integrate(S1, tf, tau)$value/ta
  p2=1-integrate(S2, tf, tau)$value/ta
  z0=qnorm(1-alpha); z1=qnorm(1-beta); R=lambda1/lambda2
  ans=r*ta-(1+omega)*(z0+z1)^2*(1/p1+1/(omega*p2))/log(delta)^2}
  ta=uniroot(root, lower=1, upper=10)$root
  n=ceiling(r*ta);ans=list(c(ta=round(ta,2), n=n))
  return(ans)}
Duration(kappa=1.22,m1=9,delta=0.583,alpha=0.05,beta=0.1,r=74, tf=3,omega=1)
     ta      n
   5.99    444
Duration(kappa=1.22,m1=9,delta=0.583,alpha=0.05,beta=0.1,r=100,tf=3,omega=1)
     ta      n
   4.89    490
```

5

Survival Trial Design under the Proportional Hazards Model

5.1 Introduction

The sample size calculation discussed in the previous chapter is restricted under the assumption of the Weibull distribution, which has a monotonic hazard function and may not be suitable for the existing historical data for planning the study. To avoid a parametric survival distribution assumption, a proportional hazards (PH) model is usually used to derive the sample size calculation with the well-known nonparametric log-rank test. The methods for sample size calculation under the proportional hazards model have been discussed extensively in the literature, e.g., by Schoenfeld (1981, 1983), Freedman (1982), Collett (2003), and many others. Their extension to a more general survival model has also been studied recently. Gangnon and Kosorok (2004) derived a sample size formula for trial designs with clustered survival data; Zhang and Quan (2009) discussed sample size calculation for the log-rank test with a time lag in the treatment effect; Wang (2013) derived a sample size formula under a semiparametric model; and Lakatos (1986, 1988) provided a sample size calculation for complex survival trial designs by using the Markov chains approach to account for loss to follow-up, noncompliance, and nonproportional hazards models. Ahnn et al. (1995, 1998) extended the Schoenfeld and Lakatos formulae to multiple treatment groups. Barthel et al. (2004) derived a sample size calculation for comparing more than two treatment groups under piecewise exponential models, allowing for nonproportional hazards, loss to follow-up, and cross-over. Among these methods, the sample size formula derived by Schoenfeld (1981, 1983) is most commonly used in clinical trial practice. In this book, we will restrict our discussion to two-arm survival trial design, which is essential for most cancer clinical trials. For trial designs with more than two treatment groups, we refer the reader to the works by Ahnn et al. (1995, 1998), Barthel et al. (2004), Halabi and Singh (2008), Jung et al. (2008), and others.

5.2   Proportional Hazards Model

We assume that there are two treatment groups, the control and experimental groups, which are designated by groups 1 and 2, respectively. We also assume that the hazard functions of the two groups satisfy the proportional hazards (PH) model

$$\lambda_2(t) = \delta\lambda_1(t),$$

or equivalently, the survival distributions of the two groups satisfy

$$S_2(t) = [S_1(t)]^\delta,$$

where δ is the unknown hazard ratio, which is a measurement of treatment effect between the two groups, and $\delta < 1$ indicates an improvement in survival in the experimental group vs. the control group.

We illustrate proportional hazards model by following the lung cancer clinical trial (Piantadosi, 1997). This clinical trial tested the benefit of adding adjuvant chemotherapy to patients with surgically resected lung cancer. A total of 172 patients were randomized to receive either radiotherapy or radiotherapy plus chemotherapy between 1979 and 1985. Figure 5.1 presents disease-free survival distributions from this randomized lung cancer trial. The score test (Grambsch and Therneau, 1994) shows that the proportionality assumption of the disease-free survival distributions is not rejected ($p = 0.11$).

A two-sided hypothesis for the difference in the survival distributions of the experimental treatment group and the control group is represented by

$$H_0 : S_1(t) = S_2(t) \quad \text{vs.} \quad H_1 : S_1(t) \neq S_2(t).$$

Under the PH model, this hypothesis is equivalent to the following hypothesis for the hazard ratio:

$$H_0 : \delta = 1 \quad \text{vs.} \quad H_1 : \delta \neq 1. \tag{5.1}$$

A well-known test statistic for testing the above hypothesis is the log-rank test, which was introduced in Section 2.4 of Chapter 2. Using the same notation, the log-rank score is given by

$$U = \sum_{j=1}^{k} (d_{1j} - e_{1j}),$$

and its variance estimate under the null hypothesis is given by

$$V = \sum_{j=1}^{k} \frac{n_{1j}n_{2j}d_j(n_j - d_j)}{n_j^2(n_j - 1)}.$$

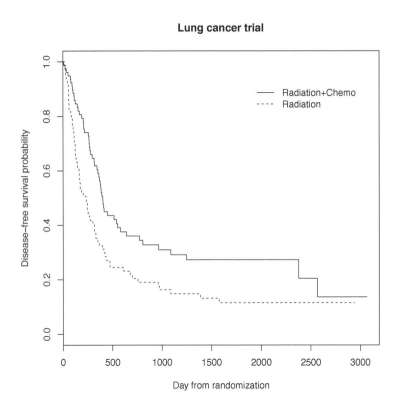

FIGURE 5.1: Disease-free survival by treatment group from a randomized lung cancer clinical trial.

The log-rank test is then given by

$$L = \frac{U}{\sqrt{V}}.$$

The asymptotic distribution of the log-Rank test under the fixed alternative has a rather complex form. In the literature, the asymptotic distribution of the log-rank test is usually derived under the local alternative, which is discussed in the next section.

5.3   Asymptotic Distribution of the Log-Rank Test

We will first introduce some notation. Let T be the failure time and C be the censoring time. Let us denote $f(t)$ and $S(t)$ as the probability density function and survival distribution of the failure time T, respectively, and denote $g(t)$ and $G(t)$ as the probability density function and survival distribution of the censoring time C, respectively, with $t \in [0, \tau]$, where $\tau > 0$ is a finite time point at which the study ends. Now let us consider the following regularity conditions:

(A1) T is independent of C.

(A2) $S(t)$ and $G(t)$ are continuously differentiable in $t \in (0, \tau]$.

(A3) $f(t)$ and $g(t)$ are uniformly bounded in $t \in (0, \tau]$.

(A4) $P(C \geq \tau) = P(C = \tau) > 0$.

(A5) $P(T > \tau) > 0$.

(A6) $P(T \leq C) > 0$.

Condition (A1) is the assumption of an independent censorship model. Conditions (A2) and (A3) are technical assumptions that are needed in the derivation of an asymptotic distribution. Condition (A4) implies that any patients alive at the end of the study are considered to be censored. Condition (A5) indicates that the probability of an individual surviving after τ is positive. Condition (A6) implies that there is a positive probability of observing a failure (Wang, 2013).

For notational convenience, we write the PH model as $\lambda_1(t) = \lambda_2(t)e^\gamma$, where $\gamma = -\log(\delta)$ is the negative log hazard ratio. To derive the asymptotic distribution of the log-rank test, we consider a null hypothesis $H_0 : \lambda_1(t) = \lambda_2(t)$ and a sequence of local alternatives: $H_{1n} : \lambda_1(t) = \lambda_1^{(n)}(t) = \lambda_2(t)e^{\gamma_{1n}}$, where $\gamma = \gamma_{1n} = b/\sqrt{n}$, $b < \infty$. Then, the asymptotic distribution of the log-rank test under the null and local alternative hypotheses can be summarized in the following theorem.

Theorem 5.1 *Under regularity conditions (A1)-(A6), the following results hold:*

Under the null hypothesis $H_0 : \gamma = 0$,

(i) $n^{-1/2}U \xrightarrow{D} N(0, \sigma^2)$, as $n \to \infty$,

(ii) $L = U/\sqrt{V} \xrightarrow{D} N(0, 1)$, as $n \to \infty$.

Under the local alternative $H_{1n} : \gamma = \gamma_{1n} = b/\sqrt{n}$, where $b < \infty$,

(i) $n^{-1/2}U \xrightarrow{D} N(b\sigma^2, \sigma^2)$, as $n \to \infty$,

(ii) $L = U/\sqrt{V} \xrightarrow{D} N(b\sigma, 1)$, as $n \to \infty$,

where $b = \sqrt{n}\gamma = -\sqrt{n}\log(\delta)$ and σ^2 is defined by equation (5.6).

To demonstrate the theorem, let $\{(T_{ij}, C_{ij}), j = 1, \ldots, n_i, i = 1, 2\}$ denote independent and identically distributed samples of (T, C) for the control group $(i = 1)$ and treatment group $(i = 2)$, and assume that the censoring distributions of the two groups are the same. The observed failure time and failure indicator are $X_{ij} = T_{ij} \wedge C_{ij}$ and $\Delta_{ij} = I(T_{ij} \leq C_{ij})$, respectively. We will use the following counting process notation:

$$
\begin{aligned}
N_{ij}(t) &= \Delta_{ij}I(X_{ij} \leq t), \\
N_i(t) &= \sum_{j=1}^{n_i} N_{ij}(t), \\
N(t) &= N_1(t) + N_2(t), \\
Y_{ij}(t) &= I(X_{ij} \geq t), \\
Y_i(t) &= \sum_{j=1}^{n_i} Y_{ij}(t), \\
Y(t) &= Y_1(t) + Y_2(t), \\
M_i(t) &= N_i(t) - \int_0^t Y_i(u)d\Lambda_i(u), \\
M(t) &= M_1(t) + M_2(t),
\end{aligned}
$$

where $\Lambda_i(t)$ is the cumulative hazard function for the ith group. Then $M_i(t)$ is a martingale with respect to the filtration $\mathcal{F}_t = \sigma\{N_{ij}(s), Y_{ij}(s+) : 0 \leq s \leq t, j = 1, \ldots, n_i, i = 1, 2\}$. The log-rank score statistic can be represented using the counting process notation as follows:

$$
\begin{aligned}
U &= \sum_{j=1}^{k}(d_{1j} - e_{1j}) \\
&= \sum_{j=1}^{n_1}\int_0^\infty dN_{1j}(u) - \sum_{i=1}^{2}\sum_{j=1}^{n_2}\int_0^\infty \frac{Y_1(u)}{Y(u)}dN_{ij}(u) \\
&= \sum_{j=1}^{n_1}\int_0^\infty \frac{Y_2(u)}{Y(u)}dN_{1j}(u) - \sum_{j=1}^{n_2}\int_0^\infty \frac{Y_1(u)}{Y(u)}dN_{2j}(u) \\
&= \int_0^\infty \left\{ \frac{Y_2(u)}{Y(u)}dN_1(u) - \frac{Y_1(u)}{Y(u)}dN_2(u) \right\}.
\end{aligned} \tag{5.2}
$$

Theorem 5.1 can then be shown as follows:

Proof 5.1 *Generally, we consider the following weighted log-rank score statistic:*

$$
U_w = \int_0^\infty W(u)\left\{ \frac{Y_2(u)}{Y(u)}dN_1(u) - \frac{Y_1(u)}{Y(u)}dN_2(u) \right\},
$$

where the weight function $W(t)$ is a bounded nonnegative $\mathcal{F}_t$ predictable process, and $W(t) \xrightarrow{P} w(t)$. Substituting the martingale $M_i(t)$ into the expression of U_w, we have

$$
\begin{aligned}
U_w &= \int_0^\infty W(u)\left\{ \frac{Y_2(u)}{Y(u)}dM_1(u) - \frac{Y_1(u)}{Y(u)}dM_2(u) \right\} \\
&+ \int_0^\infty W(u)\frac{Y_1(u)Y_2(u)}{Y(u)}\{d\Lambda_1(u) - d\Lambda_2(u)\}.
\end{aligned}
$$

Under the null hypothesis $H_0 : \Lambda_1(t) = \Lambda_2(t) = \Lambda(t)$, this reduces to

$$
U_w = \int_0^\infty W(u)\left\{ \frac{Y_2(u)}{Y(u)}dM_1(u) - \frac{Y_1(u)}{Y(u)}dM_2(u) \right\}.
$$

By the martingale properties, $EU_w = 0$, and

$$
\begin{aligned}
n^{-1}EU_w^2 &= n^{-1}E\int_0^\infty W^2(u)\left\{ \frac{Y_2^2(u)}{Y^2(u)}Y_1(u)d\Lambda(u) + \frac{Y_1^2(u)}{Y^2(u)}Y_2(u)d\Lambda(u) \right\} \\
&= E\int_0^\infty W^2(u)\frac{Y_1(u)Y_2(u)}{nY(u)}d\Lambda(u).
\end{aligned}
$$

As $W(t) \xrightarrow{P} w(t)$ and

$$
\frac{Y_1(t)Y_2(t)}{nY(t)} = \frac{n_1n_2}{n^2}\frac{\{Y_1(t)/n_1\}\{Y_2(t)/n_2\}}{Y(t)/n} \xrightarrow{P} w_1w_2\frac{\pi_1(t)\pi_2(t)}{\pi(t)}, \tag{5.3}
$$

we have

$$n^{-1}EU_w^2 \xrightarrow{P} \omega_1\omega_2 \int_0^\infty w^2(u)\frac{\pi_1(u)\pi_2(u)}{\pi(u)}\lambda(u)du = \sigma_w^2,$$

where $\pi_i(t) = P(X_{ij} \geq t), \omega_i = \lim_{n\to\infty} n_i/n, i = 1, 2,$ *and* $\pi(t) = \omega_1\pi_1(t) + \omega_2\pi_2(t)$. *The asymptotic variance* σ_w^2 *can be consistently estimated by*

$$\hat{\sigma}_w^2 = n^{-1}\int_0^\infty W^2(u)\frac{Y_1(u)Y_2(u)}{Y(u)}d\hat{\Lambda}(u)$$
$$= n^{-1}\int_0^\infty W^2(u)\frac{Y_1(u)Y_2(u)}{Y^2(u)}dN(u).$$

Thus, by the martingale central limit theorem, under the null hypothesis, we have shown that

$$n^{-1/2}U_w \xrightarrow{D} N(0, \sigma_w^2).$$

By Slutsky's theorem, it follows that

$$L_w = n^{-1/2}U_w/\hat{\sigma}_w \xrightarrow{D} N(0, 1).$$

To drive the asymptotic distribution of the weighted log-rank test under the alternative, consider a sequence of contiguous time-varying proportional hazards alternatives $H_1^{(n)}$: $\lambda_1(t) = \lambda_1^{(n)}(t) = \lambda_2(t)e^{\gamma_{1n}\theta(t)}$, where γ_{1n} is a sequence of constants satisfying $n^{1/2}\gamma_{1n} = b < \infty$ and $\theta(t)$ is a known function of time, which takes into account nonproportionality, and let $M_1^{(n)}(t) = N_1(t) - \int_0^t Y_1(u)\lambda_1^{(n)}(u)du$. Then, $U_w = U_{1w} + U_{2w}$, where

$$U_{1w} = \int_0^\infty W(u)\left\{\frac{Y_2(u)}{Y(u)}dM_1^{(n)}(u) - \frac{Y_1(u)}{Y(u)}dM_2(u)\right\}$$

and

$$U_{2w} = \int_0^\infty W(u)\frac{Y_1(u)Y_2(u)}{Y(u)}\{\lambda_1^{(n)}(u) - \lambda_2(u)\}du.$$

As $\gamma_{1n} \to 0$, $H_1^{(n)} \to H_0$ *and* $\lambda_1^{(n)}(t) \to \lambda_2(t)$, *again by the martingale central limit theorem,* U_{1w} *converges in its distribution to a normal variable with mean* $EU_{1w} = 0$ *and variance*

$$n^{-1}EU_{1w}^2 = n^{-1}E\int_0^\infty W^2(u)\left\{\frac{Y_2^2(u)}{Y^2(u)}Y_1(u)\lambda_1^{(n)}(u) + \frac{Y_1^2(u)}{Y^2(u)}Y_2(u)\lambda_2(u)\right\}du$$
$$\xrightarrow{P} \omega_1\omega_2\int_0^\infty w^2(u)\left\{\omega_2\frac{\pi_2^2(u)\pi_1(u)}{\pi^2(u)}\lambda_2(u) + \omega_1\frac{\pi_1^2(u)\pi_2(u)}{\pi^2(u)}\lambda_2(u)\right\}du$$
$$= \omega_1\omega_2\int_0^\infty w^2(u)\frac{\pi_1(u)\pi_2(u)}{\pi(u)}\lambda_2(u)du = \sigma_w^2. \tag{5.4}$$

Furthermore, substituting $\lambda_1^{(n)}(t) = \lambda_2(t)e^{\gamma_{1n}\theta(t)}$ *into* U_{2w}, *we obtain*

$$n^{-1/2}U_{2w} = n^{-1/2}\int_0^\infty W(u)\frac{Y_1(u)Y_2(u)}{Y(u)}\{e^{\gamma_{1n}\theta(u)} - 1\}\lambda_2(u)du.$$

By a Taylor series expansion,

$$e^{\gamma_{1n}\theta(u)} = 1 + \gamma_{1n}\theta(u) + O_p(\gamma_{1n}^2).$$

As $\gamma_{1n} \to 0$, $n^{1/2}\gamma_{1n} = b$, $e^{\gamma_{1n}\theta(u)} \to 1$, and $n^{1/2}O_p(\gamma_{1n}^2) = O_p(n^{-1/2})$, using equation (5.3), we have

$$n^{-1/2}U_{2w} \xrightarrow{P} b\omega_1\omega_2 \int_0^\infty w(u)\theta(u)\frac{\pi_1(u)\pi_2(u)}{\pi(u)}\lambda_2(u)du = \mu_w. \qquad (5.5)$$

Thus, under the contiguous alternative $H_1^{(n)}$, the weighted log-rank test is asymptotically normal distributed with mean μ_w/σ_w and unit variance, that is

$$L_w = n^{-1/2}U_w/\hat{\sigma}_w \xrightarrow{D} N(\mu_w/\sigma_w, 1).$$

The standard log-rank test is a special case of the weighted log-rank test with weight function $W(t) = 1$. Under the proportional hazard model, that is when $\theta(t) = 1$, by equations (5.5) and (5.4), the asymptotic variance and mean of the standard log-rank test are given by

$$\sigma^2 = \omega_1\omega_2 \int_0^\infty \frac{\pi_1(u)\pi_2(u)}{\pi(u)}\lambda_2(u)du \qquad (5.6)$$

and

$$\mu = b\omega_1\omega_2 \int_0^\infty \frac{\pi_1(u)\pi_2(u)}{\pi(u)}\lambda_2(u)du = b\sigma^2.$$

The variance estimate is given by

$$\hat{\sigma}^2 = n^{-1} \int_0^\infty \frac{Y_1(u)Y_2(u)}{Y^2(u)}dN(u),$$

which is a consistent estimate of σ^2 and is equal to the variance estimate $n^{-1}V$ (assuming continuous failure time; thus, there are no tied failure times).

As we have shown, the log-rank test under the null hypothesis follows a standard normal distribution. For testing a one-sided hypothesis $H_0 : \delta \geq 1$ vs. $H_1 : \delta < 1$, a large value of the log-rank test indicates a strong evidence against the null hypothesis, thus, we reject H_0 if $L > z_{1-\alpha}$; and for a two-sided hypothesis $H_0 : \delta = 1$ vs. $H_1 : \delta \neq 1$, we reject H_0 if $|L| > z_{1-\alpha/2}$.

5.4   Schoenfeld Formula

A sample size that is too small can lead to an underpowered study and is to be avoided. When the sample size is too large, one may fail to conduct or finish the study, thereby wasting money and resources. Thus, it is preferable to accurately determine the sample size required for the study. Among the available sample size formula in the literature, the Schoenfeld formula is widely used in clinical trial design. In this section, we will derive the Schoenfeld formula under the proportional hazards model.

Assume that there are n patients who are allocated between the control and treatment groups, which are designated groups 1 and 2, respectively. Let D be the set of identifiers in the two groups who died, and let t_j be the death time of the jth patient in either group. We assume that the $\{t_j\}$ are distinct. Let y_j be an indicator variable of the control group, that is, $y_j = 1$ if the jth subject belongs to the control group and $y_j = 0$ if the jth subject belongs to the treatment group. If we define $n_i(t)$ to be the number at risk just before time t in group i, then, the log-rank score (2.6) can be expressed as

$$U = \sum_{j \in D} \{y_j - p(t_j)\},$$

where $p(t_j) = n_1(t_j)/\{n_1(t_j) + n_2(t_j)\}$, and the log-rank test is given by

$$L = \frac{\sum_{j \in D} \{y_j - p(t_j)\}}{[\sum_{j \in D} p(t_j)\{1 - p(t_j)\}]^{1/2}}.$$

As shown in section 2.6, conditional on $n_1(t_j)$ and $n_2(t_j)$, the $\{y_j\}$ are a sequence of uncorrelated Bernoulli random variables with means

$$\mu_j = \frac{n_1(t_j)\lambda_1(t_j)}{n_1(t_j)\lambda_1(t_j) + n_2(t_j)\lambda_2(t_j)}$$

and variances $\mu_j(1 - \mu_j)$, where $\lambda_i(t)$ is the hazard function of group i. To derive the asymptotic distribution, we define function $\pi(t)$ to be the probability of a subject being at risk at time t in the group 1 and $V(t)$ the probability of observing an event at time t, given as

$$\pi(t) \quad = \quad \frac{w_1 S_1(t) G(t)}{w_1 S_1(t) G(t) + w_2 S_2(t) G(t)} = \frac{w_1 S_1(t)}{w_1 S_1(t) + w_2 S_2(t)} \qquad (5.7)$$

and

$$V(t) \quad = \quad \{w_1 \lambda_1(t) S_1(t) + w_2 \lambda_2(t) S_2(t)\} G(t), \qquad (5.8)$$

where $S_i(t)$ is the survival distribution of group i, w_i is the proportion of subjects assigned to group i, and $G(t)$ is the common survival distribution of the censoring time for the two groups. If we assume a proportional hazards model, then $\delta = \lambda_2(t)/\lambda_1(t)$ is a constant. Consider the local alternatives $\gamma = -\log(\delta) = b/\sqrt{n}$ with $b < \infty$; then, by a Taylor expansion at $\gamma = 0$

$$\mu_j \quad = \quad \frac{n_1(t_j)e^{\gamma}}{n_1(t_j)e^{\gamma} + n_2(t_j)}$$

$$= \quad \frac{n_1(t_j)}{n_1(t_j) + n_2(t_j)} + \frac{n_1(t_j)n_2(t_j)}{[n_1(t_j) + n_2(t_j)]^2}\gamma + O_p(n^{-1}),$$

or

$$\mu_j - p(t_j) = p(t_j)\{1 - p(t_j)\}\gamma + O_p(n^{-1}).\tag{5.9}$$

Replacing $p(t_j)$ by its limit $\pi(t_j)$ and γ by $bn^{-1/2}$, we have

$$n^{-1/2}\sum_{j\in D}\{\mu_j - p(t_j)\} = bn^{-1}\sum_{j\in D}p(t_j)\{1 - p(t_j)\} + O_p(n^{-1/2})$$

$$\xrightarrow{P} b\int_0^\infty \pi(t)\{1 - \pi(t)\}V(t)dt,\tag{5.10}$$

and

$$n^{-1}\sum_{j\in D}p(t_j)\{1 - p(t_j)\} \xrightarrow{P} \int_0^\infty \pi(t)\{1 - \pi(t)\}V(t)dt = \sigma^2.\tag{5.11}$$

The log-rank test L can be written as

$$
\begin{aligned}
L &= \frac{\sum_{j\in D}\{y_j - p(t_j)\}}{[\sum_{j\in D}p(t_j)\{1 - p(t_j)\}]^{1/2}} \\
&= \frac{\sum_{j\in D}\{y_j - \mu_j\}}{[\sum_{j\in D}\mu_j(1 - \mu_j)]^{1/2}} \times \frac{[\sum_{j\in D}\mu_j(1 - \mu_j)]^{1/2}}{[\sum_{j\in D}p(t_j)\{1 - p(t_j)\}]^{1/2}} \\
&\quad + \frac{\sum_{j\in D}\{\mu_j - p(t_j)\}}{[\sum_{j\in D}p(t_j)\{1 - p(t_j)\}]^{1/2}} \\
&= I_1 \times I_2 + I_3.
\end{aligned}
$$

By theorem 5.1, the first term, I_1, has a limiting standard normal distribution. From equations (5.10) and (5.11), the third term, I_3, converges in probability to

$$I_3 = \frac{n^{-1/2}\sum_{j\in D}\{\mu_j - p(t_j)\}}{[n^{-1}\sum_{j\in D}p(t_j)\{1 - p(t_j)\}]^{1/2}} \xrightarrow{P} b\sigma,$$

and using equation (5.9), the second term converges in probability to

$$I_2 = \frac{[\sum_{j\in D}\mu_j(1 - \mu_j)]^{1/2}}{[\sum_{j\in D}p(t_j)\{1 - p(t_j)\}]^{1/2}} \xrightarrow{P} 1.$$

Thus, we have shown that the log-rank test L is asymptotically normal distributed with unit variance and mean $E = b\sigma$. Let

$$P = \int_0^\infty V(t)dt = \omega_1 p_1 + \omega_2 p_2,$$

where $p_i = \int_0^\infty \lambda_i(t)S_i(t)G(t)dt$ and ω_1 and $\omega_2(= 1 - \omega_1)$ are the proportions of subjects assigned to treatment groups 1 and 2, respectively. Under the contiguous alternative, $\pi(t) \to \omega_1$ since $S_2(t) \to S_1(t)$, then $\sigma^2 \simeq \omega_1\omega_2 P$ and $E \simeq b(\omega_1\omega_2 P)^{1/2}$. Thus, we reject the null hypothesis H_0 with a two-sided type I error α if $|L| > z_{1-\alpha/2}$. The power $1 - \beta$ of the log-rank test L under the contiguous alternative H_{1n} satisfies the following:

$$1 - \beta = P(|L| > z_{1-\alpha/2}|H_{1n}) \simeq \Phi\{E - z_{1-\alpha/2}\}.$$

That is,

$$E = z_{1-\alpha/2} + z_{1-\beta}.$$

Replacing b by $-n^{1/2}\log(\delta)$ in the expression of E and solving $d = nP$, the total number of events is given by

$$d = \frac{(z_{1-\alpha/2} + z_{1-\beta})^2}{\omega_1\omega_2[\log(\delta)]^2}. \tag{5.12}$$

and the total sample size n for the two groups is given by

$$n = \frac{(z_{1-\alpha/2} + z_{1-\beta})^2}{\omega_1\omega_2[\log(\delta)]^2 P}. \tag{5.13}$$

Example 5.1 *Sample size calculation under the exponential model*

To illustrate sample size calculation using the Schoenfeld formula, we assume that the overall survival is exponentially distributed for both the standard and treatment groups. Assume that the 3-year survival probability of the standard group is 50% and that the investigators expect the experimental treatment to improve the 3-year survival probability to 60%. Then, the trial can be designed to detect a hazard ratio $\delta = \log(0.6)/\log(0.5) = 0.737$ for the one-sided hypothesis

$$H_0 : \delta \geq 1 \quad vs. \quad H_1 : \delta < 1.$$

Given a type I error of 0.05 and power of 90%, under the equal allocation $\omega_1 = \omega_2 = 0.5$, the total number of deaths required for the study can be calculated by

$$d = \frac{(z_{1-\alpha} + z_{1-\beta})^2}{\omega_1\omega_2[\log(\delta)]^2},$$

where $z_{1-0.05} = 1.645$, $z_{1-0.1} = 1.28$, and $\delta = 0.737$. Thus, we obtain $d = 368$. For the sample size calculation, we further assume a uniform accrual with accrual period $t_a = 5$ (years) and follow-up $t_f = 3$ (years), with no subjects being lost to follow-up. Under the exponential model and uniform accrual, the probability of death for each group is given by

$$p_i = 1 - \frac{1}{\lambda_i t_a}\left\{e^{-\lambda_i t_f} - e^{-\lambda_i(t_a+t_f)}\right\}, \quad i = 0, 1,$$

where $\lambda_i = -\log S_i(3)/3, i = 1, 2$, with $S_1(3) = 50\%$ and $S_2(3) = 60\%$. Hence, $p_1 = 0.704$ and $p_2 = 0.596$, and $P = 0.5 \times 0.704 + 0.5 \times 0.596 = 0.65$. Thus, by using the Schoenfeld formula, the total sample size of the two groups is given as $n = 368/0.65 \simeq 567$.

Remark 1: The Schoenfeld formula has been implemented in the commercially available software EAST 6, but its use is limited to the piecewise exponential model.

Remark 2: The power of the log-rank test is $1 - \beta \simeq \Phi\{|\log(\delta)|\sqrt{\omega_1\omega_2 d} - z_{1-\alpha/2}\}$, which depends on the total number of events d. Thus, the total of number of events determines the study power for the survival trial, not the total number of subjects.

Remark 3: The number of events formula (5.12) has several advantages over the sample size formula (5.13). First, it is a free assumption of the underlying survival distribution, censoring distribution, and accrual distribution. Thus, it can be applied to any PH model for study design and does not need to specify the survival distribution (to avoid possible misspecification) or the censoring distribution, which is usually difficult to know at the design stage. Second, it can be used to calculate the information time for trial monitoring. For example, if an interim analysis is planned with a number of d_0 events observed, then the information time for the interim analysis can be calculated by $t^* = d_0/d$, where d is the projected number of events calculated by (5.12). Thus, trial design based on formula (5.12) is much easier, more flexible and reliable. The only disadvantage is that trial management is more difficult or impractical when based on the number of events rather than the number of patients.

5.5   Rubinstein Formula

The Schoenfeld formula has been widely used to calculate the number of events and sample size of randomized two-arm clinical trials with time-to-event endpoints. It is common practice in randomized trials to allocate equal sample sizes to the treatment groups to gain higher statistical power. However, in some situations, despite the loss of power, investigators may still prefer an unbalanced design. For example, when the trial is designed to compare the experimental treatment to the standard therapy, the investigators want to gain more experience with or collect as much safety and efficacy data as possible on the experimental treatment. For unbalanced trial designs, we will show in Example 5.2 that the sample size calculated by the Schoenfeld formula tends to be either underestimated or overestimated, depending on the sample size allocation ratio of the treatment group and control group. A variant on the formula for the expected number of events is as follows:

$$d_1^{-1} + d_2^{-1} = \frac{[\log(\delta)]^2}{(z_{1-\alpha/2} + z_{1-\beta})^2}.$$

This was first derived by Rubinstein et al. (1981) based on the maximum likelihood test under the exponential model. Wu and Xiong (2015) derived the same formula under the Weibull model. It has been used for clinical trial designs for the log-rank test (Cantor, 1992; Case and Morgan, 2001). However, the formula has not been validated for the log-rank test.

To verify that this formula is also valid for the log-rank test under the PH model, we consider a sequence of local alternatives $H_{1n} : \gamma = \gamma_{1n} = b/\sqrt{n}$, where $b < \infty$. Under the local alternative H_{1n}, we have shown that the log-rank test L is asymptotically normal with unit variance and mean $b\sigma$, where $n\sigma^2 = w_1 w_2 (n_1 p_1 + n_2 p_2)$ is the asymptotic variance of the log-rank score U. As $p_1 \simeq p_2$, under the local alternative, we then have

$$\left(\frac{1}{n_1 p_1} + \frac{1}{n_2 p_2} \right)^{-1} \simeq w_1 w_2 (n_1 p_1 + n_2 p_2).$$

Thus, replacing $n\sigma^2$ by $\tilde{\sigma}^2 = (d_1^{-1} + d_2^{-1})^{-1}$, where $d_i = n_i p_i$, and given a type I error of α, the power $(1 - \beta)$ of the log-rank test L satisfies the following:

$$1 - \beta = P(|L| > z_{1-\alpha/2} | H_{1n}) \simeq \Phi(|\log(\delta)| \tilde{\sigma} - z_{1-\alpha/2}).$$

Hence, the expected number of events in each group satisfies the following equation for the log-rank test:

$$d_1^{-1} + d_2^{-1} = \frac{[\log(\delta)]^2}{(z_{1-\alpha/2} + z_{1-\beta})^2}. \tag{5.14}$$

We call this the Rubinstein formula hereafter. Substituting $d_i = n_i p_i$, the total sample size can be calculated by

$$n = \frac{(z_{1-\alpha/2} + z_{1-\beta})^2 P}{w_1 w_2 [\log(\delta)]^2 p_1 p_2}. \tag{5.15}$$

where $P = w_1 p_1 + w_2 p_2$. The Rubinstein formula is particularly useful because it shows the number of events required in each group and is more accurate than the Schoenfeld formula, particular for an unbalanced design. We will discuss its application in later chapters.

Example 5.2 *Continuation of Example 5.1*

The Rubinstein formula (5.15) can be written as

$$n_R = d_S P / (p_1 p_2),$$

where $d_S = (z_{1-\alpha} + z_{1-\beta})^2 / \{w_1 w_2 [\log(\delta)]^2\}$ is the total number of events calculated by the Schoenfeld formula. Under the same model assumptions and design parameters as in Example 5.1, the total sample size calculated by the Rubinstein formula is given by $n_R = d_S P / (p_1 p_2) = 368 \times 0.65 / (0.704 \times 0.596) \simeq 571$, and the total number of deaths is given by $d_R = n_R P = 571 \times 0.65 \simeq 372$; these are close to the results calculated by the Schoenfeld formula under this balanced design (with equal treatment allocation).

5.6　Freedman Formula

Another widely used formula for sample size calculation is that of Freedman (1982). Let us assume that there are n patients who are allocated between the control and treatment groups, which are designated groups 1 and 2, respectively. Assume the total number of events for the two groups are d and all event times are distinct. Without a loss of generality, we assume that $k = 1, \ldots, d$ identifies the patients who had an event. Let y_k be an indicator variable of the control group, that is, $y_k = 1$ if the kth subject belongs to the control group and $y_k = 0$ if the kth subject belongs to the treatment group. If we define n_{1k} and n_{2k} as the numbers at risk just before the kth death in the control and treatment groups, respectively, then the log-rank test statistic (2.8) can be expressed as

$$L = \sum_{k=1}^{d} \left(y_k - \frac{n_{1k}}{n_{1k} + n_{2k}} \right) \Big/ \left[\sum_{k=1}^{d} \frac{n_{1k} n_{2k}}{(n_{1k} + n_{2k})^2} \right]^{1/2}.$$

Conditional on n_{1k} and n_{2k}, the $\{y_k\}$ are a sequence of uncorrelated Bernoulli random variables with means

$$\mu_k = \frac{n_{1k} \lambda_{1k}}{n_{1k} \lambda_{1k} + n_{2k} \lambda_{2k}}$$

and variances $\mu_k(1 - \mu_k)$, where λ_{1k} and λ_{2k} are the hazards just before the kth death in the control and treatment groups, respectively. To obtain the asymptotic distribution of the log-rank test L, assume $\theta = \lambda_{1k}/\lambda_{2k}$ is a constant and consider a sequence of contiguous alternatives $\gamma = O(n^{-1/2})$, where $\gamma = \log(\theta)$. Then, one can show that by expanding μ_k in terms of γ in a Taylor series about zero, we have

$$L = \sum_{k=1}^{d} (y_k - \mu_k) \Big/ \left[\sum_{k=1}^{d} \mu_k(1 - \mu_k) \right]^{1/2} + E + O_p(n^{-1/2}),$$

where

$$E = \sum_{k=1}^{d} \left(\mu_k - \frac{n_{1k}}{n_{1k} + n_{2k}} \right) \Big/ \left[\sum_{k=1}^{d} \frac{n_{1k} n_{2k}}{(n_{1k} + n_{2k})^2} \right]^{1/2}.$$

Thus, L is approximately normal distributed with unit variance and mean E given by

$$E = \sum_{k=1}^{d} \left(\frac{\phi_k \theta}{1 + \phi_k \theta} - \frac{\phi_k}{1 + \phi_k} \right) \Big/ \left[\sum_{k=1}^{d} \frac{\phi_k}{(1 + \phi_k)^2} \right]^{1/2},$$

where $\phi_k = n_{1k}/n_{2k}$ and $\theta = \lambda_{1k}/\lambda_{2k}$. If we further assume that $\phi_k = \phi$ independent of k, then E reduces to

$$E = \sqrt{d}\frac{\sqrt{\phi}(\theta - 1)}{1 + \phi\theta}.$$

Thus, given a two-sided type I error of α, the study power of $1 - \beta$ satisfies the following:

$$
\begin{aligned}
1 - \beta &= P(|L| > z_{1-\alpha/2}|H_1) \\
&\simeq P(L - E > z_{1-\alpha/2} - E|H_1) \\
&\simeq \Phi(E - z_{1-\alpha/2}).
\end{aligned}
$$

It follows that

$$E = z_{1-\alpha/2} + z_{1-\beta}.$$

Thus, solving for d, the required number of events for the trial is given by

$$d = \frac{(z_{1-\alpha/2} + z_{1-\beta})^2(1 + \phi\theta)^2}{\phi(1 - \theta)^2}. \tag{5.16}$$

This formula was first derived by Freedman (1982). Using standard notation, let $\delta = 1/\theta$ be the hazard ratio of the treatment to the control and let $\omega = 1/\phi$ be the sample size ratio n_2/n_1. By substituting them into formula d in equation (5.16), we obtain

$$d = \frac{(z_{1-\alpha/2} + z_{1-\beta})^2(1 + \omega\delta)^2}{\omega(1 - \delta)^2}. \tag{5.17}$$

To calculate the required sample size, let p_1 and p_2 be the probabilities of failure for the control and treatment groups, respectively. Then, the total sample size of the two groups is given by

$$n = \frac{(z_{1-\alpha/2} + z_{1-\beta})^2(1 + \omega\delta)^2}{\omega(1 - \delta)^2 P}, \tag{5.18}$$

where $P = \omega_1 p_1 + \omega_2 p_2$ and $\omega_1 = 1/(1+\omega)$ and $\omega_2 = \omega/(1+\omega)$ are the sample size allocation ratio for the control and treatment, respectively.

Remark 1: The original Freedman formula was derived under simultaneous entry. This limitation is unnecessary. We have extended the formula so that it can be used for the trial design with staggered entry.

Remark 2: The Freedman formula has been implemented in the commercially available software nQuery, but its use is limited to the exponential model only.

Example 5.3 *Continuation of Example 5.1*

Again, under the same model assumption and design parameters as in

Example 5.1, the total number of deaths calculated using the Freedman formula is given by

$$d_F = \frac{(z_{1-\alpha} + z_{1-\beta})^2 (1 + \omega\delta)^2}{\omega(\delta - 1)^2},$$

where $\omega = 1$. Then, we have $d_F = 374$ and sample size $n_F = 374/0.65 = 576$. Thus, for this balanced design, the sample sizes calculated from the Schoenfeld, Rubinstein, and Freedman formulae are $n_S = 567$, $n_R = 570$, and $n_F = 576$, respectively, which are close to one another.

    Now consider an unequal allocation with 30% of patients randomized to the control group and 70% to the treatment group, that is, $\omega_1 = 0.3$ and $\omega_2 = 0.7$. Then, the failure probability $P = 0.3 \times 0.704 + 0.7 \times 0.596 = 0.628$. Thus, the total number of deaths and the sample size are $d_S = 438$ and $n_S = 438/0.628 \simeq 698$, respectively, by using the Schoenfeld formula. The total sample size calculated using the Rubinstein formula is given by $n_R = d_S P/(p_1 p_2) = 438 \times 0.628/(0.704 \times 0.596) \simeq 656$, and the total number of deaths is given by $d_R = n_R P = 656 \times 0.628 \simeq 412$. By using the Freedman formula, the total number of deaths is $d_F = 393$ and the sample size is $n_F = 625$. Thus, for an unbalanced design, relatively large discrepancies are observed among the sample sizes calculated by the three formulae. A simulation study with 10,000 runs showed that the empirical powers of the log-rank test for sample sizes $n_S = 698$, $n_R = 656$ and $n_F = 626$ are 0.915, 0.896 and 0.884, respectively. Thus, the Schoenfeld formula overestimated the sample size, and the Freedman formula underestimated the sample size, whereas the Rubinstein formula gave the most accurate sample size estimation. The R function 'SizeSRF' given below is for sample size calculation using the Schoenfeld, Rubinstein, and Freedman formulae for this example.

```
############################ Input parameters ############################
### s1 and s2 are the survival probability at landmark time point x;    ###
### ta and tf are the accrual and follow-up duration;                   ###
### alpha and beta are the type I error and type II error;              ###
### omega1 is the sample size allocation ratio for the control group.    ###
##########################################################################
SizeSRF=function(s1, s2, x, ta, tf, alpha, beta, omega1)
{lambda1=-log(s1)/x; lambda2=-log(s2)/x
 p1=1-(exp(-lambda1*tf)-exp(-lambda1*(ta+tf)))/(ta*lambda1)
 p2=1-(exp(-lambda2*tf)-exp(-lambda2*(ta+tf)))/(ta*lambda2)
 omega2=1-omega1; omega=1/omega1-1
 P=omega1*p1+omega2*p2; delta=lambda2/lambda1
 z0=qnorm(1-alpha); z1=qnorm(1-beta)
 dS=ceiling((z0+z1)^2/(omega1*omega2*log(delta)^2))
 nR=ceiling((z0+z1)^2*P/(omega1*omega2*p1*p2*log(delta)^2))
 dF=ceiling((z0+z1)^2*(1+omega*delta)^2/(omega*(delta-1)^2))
 nS=ceiling(dS/P); nF=ceiling(dF/P); dR=ceiling(nR*P)
 ans=list(c(dS=dS,nS=nS,dR=dR,nR=nR,dF=dF,nF=nF))
 return(ans)}
SizeSRF(s1=0.5,s2=0.6,x=3,ta=5,tf=3,alpha=0.05,beta=0.1,omega1=0.5)
 dS  nS  dR  nR  dF  nF
368 567 371 570 374 576
SizeSRF(s1=0.5,s2=0.6,x=3,ta=5,tf=3,alpha=0.05,beta=0.1,omega1=0.3)
```

dS nS dR nR dF nF
438 698 413 656 393 626

5.7   Comparison

So far, we have discussed the three most popular sample size calculation methods for survival trial design. Example 5.3 has shown that all three methods work well for a balanced design with a moderate hazard ratio and that the Rubinstein formula outperforms the Schoenfeld and Freedman formulae for an unbalanced design. To confirm this finding, a comparison of the three methods of sample size calculation was conducted under exponential models, where the 2-year survival probability for the control ($i = 1$) and treatment ($i = 2$) groups are given as in Table 5.1. We supposed that the trial was intended

TABLE 5.1: Comparison of sample sizes and empirical powers by using the Schoenfeld (S), Rubinstein (R), and Freedman (F) formulae under the exponential model, assuming a uniform accrual with accrual period $t_a = 5$, follow-up $t_f = 3$, a one-sided type I error of 5%, and power of 90%

\multicolumn{4}{c}{Design parameters}				Sample size			Empirical power		
ω_1	$S_1(2)$	$S_2(2)$	δ	S	R	F	S	R	F
0.5	0.1	0.25	0.602	137	136	142	.901	.893	.906
	0.2	0.35	0.652	198	198	204	.902	.902	.907
	0.3	0.45	0.663	225	224	230	.904	.897	.907
	0.4	0.55	0.653	223	224	230	.900	.900	.908
	0.5	0.65	0.622	202	203	210	.895	.905	.910
	0.6	0.75	0.563	164	168	173	.897	.907	.910
	0.7	0.85	0.456	116	124	129	.895	.915	.934
	0.8	0.95	0.230	55	79	76	.874	.956	.948
0.3	0.1	0.25	0.602	164	161	139	.908	.907	.863
	0.2	0.35	0.652	238	233	206	.910	.904	.873
	0.3	0.45	0.663	272	263	237	.916	.897	.871
	0.4	0.55	0.653	273	259	236	.912	.896	.875
	0.5	0.65	0.622	250	232	213	.913	.897	.873
	0.6	0.75	0.563	208	187	173	.917	.897	.875
	0.7	0.85	0.456	153	132	123	.934	.894	.881
	0.8	0.95	0.230	84	73	67	.942	.912	.893
0.7	0.1	0.25	0.602	162	163	203	.890	.890	.940
	0.2	0.35	0.652	233	238	282	.893	.898	.935
	0.3	0.45	0.663	262	272	315	.886	.904	.936
	0.4	0.55	0.653	259	274	313	.883	.903	.930
	0.5	0.65	0.622	231	251	285	.884	.907	.935
	0.6	0.75	0.563	184	212	240	.880	.922	.942
	0.7	0.85	0.456	126	163	182	.865	.933	.958
	0.8	0.95	0.230	54	114	116	.789	.979	.978

to detect a 15% increase in the 2-year survival probability (a one-sided test). We assumed a uniform accrual with accrual time $t_a = 5$ years and follow-up time $t_f = 3$ years, one-sided type I error of 0.05, and power of 90%. The sample sizes were calculated for each design scenario and are recorded in Table 5.1. The empirical powers were calculated based on 10,000 simulation runs. For equal-allocation designs ($\omega_1 = 0.5$), all three methods gave an accurate estimation of the sample size when the hazard ratio was close to the null hypothesis ($\delta > 0.5$). However, when the hazard ratio was far away from the null hypothesis ($\delta \leq 0.25$), the Schoenfeld formula underestimated the sample size, whereas both the Rubinstein and Freedman formulae overestimated the sample size. Because all three formulae were derived under the local alternative, they would be expected to perform well when the hazard ratio was close to 1 and perform worse when the hazard ratio was far away from 1. For unequal-allocation designs ($\omega_1 \neq 0.5$), the Schoenfeld formula still worked well when the hazard ratio was close to 1, but as the hazard ratio moved away from 1, the formula began to overestimate the sample size when more patients were assigned to the treatment group ($\omega_1 = 0.3$) and to underestimate the sample size when more patients were assigned to the control group ($\omega_1 = 0.7$). The Rubinstein formula provided an accurate estimation of the sample size, except when the hazard ratio was small ($\delta \leq 0.25$). The Freedman formula did not work well for unbalanced trial designs. The R function 'pow' is given below for the power simulation.

```
########################## Input parameters ###########################
### kappa is the shape parameter for the Weibull distribution;       ###
### s1 and s2 are the survival probabilities at landmark time point x; ###
### ta and tf are the accrual and follow-up duration;                ###
### alpha and beta are the type I error and type II error;           ###
### omega1 is the sample size allocation ratio for the control group; ###
### n is the total sample size of two groups.                        ###
######################################################################
library(survival)
pow=function(kappa,s1,s2,x,ta,tf,alpha,omega1,n)
{z0=qnorm(1-alpha); lambda1=-log(s1)/x; lambda2=-log(s2)/x
 tau=tf+ta; rho1=lambda1; rho2=lambda2
 shape=kappa; scale1=1/rho1; scale2=1/rho2
 s=0; N=10000; omega2=1-omega1
 n1=ceiling(n*omega1); n2=ceiling(n*omega2)
 set.seed(3485)
 for (i in 1:N)
 {w1=rweibull(n1, shape, scale1)
  u1=runif(n1, 0, ta); xt1=pmax(0, pmin(w1,tau-u1))
  delta1 = as.numeric(w1<tau-u1)
  d1=sum(delta1); grp1=rep(1,n1)
  w2=rweibull(n2, shape, scale2)
  u2=runif(n2, 0, ta); xt2=pmax(0, pmin(w2,tau-u2))
  delta2 = as.numeric(w2<tau-u2)
  d2=sum(delta2); grp2=rep(2,n2)
  time=c(xt1,xt2); grp=c(grp1, grp2)
  censor=c(delta1, delta2)
  dat=data.frame(time,censor, grp)
  survtest = survdiff(Surv(time, censor)~grp, data = dat)
```

```
sgn=sign(survtest$obs[1]-survtest$exp[1])
Z=sgn*sqrt(survtest$chisq)
if (Z>z0) (s=s+1)}
pow=s/N; ans=round(pow, 3); return(ans)}
pow(kappa=1,s1=0.1,s2=0.25,x=2,ta=5,tf=3,alpha=0.05,omega1=0.5,n=137)
0.901
```

5.8 Sample Size Calculation under Various Models

Three sample size formulae have been introduced in this chapter, and sample size calculations under the exponential model have been illustrated. However, the exponential model may not be adequate for survival trial design. Here, we will illustrate how the sample size can be calculated under various parametric and nonparametric proportional hazards models.

Under the Parametric Model

To calculate the sample size using formula (5.13), (5.15), or (5.18), we have to calculate p_i, where $i = 1, 2$. We assume that subjects are recruited with a uniform distribution over the accrual period t_a and are followed for t_f and that the study duration is $\tau = t_a + t_f$. We further assume that no subjects are lost to follow-up. Then, the censoring distribution is uniform over the interval $[t_f, t_a + t_f]$, that is, $G(t) = 1$ if $u \leq t_f$; $= (t_a + t_f - t)/t_a$ if $t_f \leq t \leq t_a + t_f$; $= 0$ otherwise. Thus, p_i can be calculated by

$$p_i = 1 - \frac{1}{t_a} \int_{t_f}^{t_a + t_f} S_i(t)dt, \quad i = 1, 2,$$

where $S_2(t) = [S_1(t)]^\delta$.

When a parametric distribution $S_1(t)$ can be estimated from the historical data for the control group, the survival distribution of the treatment group under the alternative can be specified by PH model $S_2(t) = [S_1(t)]^\delta$. Thus, the probability of an event during the study period can be calculated by using numerical integrations as follows:

1. The Weibull distribution,

$$S(t) = e^{-\lambda t^\kappa},$$

where $\lambda > 0$ and $\kappa > 0$. It can be easily seen that if $S(t)$ is a Weibull distribution with parameters λ and κ, then $[S(t)]^\delta$ is a Weibull distribution with parameters $\lambda \delta$ and κ. Thus, given a common κ for two groups, the probability of death for treatment groups 1 and 2 can be calculated by

$$p_i = 1 - \frac{1}{t_a} \int_{t_f}^{t_a + t_f} e^{-\lambda_i t^\kappa} dt, \quad i = 1, 2,$$

where $\lambda_2 = \delta \lambda_1$.

2. The Gompertz distribution,

$$S(t) = e^{-\frac{\theta}{\gamma}(e^{\gamma t}-1)},$$

where $\theta > 0$. It can be easily seen that if $S(t)$ is a Gompertz distribution with parameters θ and γ, then $[S(t)]^\delta$ is a Gompertz distribution with parameters $\delta\theta$ and γ. Thus, given a common γ for two groups, the probability of death for treatment groups 1 and 2 can be calculated by

$$p_i = 1 - \frac{1}{t_a}\int_{t_f}^{t_a+t_f} e^{-\frac{\theta_i}{\gamma}(e^{\gamma t}-1)}\,dt, \quad i = 1, 2,$$

where $\theta_2 = \delta\theta_1$.

3. The log-normal distribution,

$$S(t) = 1 - \Phi\left(\frac{\log t - \mu}{\sigma}\right)$$

where $\sigma > 0$. One can see that if $S(t)$ is a log-normal distribution with parameters μ and σ, then $[S(t)]^\delta$ is no longer a log-normal distribution. However, the probability of death for treatment group 1 can be calculated by

$$p_1 = 1 - \frac{1}{t_a}\int_{t_f}^{t_a+t_f}\left\{1 - \Phi\left(\frac{\log t - \mu}{\sigma}\right)\right\}dt,$$

and that for treatment group 2 can be calculated by

$$p_2 = 1 - \frac{1}{t_a}\int_{t_f}^{t_a+t_f}\left\{1 - \Phi\left(\frac{\log t - \mu}{\sigma}\right)\right\}^\delta dt.$$

4. The gamma distribution,

$$S(t) = 1 - I_k(\lambda t),$$

where $k, \lambda > 0$. If $S(t)$ is a gamma distribution with parameters λ and k, $[S(t)]^\delta$ is no longer a gamma distribution. However, the probability of death for treatment group 1 can be calculated by

$$p_1 = 1 - \frac{1}{t_a}\int_{t_f}^{t_a+t_f}\left\{1 - I_k(\lambda t)\right\}dt,$$

and that for treatment group 2 can be calculated by

$$p_2 = 1 - \frac{1}{t_a}\int_{t_f}^{t_a+t_f}\left\{1 - I_k(\lambda t)\right\}^\delta dt.$$

5. The log-logistic distribution,

$$S(t) = \frac{1}{1 + \lambda t^p},$$

where $p, \lambda > 0$. If $S(t)$ is a log-logistic distribution with parameters λ and p, then $[S(t)]^{\delta}$ is no longer a log-logistic distribution. However, the probability of death for treatment group 1 can be calculated by

$$p_1 = 1 - \frac{1}{t_a} \int_{t_f}^{t_a + t_f} \left\{ \frac{1}{1 + \lambda t^p} \right\} dt,$$

and that for treatment group 2 can be calculated by

$$p_2 = 1 - \frac{1}{t_a} \int_{t_f}^{t_a + t_f} \left\{ \frac{1}{1 + \lambda t^p} \right\}^{\delta} dt.$$

Under the Nonparametric Model

All parametric distributions have a restricted assumption and may not be suitable for the historical survival data used for trial design. Furthermore, the sample size calculation may be sensitive to the underlying survival distribution assumption used for the trial design. Thus, for greater robustness, one may prefer to calculate the sample size without making any parametric survival distribution assumptions. This can be achieved by using the Kaplan-Meier estimate of the historical survival data for the standard treatment group and Simpson's rule to calculate the failure probability numerically. Specifically, the integration

$$p_i = 1 - \frac{1}{t_a} \int_{t_f}^{t_a + t_f} S_i(t) dt, \quad i = 1, 2, \qquad (5.19)$$

can be calculated numerically by using Simpson's rule as

$$p_i = 1 - \frac{1}{6} \{ S_i(t_f) + 4 S_i(0.5 t_a + t_f) + S_i(t_a + t_f) \},$$

where the survival distribution $S_1(t)$ can be the Kaplan-Meier estimate of the historical data for the standard group, and by using the relationship $S_2(t) = [S_1(t)]^{\delta}$ to calculate the survival probability p_2.

Another approach is to use the logspline method (Kooperberg and Stone, 1992). Let the integer $K \geq 3$, and the knots be $\tau_1, \ldots, \tau_K$, with $0 < \tau_1 < \cdots < \tau_K \leq A \leq \infty$, where A is a real number, let $\mathcal{S}$ be p-dimensional space with natural cubic spline functions in this space, and let $1, B_1(t), \ldots, B_p(t)$ be the basis functions of $\mathcal{S}$. The logspline density function is defined as

$$f(t; \theta) = \exp\{\theta_1 B_1(t) + \cdots + \theta_p B_p(t) - C(\theta)\}, \quad 0 < t < A \leq \infty,$$

where

$$C(\theta) = \log \left[\int_0^A \exp\{\theta_1 B_1(t) + \cdots + \theta_p B_p(t)\} dt \right]$$

is the normalizing constant and $\theta = (\theta_1, \ldots, \theta_p)'$. The survival distribution function is then given by

$$S(t; \theta) = 1 - \int_0^t f(u, \theta) du, \quad 0 < t < A.$$

Under the assumption of the independent censorship model, a maximum likelihood estimate of θ is then obtained by maximizing the log-likelihood

$$\ell(\theta) = \sum_{j=1}^n \log \left\{ \int_{A_j} f(t; \theta) dt \right\},$$

where interval $A_j = \{X_j\}$ if $\Delta_j = 1$ and $A_j = (X_j, A)$ if $\Delta_j = 0$ on the basis of the censored survival data $\{(X_j, \Delta_j), j = 1, \ldots, n\}$. The maximum likelihood estimate $\hat{\theta} = \arg \max_\theta \ell(\theta)$ can be obtained using the Newton-Raphson iterative procedure. The corresponding maximum likelihood estimates of f and S are given by $\hat{f} = f(t; \hat{\theta})$ and $\hat{S} = S(t; \hat{\theta})$. For details, see Kooperberg and Stone (1992). This procedure has been implemented in R by using the function 'oldlogspline.' Once the survival function has been estimated by using 'oldlogspline' for the historical survival data, then, by numerical integration versus the logspline survival function, we can calculate the failure probabilities p_i given by (5.19).

The major advantage of the nonparametric approach is that it does not assume a specific parametric distribution and is therefore valid for any unknown distribution of survival time. The patients chosen for the historical control group should be similar in all aspects to the patients in the control arm of the planned study. Ideally, they should have the same distribution of prognostic factors, receive identical therapy and supportive care by the same health care professionals at the same locations. Obviously, these conditions cannot all be obtained exactly, but, many of them can be achieved approximately. For example, oncology cooperative groups perform serial clinical trials studying the same cancer type by using similar eligibility criteria, physicians, hospitals, and supportive care from trial to trial, and the control treatment in a study is usually one of the treatments used in the previous clinical trial.

Nonuniform accrual

The most common assumption of patient entry distribution is uniform distribution over an interval $[0, t_a]$, where t_a is the accrual period of the trial. The uniform accrual assumes that patients enter the study at a constant rate over the accrual period. However, in practice, particularly for a large trial with a long accrual period, the accrual rate may not be constant; the accrual rates could be higher in the early or later period of accrual. The sample size will be affected by the accrual pattern. To incorporate different accrual distributions in the sample size calculation, we adopt an increasing and decreasing accrual distribution as defined by Maki (2006). Assume the accrual period is t_a, the follow-up is t_f, and the study duration is $\tau = t_a + t_f$; we can then calculate the sample size by using the same sample size formula by numerical integration.

1. Increasing accrual: The density function $a(t)$ of the entry time and the corresponding survival distribution function $G(t)$ of the administrative censoring time are given by

$$a(t) = \begin{cases} \frac{2t}{t_a^2} & \text{if } 0 < t \le t_a \\ 0 & \text{otherwise} \end{cases} \qquad G(t) = \begin{cases} 1 & \text{if } t \le t_f \\ \frac{(t_a + t_f - t)^2}{t_a^2} & \text{if } t_f < t \le \tau \\ 0 & \text{if } t > \tau \end{cases}$$

2. Decreasing accrual: Density function $a(t)$ of entry time and the corresponding survival distribution function $G(t)$ of administrative censoring time are given by

$$a(t) = \begin{cases} \frac{2(t_a - t)}{t_a^2} & \text{if } 0 < t \le t_a \\ 0 & \text{otherwise} \end{cases} \qquad G(t) = \begin{cases} 1 & \text{if } t \le t_f \\ 1 - \frac{(t_f - t)^2}{t_a^2} & \text{if } t_f < t \le \tau \\ 0 & \text{if } t > \tau \end{cases}$$

Loss to follow-up

In survival trials, it is expected that some patients will be lost to follow-up due to their relocation or ceasing to return for follow-up visits, etc. When loss to follow-up is considered in the sample size calculation, the most common assumption is independent censorship. This model assumes that the probability of being censored is independent of the probability of failure and that patients are lost at random through the duration of the trial. Thus, there is a constant hazard of patients becoming lost to follow-up, and the times to loss to follow-up are exponentially distributed (Yatman and Skene, 1991). Furthermore, the rates of loss to follow-up are expected to be identical in the two groups. If the reason for the loss to follow-up is related to the treatment group assignment, serious problems of interpretation can arise. Hence, we can combine the loss to follow-up censoring with administrative censoring in the sample size calculation. For example, let C_1 and C_2 be the variables for administrative censoring and loss to follow-up, respectively; then, the overall censoring variable is $C = C_1 \wedge C_2$. Thus, the overall censoring distribution is $G(t) = P(C > t) = P(C_1 \wedge C_2 > t) = P(C_1 > t)P(C_2 > t) = G_1(t)G_2(t)$. Under the independent censoring assumption, T and C are independent, and the probability of failure can be calculated as

$$\begin{aligned} p &= E(\Delta) = P(T < C) \\ &= \int_0^\infty P(C > T | T = t) f(t) dt \\ &= \int_0^\infty P(C > t) f(t) dt \\ &= \int_0^\infty G_1(t) G_2(t) S(t) d\Lambda(t). \end{aligned} \tag{5.20}$$

Therefore, the sample size calculations can be adjusted using the overall censoring distribution. For example, under uniform accrual, the total censoring is a combination of both the administrative censoring and the loss to follow-up censoring. Consider a special case where both the failure time and the loss to follow-up time are exponentially distributed with hazard rates of λ and η, respectively, with uniform accrual over an interval $[0, t_a]$ and follow-up duration t_f. Then the survival distribution functions of the administrative censoring and loss to follow-up censoring are $G_1(t) = 1$ if $t \leq t_f$; $= (t_a + t_f - t)/t_a$ if $t_f \leq t \leq t_a + t_f$; $= 0$ otherwise, and $G_2(t) = e^{-\eta t}(t > 0)$, respectively. Thus, the probability of failure during the study is given by

$$
\begin{aligned}
p &= \lambda \int_0^{t_f} e^{-(\lambda+\eta)t} dt + \frac{\lambda}{t_a} \int_{t_f}^{t_a+t_f} (t_a + t_f - t) e^{-(\lambda+\eta)t} dt \\
&= \frac{\lambda}{(\lambda+\eta)} \left\{ 1 - \frac{e^{-(\lambda+\eta)t_f} - e^{-(\lambda+\eta)(t_a+t_f)}}{(\lambda+\eta)t_a} \right\}.
\end{aligned}
$$

The sample size can be adjusted based on the probabilities of an event for each group given above. Let ξ be the indicator of loss to follow-up and let C_1 and C_2 be the variables for administrative censoring and loss to follow-up. Then, the probability of loss to follow-up can be calculated by

$$
\begin{aligned}
p_L &= E(\xi|\lambda, \eta) = P(C_2 < T \wedge C_1) \\
&= \int_0^{\infty} P(T \wedge C_1 > t) f_{C_2}(t) dt \\
&= \int_0^{\infty} S(t) G_1(t) f_{C_2}(t) dt \\
&= \frac{\eta}{(\lambda+\eta)} \left\{ 1 - \frac{e^{-(\lambda+\eta)t_f} - e^{-(\lambda+\eta)(t_a+t_f)}}{(\lambda+\eta)t_a} \right\}.
\end{aligned}
$$

However, complicated numerical integrations may be needed for a general distribution of loss to follow-up. For increasing and decreasing accrual distributions, numeric integration can be used to calculate the failure probability p by using formula (5.20).

    Examples of sample size calculations for uniform and non-uniform accruals under the Weibull distribution are given in Table 5.2. The R function 'Size' is given below for the sample size calculation under the uniform accrual and exponential loss to follow-up. The results show that an increasing (decreasing) accrual requires more (fewer) patients compared to a uniform accrual.

```
######################### Input parameters ############################
### kappa is the shape parameter of the Weibull distribution;       ###
### lambda1 is the hazard parameter for the control group;          ###
### HR is inverse of the hazard ratio; p is the allocation ratio of control;###
### ta and tf are the accrual time and follow-up duration;          ###
### eta is the hazard rate of exponential loss to follow-up;        ###
### alpha and beta are the type I error and type II error.          ###
######################################################################
```

TABLE 5.2: Sample size calculation using the Schoenfeld formula for the Weibull-distributed failure time ($\lambda_1 = 0.5$) under uniform, increasing, and decreasing accrual distributions with a common exponential loss to follow-up distribution ($\eta=0.1$) for both control and treatment groups for various hazard ratios, with an accrual duration $t_a = 5$ and follow-up time $t_f = 3$, two-sided type I error of 5%, and power of 90%

	Uniform			Increasing			Decreasing		
	κ			κ			κ		
δ^{-1}	0.5	1	2	0.5	1	2	0.5	1	2
1.2	2207	1648	1440	2275	1695	1441	2143	1603	1439
1.3	1092	807	698	1126	832	699	1059	784	697
1.4	679	498	426	701	514	426	659	483	425
1.5	478	348	294	493	359	295	463	337	294
1.6	363	262	220	374	271	220	351	254	219
1.7	290	208	173	299	216	173	281	201	173
1.8	240	172	141	248	178	142	233	166	141
1.9	205	146	119	212	152	119	198	141	119
2.0	178	127	102	184	132	103	173	122	102

```
Size=function(kappa,lambda1,HR,eta,p,ta,tf,alpha,beta)
{z0=qnorm(1-alpha/2)
 z1=qnorm(1-beta)
 lambda2=lambda1/HR
 tau=tf+ta
 S1=function(t){exp(-lambda1*t^kappa)}
 S2=function(t){exp(-lambda2*t^kappa)}
 h1=function(t){kappa*lambda1*t^(kappa-1)}
 h2=function(t){kappa*lambda2*t^(kappa-1)}
 G=function(t){1-punif(t, tf, tau)}
 H=function(t){exp(-eta*t)}
 f1=function(t){H(t)*G(t)*S1(t)*h1(t)}
 f2=function(t){H(t)*G(t)*S2(t)*h2(t)}
 p1=integrate(f1, 0, tau)$value
 p2=integrate(f2, 0, tau)$value
 P=p*p1+(1-p)*p2
 n=ceiling((z0+z1)^2/(p*(1-p)*log(HR)^2*P))
 return(n)}
Size(kappa=0.5,lambda1=0.5,HR=1.2,eta=0.1,p=0.5,ta=5,tf=3,alpha=0.05,beta=0.1)
2207
Size(kappa=1,lambda1=0.5,HR=1.2,eta=0.1,p=0.5,ta=5,tf=3,alpha=0.05,beta=0.1)
1648
Size(kappa=2,lambda1=0.5,HR=1.2,eta=0.1,p=0.5,ta=5,tf=3,alpha=0.05,beta=0.1)
1440
```

The PBC trial

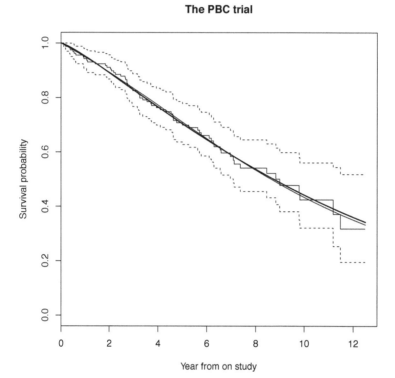

FIGURE 5.2: The step function is the Kaplan-Meier survival curve and the dotted lines are the 95% confidence limits. The solid curves are the fitted logspline survival distribution (thin line) and the Weibull distribution (wide line).

5.9   Example

Example 5.4 *Continuation of the PBC trial example*

Suppose a new treatment is now available and investigators want to design a new randomized phase III trial using the DPCA-arm of the PBC trial as a control group. The survival distribution of the DPCA-arm of the PBC trial can be estimated by a Kaplan-Meier curve, the Weibull distribution and a logspline curve by using the R function 'oldlogspline' (Figure 5.2).

The Weibull distribution fits the survival distribution well, with an estimated shape parameter $\hat{\kappa} = 1.22$ and median survival time $\hat{m}_1 = 9$ (years). We assume that the failure time of patients on the new trial follows the Weibull

Example 87

distribution with shape parameter $\kappa = 1.22$ and median survival time m_2; hence the survival distributions of the two groups satisfy the PH model assumption. Let $\delta = (m_1/m_2)^\kappa$ be the hazard ratio. The study aim is to test the following two-sided hypothesis:

$$H_0 : \delta = 1 \quad vs. \quad H_0 : \delta \neq 1$$

with a significance level of $\alpha = 0.05$ and power of $1 - \beta = 90\%$ to detect an alternative hazard ratio $\delta = 0.583$, which is calculated by increasing the median survival time of the treatment group by 5 years relative to that of the control group. To calculate the sample size, we assume that the accrual period is $t_a = 6$ years, the follow-up is $t_f = 3$ years, no patient is lost to follow-up, with an equal allocation ($\omega_1 = \omega_2 = 0.5$). We will calculate the sample size by using the Schoenfeld formula. First, under the Weibull model, the probability of death can be calculated by

$$p_i = 1 - \frac{1}{t_a} \int_{t_f}^{t_a + t_f} e^{-\log(2)(\frac{t}{m_i})^\kappa} dt, \quad i = 1, 2.$$

By numerical integration using R function 'integrate,' we obtain $p_1 = 0.341$ and $p_2 = 0.218$. Thus, the required total sample size of the two groups is $n = 519$.

Second, if we feel that the Weibull distribution assumption may be unreliable, the study design can be performed by using the Kaplan-Meier estimate without a parametric model assumption. The probability of failure can be calculated numerically by using Simpson's rule as follows:

$$p_i = 1 - \frac{1}{6}\{S_i(t_f) + 4S_i(0.5t_a + t_f) + S_i(t_a + t_f)\},$$

where the survival distribution $S_1(t)$ can be the Kaplan-Meier estimate for the historical data for the control group, and by using the PH assumption $S_2(t) = [S_1(t)]^\delta$ to calculate the failure probability p_2. From the Kaplan-Meier estimate, we have $S_1(3) = 0.826$, $S_1(6) = 0.661$, and $S_1(9) = 0.478$. Thus, $p_1 = 1 - (0.826 + 4 \times 0.661 + 0.478)/6 = 0.342$ and $p_2 = 1 - (0.826^{0.583} + 4 \times 0.661^{0.583} + 0.478^{0.583})/6 = 0.219$, which are very close to the values calculated under the Weibull model. The required total sample size of the two groups is $n = 517$

Finally, a spline version of the survival distribution fitted using the 'old-logspline' function, e.g., $S_1(t)$, can be used to calculate the probability of death as

$$p_i = 1 - \frac{1}{t_a} \int_{t_f}^{t_a + t_f} S_i(t)dt, \quad i = 1, 2, \tag{5.21}$$

where $S_2(t) = [S_1(t)]^\delta$. By numerical integration, we have $p_1 = 0.348$ and $p_2 = 0.223$, which are also close to the values calculated under the Weibull *model and Kaplan-Meier survival curve. The required sample size calculated under the spline survival distribution is n = 508.*

If we assume that the time of loss to follow-up time is exponentially distributed with a hazard rate $\eta = 0.025$ for both the control and treatment groups, then the sample sizes calculated under the Weibull distribution, Kaplan-Meier curve, and log-spline curve by using the R function 'SizeSch' are 563, 561, and 552, respectively (see Appendix D).

Note: If we use the Kaplan-Meier curve for sample size calculation with an exponential loss to follow-up distribution $e^{-\eta t}$ and uniform accrual with administrative censoring distribution $G(t)$, by integrating by parts, we can show that

$$
\begin{aligned}
p &= \int_0^\infty e^{-\eta t} G(t) S(t) d\Lambda(t) \\
&= 1 - \eta \int_0^{t_f} e^{-\eta t} S(t) dt \\
&\quad - \frac{1}{t_a} \left[(1 + \tau\eta) \int_{t_f}^\tau e^{-\eta t} S(t) dt - \eta \int_{t_f}^\tau t e^{-\eta t} S(t) dt \right].
\end{aligned}
$$

Thus, by apply Simpson's rule to the integrations $\int_0^{t_f} e^{-\eta t} S(t) dt$, $\int_{t_f}^\tau e^{-\eta t} S(t) dt$ and $\int_{t_f}^\tau t e^{-\eta t} S(t) dt$, one can calculate the failure probability based on the Kaplan-Meier curve.

5.10   Optimal Properties of the Log-Rank Test

5.10.1   Optimal Sample Size Allocation

In a randomized clinical trial, to achieve the maximum power for the study, it is important to know the optimal sample size allocation ratio ($\zeta = \omega_1/\omega_2$). The Schoenfeld formula $d = (z_{1-\alpha} + z_{1-\beta/2})^2/\omega_1\omega_2[\log(\delta)]^2$ predicts the highest power (or, equivalently, gives the maximum number of events) when equal sample size allocation is used for the study design ($\zeta = 1$). It is desirable to know the optimal sample size ratio for the Rubinstein formula (5.15). For equal allocation of sample sizes (i.e., $\zeta = 1$) or equal allocation of events (i.e., $\zeta = p_2/p_1$, or $\omega_1 p_1 = \omega_2 p_2$), it is easy to check that the sample size obtained by formula (5.15) reduces to

$$
n = \frac{2(z_{1-\alpha/2} + z_{1-\beta})^2}{[\log(\delta)]^2}(p_1^{-1} + p_2^{-1}), \tag{5.22}
$$

which is not the minimum sample size. It can be shown that the optimal sample size for formula (5.15) is located at the ratio of

$$\hat{\zeta} = \sqrt{\frac{p_2}{p_1}},$$

(see Appendix C) and the minimum sample size achieved at the optimal allocation ratio $\hat{\zeta}$ is given by

$$n = \frac{(z_{1-\alpha/2} + z_{1-\beta})^2}{[\log(\delta)]^2}(p_1^{-1/2} + p_2^{-1/2})^2. \tag{5.23}$$

Thus, the optimal sample size ratio of formula (5.15) satisfies the following:

$$\frac{p_2}{p_1} < \hat{\zeta} < 1 \quad \text{or} \quad 1 < \hat{\zeta} < \frac{p_2}{p_1},$$

which implies that the optimal sample size ratio is located within an equal allocation of events and an equal allocation of sample sizes, as predicted by Hsieh (1992) from a power simulation of the log-rank test. Under the optimal sample size ratio, the events ratio η is given by

$$\eta = \frac{\omega_1 p_1}{\omega_2 p_2} = \hat{\zeta}\frac{p_1}{p_2} = \sqrt{\frac{p_1}{p_2}} = \frac{1}{\hat{\zeta}},$$

which is the reciprocal of the optimal sample size ratio. It can also be shown that the sample size ratio minimizing the expected total number of events $d = nP$ for the formula (5.15) is given by

$$\tilde{\zeta} = \frac{p_2}{p_1},$$

(see Appendix C) and the minimum expected total number of events is given by

$$d = \frac{4(z_{1-\alpha/2} + z_{1-\beta})^2}{[\log(\delta)]^2}.$$

Thus, the minimum expected total number of events is achieved when an equal allocation of events ($\zeta = p_2/p_1$) is used for the randomization. The total sample size with the minimum expected total number of events is given by formula (5.22).

Simulations were conducted to study the power of the log-rank test when the sample size ratio was equal to the equal events allocation ratio ($\zeta = p_2/p_1$), optimal sample size ratio ($\zeta = \hat{\zeta}$) and equal sample size ratio ($\zeta = 1$). The results showed that the power curves are flat over the interval $(1, p_2/p_1)$ or $(p_2/p_1, 1)$, which is consistent with the findings of Hsieh (1992) and Kalish and Harrington (1988). Thus, both equal sample size allocation and equal event allocation are nearly optimal. However, it is usually impractical to perform randomization to yield equal numbers of events in two groups. Thus, equal sample size allocation is still recommended.

5.10.2   Optimal Power

We have shown in Chapter 5 that under the local alternative $H_1^{(n)} : \lambda_1^{(n)}(t) = \lambda_2(t)e^{\gamma_{1n}\theta(t)}$, the weighted log-rank test $L_w \overset{D}{\longrightarrow} N(\mu_w/\sigma_w, 1)$, where

$$\mu_w = b\omega_1\omega_2 \int_0^\infty w(t)\theta(t)h(t)dt$$

and

$$\sigma_w^2 = \omega_1\omega_2 \int_0^\infty w^2(t)h(t)dt,$$

where $h(t) = \pi_1(t)\pi_2(t)\lambda_2(t)/\pi(t)$. Thus, the power of the weighted log-rank test is given by

$$1 - \beta \simeq \Phi\{\mu_w/\sigma_w - z_{1-\alpha}\}.$$

Hence, as μ_w/σ_w increases, the power of the weighted log-rank test increases. By the Cauchy-Schwartz inequality, we obtain the following inequality:

$$\int_0^\infty w(t)\theta(t)h(t)dt \leq \left\{ \int_0^\infty w^2(t)h(t)dt \int_0^\infty \theta^2(t)h(t)dt \right\}^{1/2},$$

with equality if and only if $w(t) \propto \theta(t)$. Thus, μ_w/σ_w is maximized when $w(t) \propto \theta(t)$. That is, the optimal weight function is proportional to the log hazard ratio $\theta(t)$. For the standard log-rank test, $w(t) = 1$, and the maximum power is achieved when $\theta(t)$ is a constant. Therefore, the log-rank test is an optimal test against the proportional hazards alternative $H_1^{(n)} : \lambda_1^{(n)}(t) = \lambda_2(t)e^{\gamma_{1n}}$.

5.11   Precise Formula

The Schoenfeld formula is derived under the local alternative $\gamma = O(n^{-1/2})$, where $\gamma = -\log(\delta)$. We call this a first-order local alternative, which implies that the log hazard ratio between the treatment groups decreases to 0 at the rate of $n^{-1/2}$. Thus, it is expected that when the alternative hypothesis value is far away from that of the null hypothesis, the formula may not work so well. To refine the Schoenfeld formula, we will derive the sample size formula under an ϵ-order local alternative, that is, $\gamma = O(n^{-\epsilon})$, where $\epsilon > 0$ is any positive real number.

    Assume that there are n patients who are allocated between the control and treatment groups, which are designated groups 1 and 2, respectively. Let D be the set of identifiers of those patients who died in the two groups, and let t_j be the death time of the jth patient in either group. We assume that the

$\{t_j\}$ are distinct. Let y_j be an indicator variable of the control group, that is $y_j = 1$ if j^{th} subject belongs to the control group and $y_j = 0$ if the jth subject belongs to the treatment group. Let us define $n_i(t)$ to be the number at risk just before time t in group i. Then, the log-rank test L can be written as

$$
\begin{aligned}
L &= \frac{\sum_{j \in D}\{y_j - p(t_j)\}}{[\sum_{j \in D} p(t_j)\{1 - p(t_j)\}]^{1/2}} \\
&= \frac{\sum_{j \in D}\{y_j - \mu_j\}}{[\sum_{j \in D} \mu_j(1 - \mu_j)]^{1/2}} \times \frac{[\sum_{j \in D} \mu_j(1 - \mu_j)]^{1/2}}{[\sum_{j \in D} p(t_j)\{1 - p(t_j)\}]^{1/2}} \\
&\quad + \frac{\sum_{j \in D}\{\mu_j - p(t_j)\}}{[\sum_{j \in D} p(t_j)\{1 - p(t_j)\}]^{1/2}} \\
&= I_1 \times I_2 + I_3.
\end{aligned}
$$

By theorem 5.1, the first term I_1 has a limiting standard normal distribution. As

$$
\begin{aligned}
\mu_j - p(t_j) &= \frac{n_1(t_j)}{n_1(t_j) + n_2(t_j)\delta} - \frac{n_1(t_j)}{n_1(t_j) + n_2(t_j)} \\
&= \frac{n_1(t_j)n_2(t_j)(1 - \delta)}{[n_1(t_j) + n_2(t_j)][n_1(t_j) + n_2(t_j)\delta]} \\
&= \frac{p(t_j)\{1 - p(t_j)\}(1 - \delta)}{[p(t_j) + \{1 - p(t_j)\}\delta]},
\end{aligned}
$$

by substituting $\lambda_2(t) = \delta\lambda_1(t)$ and $S_2(t) = [S_1(t)]^\delta$ into $\pi(t)$ and $V(t)$ (defined by equations (5.7) and (5.8), respectively) and replacing $p(t_j)$ by its limit $\pi(t_j)$, and after some simplifications (using equations given in Appendix F), we have

$$
\begin{aligned}
n^{-1} \sum_{j \in D}\{\mu_j - p(t_j)\} &\xrightarrow{P} (1 - \delta) \int_0^\infty \frac{\pi(t)(1 - \pi(t))}{[\pi(t) + \{1 - \pi(t)\}\delta]} V(t) dt \\
&= \omega_1 \omega_2 (1 - \delta) \int_0^\infty \frac{\lambda_1(t)[S_1(t)]^\delta G(t)}{[\omega_1 + \omega_2[S_1(t)]^{\delta-1}]} dt \\
&= \mu(\delta),
\end{aligned}
$$

and

$$
\begin{aligned}
n^{-1} \sum_{j \in D} p(t_j)\{1 - p(t_j)\} &\xrightarrow{P} \int_0^\infty \pi(t)(1 - \pi(t))V(t) dt \\
&= \omega_1 \omega_2 \int_0^\infty \frac{[S_1(t)]^\delta\{\omega_1 + \omega_2\delta[S_1(t)]^{\delta-1}\}\lambda_1(t)G(t)}{\{\omega_1 + \omega_2[S_1(t)]^{\delta-1}\}^2} dt \\
&= \sigma^2(\delta).
\end{aligned}
$$

Thus, the third term, I_3, converges to

$$
\frac{\sum_{j \in D}\{\mu_j - p(t_j)\}}{[\sum_{j \in D} p(t_j)\{1 - p(t_j)\}]^{1/2}} - \sqrt{n}e(\delta) \xrightarrow{P} 0,
$$

where $e(\delta) = \mu(\delta)/\sigma(\delta)$, and under the ϵ-order local alternative, we have

$$I_2 = \frac{[\sum_{j \in D} \mu_j(1 - \mu_j)]^{1/2}}{[\sum_{j \in D} p(t_j)\{1 - p(t_j)\}]^{1/2}} \xrightarrow{P} 1.$$

Now by applying Slutsky's theorem, we can show that the log-rank test L is asymptotically normal distributed with unit variance and mean $\sqrt{n}e(\delta)$. Then, given a two-sided type I error of α, the study power of $1 - \beta$ satisfies the following:

$$
\begin{aligned}
1 - \beta &= P(|L| > z_{1-\alpha/2}|H_1) \\
&\simeq \Phi(\sqrt{n}e(\delta) - z_{1-\alpha/2}),
\end{aligned}
$$

and it follows that

$$\sqrt{n}e(\delta) = z_{1-\alpha/2} + z_{1-\beta}.$$

Solving for n, the required number of subjects for the trial is given by

$$n = \frac{(z_{1-\alpha/2} + z_{1-\beta})^2 \sigma^2(\delta)}{\mu^2(\delta)}. \tag{5.24}$$

Now by substituting $\mu(\delta)$ and $\sigma^2(\delta)$ in equation (5.24), we obtain the following precise sample size formula:

$$n = \frac{(z_{1-\alpha/2} + z_{1-\beta})^2 \int_0^\infty \frac{[S_1(t)]^\delta [\omega_1 + \omega_2 \delta [S_1(t)]^{\delta-1}]}{[\omega_1 + \omega_2 [S_1(t)]^{\delta-1}]^2} \lambda_1(t)G(t)dt}{\omega_1 \omega_2 (1-\delta)^2 \left\{ \int_0^\infty \frac{[S_1(t)]^\delta}{[\omega_1 + \omega_2 [S_1(t)]^{\delta-1}]} \lambda_1(t)G(t)dt \right\}^2}. \tag{5.25}$$

Remark 1: The precise formula (5.25) was also derived by Dr. Xiaoping Xiong for the log-rank test using a different approach (personal communication).

Example 5.5 *Continuation of Example 5.1*

We will use Example 5.1 to illustrate sample size calculation by the precise formula (5.25), where $\lambda_1(t) = \lambda_1$, $S_1(t) = e^{-\lambda_1 t}$ and $G(t)$ is a uniform distribution over $[t_f, t_a + t_f]$. By using the following R function 'SizeP,' the total sample size required to detect a moderate hazard ratio $\delta = 0.737$ is calculated as $n = 568$, which is almost identical to the sample size calculated using the Schoenfeld formula.

```
############################## Input parameters ##############################
### lambda1 is the hazard parameter for the control group;           ###
### delta is the hazard ratio; p is the allocation ratio of control;  ###
### ta and tf are the accrual and follow-up duration;                ###
### alpha and beta are the type I error and type II error.           ###
#############################################################################
SizeP=function(lambda1, delta, p, ta, tf, alpha, beta)
```

```
{S1=function(t){exp(-lambda1*t)}
 S2=function(t){S1(t)^delta}
 G=function(t){1-punif(t, tf, tau)}
 m1=function(t){
   (S1(t)^delta)*(p+(1-p)*delta*S1(t)^(delta-1))/(p+(1-p)*S1(t)^(delta-1))^2}
 m2=function(t){(S1(t)^delta)*(delta-1)/(p+(1-p)*S1(t)^(delta-1))}
 f1=function(t){m1(t)*G(t)*lambda1}
 f2=function(t){m2(t)*G(t)*lambda1}
 tau=ta+tf
 Num=integrate(f1, 0, tau)$value
 Den=integrate(f2, 0, tau)$value
 z0=qnorm(1-alpha); z1=qnorm(1-beta)
 n=(z0+z1)^2*Num/(p*(1-p)*Den^2)
 ans=ceiling(n); return(ans)}
SizeP(lambda1=0.231, delta=0.737, p=0.5, ta=5, tf=3, alpha=0.05, beta=0.1)
568
```

5.12   Exact Formula

In the previous sections, the sample size formulae, such as the Schoenfeld formula and precise formula (5.25), were derived under the local alternatives, which implies that the log hazard ratio between the treatment groups decreases to 0 at the rate of $n^{-1/2}$ or $n^{-\epsilon}$, where n is the total sample size. There are two issues relating to this approach. The theoretical issue is that the accuracy of the formula derived under the local alternative is not guaranteed when the alternative departs from the null. The practical issue is that the alternative hypothesis is always fixed, and does not change as the sample size changes (Chow et al., 2003). Thus, it is important to derive a sample size formula for the log-rank test under the fixed alternative.

As shown in previous section, the third term, I_3, converges to

$$\frac{\sum_{j \in D}\{\mu_j - p(t_j)\}}{[\sum_{j \in D} p(t_j)\{1 - p(t_j)\}]^{1/2}} - \sqrt{n}e(\delta) \xrightarrow{P} 0,$$

where $e(\delta) = \mu(\delta)/\sigma(\delta)$. We can further show

$$n^{-1}\sum_{j \in D}\mu_j(1 - \mu_j) = n^{-1}\sum_{j \in D}\frac{n_1(t_j)n_2(t_j)\delta}{[n_1(t_j) + n_2(t_j)\delta]^2}$$

$$= n^{-1}\sum_{j \in D}\frac{p(t_j)(1 - p(t_j))\delta}{[p(t_j) + \{1 - p(t_j)\}\delta]^2}$$

$$\xrightarrow{P} \int_0^\infty \frac{\pi(t)\{1 - \pi(t)\}\delta}{[\pi(t) + \{1 - \pi(t)\}\delta]^2}V(t)dt$$

$$= \omega_1\omega_2\delta \int_0^\infty \frac{[S_1(t)]^\delta\lambda_1(t)G(t)}{\{\omega_1 + \omega_2\delta[S_1(t)]^{\delta-1}\}}dt$$

$$= \tilde{\sigma}^2(\delta).$$

(using equations given in Appendix F) and it follows that

$$I_2 = \frac{[\sum_{j \in D} \mu_j (1 - \mu_j)]^{1/2}}{[\sum_{j \in D} p(t_j)\{1 - p(t_j)\}]^{1/2}} \xrightarrow{P} \frac{\tilde{\sigma}(\delta)}{\sigma(\delta)}.$$

Combining results from the previous section, we have shown that the log-rank test L is asymptotically normally distributed with variance $\tilde{\sigma}^2(\delta)/\sigma^2(\delta)$ and mean $\sqrt{n}e(\delta)$, where $e(\delta) = \mu(\delta)/\sigma(\delta)$. Thus, given a two-sided type I error of α, the study power of $1 - \beta$ satisfies the following:

$$
\begin{aligned}
1 - \beta &= P(|L| > z_{1-\alpha/2}|H_1) \\
&\simeq P\left(\frac{\sigma(\delta)\{L - \sqrt{n}e(\delta)\}}{\tilde{\sigma}(\delta)} > \frac{\sigma(\delta)\{z_{1-\alpha/2} - \sqrt{n}e(\delta)\}}{\tilde{\sigma}(\delta)} \Big| H_1 \right) \\
&\simeq \Phi\left(\frac{\sqrt{n}\mu(\delta) - \sigma(\delta)z_{1-\alpha/2}}{\tilde{\sigma}(\delta)} \right),
\end{aligned}
$$

and it follows that

$$\sqrt{n}\mu(\delta) - \sigma(\delta)z_{1-\alpha/2} = \tilde{\sigma}(\delta)z_{1-\beta}.$$

Thus, solving for n, we obtain the following (asymptotically) exact sample size formula

$$n = \frac{[\sigma(\delta)z_{1-\alpha/2} + \tilde{\sigma}(\delta)z_{1-\beta}]^2}{\mu^2(\delta)}, \tag{5.26}$$

where $\mu(\delta)$, $\sigma^2(\delta)$, and $\tilde{\sigma}^2(\delta)$ are given as follows:

$$
\begin{aligned}
\mu(\delta) &= \omega_1\omega_2(1 - \delta) \int_0^\infty \frac{[S_1(t)]^\delta G(t)\lambda_1(t)}{[\omega_1 + \omega_2[S_1(t)]^{\delta-1}]} dt \\
\sigma^2(\delta) &= \omega_1\omega_2 \int_0^\infty \frac{[S_1(t)]^\delta[\omega_1 + \omega_2\delta[S_1(t)]^{\delta-1}]G(t)\lambda_1(t)}{[\omega_1 + \omega_2[S_1(t)]^{\delta-1}]^2} dt \\
\tilde{\sigma}^2(\delta) &= \omega_1\omega_2\delta \int_0^\infty \frac{[S_1(t)]^\delta G(t)\lambda_1(t)}{[\omega_1 + \omega_2\delta[S_1(t)]^{\delta-1}]} dt.
\end{aligned}
$$

Remark 2: The exact formula (5.27) was also derived by Jung and Chow (2012) for a generalized log-rank test for testing the hypothesis $H_0 : \delta = \delta_0$ vs. $H_1 : \delta = \delta_1$, where $\delta_0 \geq \delta_1$, even though their formula was presented for the exponential model only.

Example 5.6 *Continuation of Example 5.1*

We will use the previous example to illustrate sample size calculation using the exact formula (5.27), where $\lambda_1(t) = \lambda_1$, $S_1(t) = e^{-\lambda_1 t}$, and $G(t)$ is a uniform distribution over $[t_f, t_a + t_f]$. By using following R function 'SizeE,' the total sample size required to detect a moderate hazard ratio $\delta = 0.737$ is *calculated as* $n = 567$, *which is almost identical to the sample sizes calculated using the Schoenfeld formula and the precise formula (5.25). We will show in the next example that formulae (5.27) and (5.25) are both more accurate than the Schoenfeld formula when the alternative is far from the null.*

```
############################ Input parameters ############################
### lambda1 is the hazard parameter for the control group;            ###
### delta is the hazard ratio; p is the allocation ratio of control;  ###
### ta and tf are the accrual and follow-up duration;                 ###
### alpha and beta are the type I error and type II error.            ###
#########################################################################
SizeE=function(lambda1, delta, p, ta, tf, alpha, beta)
{S1=function(t){exp(-lambda1*t)}
 S2=function(t){S1(t)^delta}
 G=function(t){1-punif(t, tf, tau)}
 m1=function(t){
    (S1(t)^delta)*(p+(1-p)*delta*S1(t)^(delta-1))/(p+(1-p)*S1(t)^(delta-1))^2}
 m2=function(t){delta*(S1(t)^delta)/(p+(1-p)*delta*S1(t)^(delta-1))}
 m3=function(t){(delta-1)*S1(t)^delta/(p+(1-p)*S1(t)^(delta-1))}
 f1=function(t){m1(t)*G(t)*lambda1}
 f2=function(t){m2(t)*G(t)*lambda1}
 f3=function(t){m3(t)*G(t)*lambda1}
 tau=ta+tf
 sig1=integrate(f1, 0, tau)$value
 sig0=integrate(f2, 0, tau)$value
 mu=integrate(f3, 0, tau)$value
 z0=qnorm(1-alpha)
 z1=qnorm(1-beta)
 n=(sqrt(sig1)*z0+sqrt(sig0)*z1)^2/(p*(1-p)*mu^2)
 ans=ceiling(n)
 return(ans)}
SizeE(lambda1=0.231, delta=0.737, p=0.5, ta=5, tf=3, alpha=0.05, beta=0.1)
567
```

Example 5.7 *Comparison of five sample size formulae*

    In this chapter, we have presented five sample size formulae: the Schoenfeld, Rubinstein, Freedman, precise, and exact formulae. To investigate which formula is more accurate, sample sizes will be calculated for three scenarios under the exponential distribution. Let $S_i(x)$ be the survival probability at landmark time point x for group $i = 1, 2$. In scenario 1, the survival probabilities are $S_1(x) = 20\%$ and $S_2(x) = 30\%$, where the hazard ratio $\delta = 0.748$ is relatively large. In scenario 2, the survival probabilities are $S_1(x) = 40\%$ and $S_2(x) = 60\%$, where the hazard ratio $\delta = 0.557$ is moderate. In scenario 3, the survival probabilities are $S_1(x) = 70\%$ and $S_2(x) = 90\%$, where the hazard ratio $\delta = 0.295$ is small. For each scenario characterized by a combination of accrual period t_a, follow-up time t_f, and landmark time point x, under an assumption of uniform accrual and no loss to follow-up, the sample sizes are calculated with a two-sided type I error of 5% and power of 90%. Empirical powers were simulated based on 100,000 runs. The results (Table 5.3) show that all five formulae provide accurate sample size estimation for a relative large hazard ratio ($\delta = 0.748$). For a moderate hazard ratio ($\delta = 0.557$), *the Freedman formula may slightly overestimate the sample size, whereas the other four formulae provide accurate sample size estimation. For a small hazard ratio ($\delta = 0.295$), the Schoenfeld formula underestimates the sample size, and both the Rubinstein and Freedman formulae overestimate the sample size. Overall, both the precise formula and the exact formula showed improved accuracy of sample size estimation when compared to the other three widely used formulae.*

TABLE 5.3: Comparison of the sample size and empirical power for five sample size formulae

Design	x	t_a	t_f	Schoenfeld	Rubinstein	Freedman	Precise	Exact
$S_1(x) = 20\%$	12	24	12	547(.898)	547(.902)	554(.904)	549(.903)	551(.901)
$S_2(x) = 30\%$	24	24	24	579(.901)	580(.900)	587(.904)	579(.902)	581(.901)
$\delta = .748$	12	36	12	532(.899)	532(.899)	539(.903)	535(.900)	538(.900)
	24	36	24	559(.900)	560(.899)	567(.902)	561(.902)	563(.902)
$S_1(x) = 40\%$	12	24	12	171(.899)	174(.904)	181(.915)	172(.900)	173(.903)
$S_2(x) = 60\%$	24	24	24	195(.903)	200(.907)	206(.915)	196(.902)	195(.902)
$\delta = .557$	12	36	12	159(.900)	160(.901)	161(.902)	160(.900)	161(.904)
	24	36	24	181(.902)	185(.907)	191(.917)	182(.900)	182(.903)
$S_1(x) = 70\%$	12	24	12	83(.882)	104(.939)	104(.938)	93(.915)	85(.889)
$S_2(x) = 90\%$	24	24	24	102(.871)	132(.942)	128(.935)	117(.915)	107(.892)
$\delta = .295$	12	36	12	71(.885)	87(.938)	89(.941)	78(.906)	73(.891)
	24	36	24	91(.872)	116(.940)	114(.936)	103(.915)	94(.884)

Note: The sample sizes are calculated under the exponential model with a uniform accrual, two-sided type I error of 5%, and power of 90%. The empirical powers were estimated based on 100,000 simulation runs.

6

Survival Trial Design under the Cox Regression Model

6.1 Introduction

Randomization ensures that, on average, both the known and unknown covariates are well balanced between the treatment groups. However, randomization does not guarantee such balance, particularly for a moderate-sized or small trial. Any such imbalance can give an unfair advantage to one treatment group over another if not accounted for in the analysis. Therefore, prespecifying the inclusion of important baseline covariates in the trial design and analysis will help to ensure that any chance imbalances between the treatment groups with respect to these covariates will not affect the power of the trial and bias the results for the treatment effect. In a comparison of the survival distributions for two treatment groups of a randomized trial, the Cox proportional hazards regression model (Cox, 1972) is usually used to adjust for covariates, such as age, gender, or disease stage, that may be associated with the survival outcome, thus confounding the treatment effect. The treatment group is handled as a binary covariate in the Cox regression model. The score test statistic based on the partial likelihood for the Cox regression model can be used to test the treatment effect. Schoenfeld (1983) derived a sample size formula for the score test for testing the treatment effect. Hsieh and Lavori (2000) extended Schoenfeld's result to the case of a non-binary covariate. Recently, Wang (2013) has derived a sample size formula for the score test under the fixed alternative. However, the variance of the score test under the fixed alternative is complicated and difficult to derive. Thus, the sample size formula derived by Wang does not have an explicit form for the sample size calculation. In this chapter, we will derive a sample size formula for the score test under the contiguous alternative.

6.2   Test Statistics

Let T be the failure time, C the censoring time, $X = T \wedge C$ the observed failure time, Δ the failure indicator, and Z a vector covariate of interest, e.g., a treatment group indicator or other covariate. For simplicity of derivation, we will consider the case with only a single covariate Z in the Cox proportional hazards regression model

$$\lambda(t|Z, \theta) = \lambda_0(t)e^{\theta Z},$$

where $\lambda_0(t)$ is an unknown baseline hazard function and $\theta = \log\{\lambda(t|Z = 1)/\lambda(t|Z = 0)\}$ is the log-hazard ratio for the binary covariate ($Z = 0/1$) or is associated with a one-unit change in the continuous covariate Z.

Suppose that during the accrual phase of the trial, n subjects are enrolled in the study, and let T_i and C_i denote, respectively, the event time and censoring time of the ith subject as measured from the time of study entry, with Z_i being the covariate value of the ith subject. We assume that the failure time T_i is independent of the censoring time C_i, given Z_i. Let $X_i = T_i \wedge C_i$ and $\Delta_i = I(T_i \leq C_i)$; then, the observed data for the trial are $\{X_i, \Delta_i, Z_i, i = 1, \cdots, n\}$. If we define the counting process as $N_i(t) = \Delta_i I(X_i \leq t)$ and the at-risk process as $Y_i(t) = I(X_i \geq t)$, then the partial likelihood function for the Cox regression model is

$$L(\theta) = \prod_{i=1}^{n} \frac{e^{\theta Z_i}}{\sum_{i=1}^{n} Y_j(X_i)e^{\theta Z_j}},$$

and the corresponding log partial likelihood is

$$\ell(\theta) = \sum_{i=1}^{n} \int_0^{\tau} \left\{ \theta Z_i - \log\left(\sum_{j=1}^{n} e^{\theta Z_j} Y_j(t) \right) \right\} dN_i(t),$$

where τ is the study duration. The score function $U(\theta)$ with respect to θ is

$$U(\theta) = \sum_{i=1}^{n} \int_0^{\tau} \left\{ Z_i - \frac{\sum_{j=1}^{n} e^{\theta Z_j} Z_j Y_j(t)}{\sum_{j=1}^{n} e^{\theta Z_j} Y_j(t)} \right\} dN_i(t),$$

and the Fisher information is given by

$$V(\theta) = \sum_{i=1}^{n} \int_0^{\tau} \left\{ \frac{\sum_{j=1}^{n} e^{\theta Z_j} Z_j^2 Y_j(t)}{\sum_{j=1}^{n} e^{\theta Z_j} Y_j(t)} - \left(\frac{\sum_{j=1}^{n} e^{\theta Z_j} Z_j Y_j(t)}{\sum_{j=1}^{n} e^{\theta Z_j} Y_j(t)} \right)^2 \right\} dN_i(t).$$

If we now consider the following hypothesis of interest:

$$H_0 : \theta = \theta_0 \quad \text{vs.} \quad H_1 : \theta \neq \theta_0$$

and the study is powered at alternative $\theta_1(\neq \theta_0)$, the score test based on the partial likelihood is

$$L(\theta_0) = \frac{U(\theta_0)}{\sqrt{V(\theta_0)}},$$

which can be used to test the above hypothesis.

6.3 Asymptotic Distribution of the Score Test

The asymptotic distribution of the score test or MLE test for the Cox regression model has been discussed by Cox (1972), Tsiatis (1981), Fleming and Harrington (1991), Kalbfleisch and Prentice (2002), Wang (2013), and others. To derive the asymptotic distribution of the score test, we denote $f_{T|Z}(t)$ and $S_{T|Z}(t)$ as the probability density function and survival distribution, respectively, of the failure time T, given Z, and denote $g_{T|Z}(t)$ and $G_{T|Z}(t)$ as the probability density function and survival distribution, respectively, of the censoring time C, given Z. Let us consider the following regularity conditions:

(B1) Conditional on Z, T is independent of C.

(B2) $\theta \in \Theta$, where Θ is a compact subset of the real line $(-\infty, \infty)$.

(B3) Z has bounded support.

(B4) $S_{T|Z}(t)$ and $G_{T|Z}(t)$ are continuously differentiable in $t \in (0, \tau]$.

(B5) $f_{T|Z}(t)$ and $g_{T|Z}(t)$ are uniformly bounded in $t \in (0, \tau]$.

(B6) $P(C \geq \tau) = P(C = \tau) > 0$.

(B7) $P(T > \tau) > 0$.

(B8) $P(T \leq C|Z) > 0$.

The results of the asymptotic distribution of the score test can be summarized in the following theorem (Wang, 2003):

Theorem 6.1 *Under conditions (B1)-(B8), the following results hold:*
Under the null hypothesis $H_0 : \theta = \theta_0$,
(i) $n^{-1/2}U(\theta_0) \xrightarrow{D} N(0, v(\theta_0))$, as $n \to \infty$;
(ii) $L(\theta_0) \xrightarrow{D} N(0, 1)$, as $n \to \infty$.
Under the contiguous alternative $H_{1n} : \theta_1 = \theta_{1n} = \theta_0 + n^{-1/2}b$,
(i) $n^{-1/2}U(\theta_0) \xrightarrow{D} N(bv(\theta_0), v(\theta_0))$, as $n \to \infty$;
(ii) $L(\theta_0) \xrightarrow{D} N(b\sqrt{v(\theta_0)}, 1)$, as $n \to \infty$,
where $v(\theta_0) = \lim_{n\to\infty} E_{\theta_0}\{V(\theta_0)\}$.

Proof 6.1 *First, we define*

$$\bar{Z}_n(t, \theta_0) = \frac{\sum_{i=1}^{n} e^{\theta_0 Z_i} Z_i Y_i(t)}{\sum_{i=1}^{n} e^{\theta_0 Z_i} Y_i(t)},$$

then under $H_0 : \theta = \theta_0$, the counting precess formulation of the score test is

$$U(\theta_0) = \sum_{i=1}^{n} \int_0^\tau \{Z_i - \bar{Z}_n(t, \theta_0)\} dN_i(t).$$

Let $M_{i,\theta_0}(t) = N_i(t) - \int_0^t Y_i(u) e^{Z_i \theta_0} \lambda_0(t) dt$ be the martingale, then we have

$$U(\theta_0) = \sum_{i=1}^{n} \int_0^\tau \{Z_i - \bar{Z}_n(t, \theta_0)\} dM_{i,\theta_0}(t).$$

By the martingale central limit theorem, it follows that

$$n^{-1/2} U(\theta_0) \xrightarrow{D} N(0, v(\theta_0)), \quad as \ n \to \infty,$$

where $v(\theta_0) = \lim_{n \to \infty} E_{\theta_0} \{V(\theta_0)\}$, which can be shown as

$$v(\theta_0) = \int_0^\tau \left\{ E_{\theta_0}[Z^2 Y(t) e^{Z\theta_0}] - \frac{\{E_{\theta_0}[ZY(t) e^{Z\theta_0}]\}^2}{E_{\theta_0}[Y(t) e^{Z\theta_0}]} \right\} \lambda_0(t) dt. \qquad (6.1)$$

Under the contiguous alternative $H_{1n} : \theta_1 = \theta_{1n} = \theta_0 + n^{-1/2} b$,

$$U(\theta_0) = \sum_{i=1}^{n} \int_0^\tau \{Z_i - \bar{Z}_n(t, \theta_0)\} dM_{i,\theta_{1n}}(t)$$

$$+ \sum_{i=1}^{n} \int_0^\tau \{Z_i - \bar{Z}_n(t, \theta_0)\} Y_i(t) e^{Z_i \theta_{1n}} \lambda_0(t) dt$$

$$= U_1(\theta_0) + U_2(\theta_0),$$

where $M_{i,\theta_{1n}}(t) = N_i(t) - \int_0^t Y_i(u) e^{Z_i \theta_{1n}} \lambda_0(t)$. By the martingale central limit theorem, $n^{-1/2} U_1(\theta_0)$ converges weakly to a normal variate with mean 0 and variance $v(\theta_0)$. By the Taylor expansion $e^{Z_i \theta_{1n}}$ at θ_0, we obtain

$$n^{-1/2} U_2(\theta_0) = b n^{-1} \sum_{i=1}^{n} \int_0^\tau \{Z_i - \bar{Z}_n(t, \theta_0)\} Y_i(t) e^{Z_i \theta_0} \lambda_0(t) dt + O_p(n^{-1/2}).$$

Thus, it follows that $n^{-1/2} U_2(\theta_0) \xrightarrow{P} bv(\theta_0)$. Therefore, under the contiguous alternative H_{1n}, we have

$$n^{-1/2} U(\theta_0) \xrightarrow{D} N(bv(\theta_0), v(\theta_0)), \quad as \ n \to \infty.$$

Finally, by the dominated convergence theorem,

$$\lim_{n \to \infty} E_{\theta_{1n}} \{V(\theta_0)\} = \lim_{n \to \infty} E_{\theta_0} \{V(\theta_0)\} = v(\theta_0)$$

and by Slutsky's theorem, it follows that

$$L(\theta_0) \xrightarrow{D} N(b\sqrt{v(\theta_0)}, 1), \quad as \ n \to \infty.$$

6.4 Sample Size Formula

To derive the sample size formula under the contiguous alternative $H_{1n} : \theta_1 = \theta_{1n} = \theta_0 + n^{-1/2}b$, we have shown that

$$L(\theta_0) \xrightarrow{D} N(b\sqrt{v(\theta_0)}, 1).$$

Thus, given a two-sided type I error of α, the study power $1 - \beta$ at the alternative satisfies the following:

$$1 - \beta \simeq P(|L(\theta_0)| > z_{1-\alpha/2}|H_{1n}) \simeq \Phi\{|b|v(\theta_0) - z_{1-\alpha/2}\}.$$

By substituting $b = \sqrt{n}(\theta_1 - \theta_0)$ and solving for n, we obtain the following sample size formula:

$$n = \frac{(z_{1-\alpha/2} + z_{1-\beta})^2}{(\theta_1 - \theta_0)^2 v(\theta_0)}.$$

In the special case where $\theta_0 = 0$, by equation (6.1) we have $v(0) = \mathrm{Var}(Z)P_{\theta=0}(\Delta = 1)$, where $P_{\theta=0}(\Delta = 1)$ is the probability of failure under the null hypothesis of $\theta = 0$. Thus, the total number of events required for the study is given by

$$D = \frac{(z_{1-\alpha/2} + z_{1-\beta})^2}{\mathrm{Var}(Z)\theta_1^2}, \tag{6.2}$$

where θ_1 is the log-hazard ratio per unit change of Z, $\theta_1 < 0$ indicates a better survival when the value of Z is increased and $\theta_1 > 0$ indicates a worse survival when the value of Z is increased. In particular, when the covariate is a binary variable, e.g., the group indicator of two groups, then $\mathrm{Var}(Z) = w_1 w_2$, and $\theta_1 = \log(\delta)$, where w_1 and w_2 are the proportions of patients in groups 1 and 2, respectively, and $\delta = \lambda(t|Z = 1)/\lambda(t|Z = 0)$. Thus, the total number of events can be calculated by

$$D = \frac{(z_{1-\alpha/2} + z_{1-\beta})^2}{w_1 w_2 [\log(\delta)]^2}. \tag{6.3}$$

Schoenfeld (1983) has shown that this formula applies for a two-group randomized trial when the model includes a set of additional covariates that are assumed to be independent of the treatment.

When the Cox regression model involves multiple covariates $Z_1, Z_2, \cdots, Z_k$, where Z_1 is the covariate of interest and covariates $Z_2, \cdots, Z_k$ are possible confounders of the covariate Z_1, the total number of events can be calculated by using the following formula:

$$D = \frac{(z_{1-\alpha/2} + z_{1-\beta})^2}{\mathrm{Var}(Z_1)\theta_1^2(1 - R^2)}, \tag{6.4}$$

where R is the multiple correlation coefficient of Z_1 regressed on $Z_2, \cdots, Z_k$ (Hsieh and Lavori, 2000).

Remark: The formula (6.4) can be applied to a nonrandomized trial when the data are intended to be analyzed by using the score test based on the Cox regression model.

Example 6.1 *Multiple myeloma study*

A multiple myeloma dataset (Krall et al., 1975) is used to illustrate the sample size calculation. In this dataset, 65 patients were treated with alkylating agents at West Virginia University Medical Center. During the study, 48 of the 65 patients died (note: this was not a randomized trial). The data was fitted into a Cox regression model to identify the prognostic factors (the final eight selected variables by using backward selection are recorded in the multiple myeloma data in Table 6.1). Let us assume that LOGBUN (Z_1) is the variable of interest. The standard deviation of LOGBUN is 0.3126. The coefficient estimate of the Cox regression model with a single covariate Z_1 is $\theta = 1.746$. Thus, an increasing value of LOGBUN indicates worse survival. Suppose we wanted to have 80% power with a one-sided type I error of 5% (or two-sided type I error of 10%) to detect a log-hazard ratio of $\theta_1 = 1.2$ per unit change in Z_1. By applying formula (6.2), with no other covariates, the required number of deaths would be $D = (1.645 + 0.842)^2/(0.3126^2 \times 1.2^2) = 44$. The overall death rate was $48/65 = 0.738$. Thus, the sample size required for the study is $n = 44/0.738 = 60$. Now suppose that it was considered necessary to adjust for the other covariates for possible confounding. The R^2 obtained from the regression of Z_1 on $Z_2, \ldots, Z_8$ is 0.1827. Thus applying formula (6.4), the required number of events and the required sample size are $D = 44/(1 - 0.1827) = 54$ and $n = 54/0.738 = 74$, respectively. The R function 'SizeCoxM' is given below for the sample size calculation under the Cox proportional hazard regression model.

```
############################ Input parameters ############################
### theta1 is the log-hazard ratio; alpha and beta are the type I and    ###
### type II errors and power=1-beta; dat is a subset of multiple myeloma  ###
### data set as given in Table 6.1 which is stored as a data frame with   ###
### variables time, status, Z1-Z8.                                        ###
##########################################################################
SizeCoxM=function(theta1,alpha,beta,data)
{z0=qnorm(1-alpha/2)
 z1=qnorm(1-beta)
 time=dat$time; status=dat$status
 Z1=dat$Z1; Z2=dat$Z2
 Z3=dat$Z3; Z4=dat$Z4
 Z5=dat$Z5; Z6=dat$Z6
 Z7=dat$Z7; Z8=dat$Z8
 v2=var(Z1)
 D0=ceiling((z0+z1)^2/(v2*theta1^2))
 p=sum(status)/length(status)
 N0=ceiling(D0/p)
 fit=lm(Z1~Z2+Z3+Z4+Z5+Z6+Z7+Z8)
```

```
R2=summary(fit)$r.squared
Dadj=ceiling(DO/(1-R2))
Nadj=ceiling(Dadj/p)
ans=list(c(DO=DO, NO=NO, Dadj=Dadj, Nadj=Nadj))
 return(ans)}
SizeCoxM(theta=1.2,alpha=0.10,beta=0.2,data=dat)
DO   NO Dadj Nadj #DO and NO are unadjusted number of events and sample size#
44   60   54   74 #Dadj and Nadj are adjusted number of events and sample size#
```

Example 6.2 *International Non-Hodgkin's Lymphoma Prognostic Factors Project*

In this initial screening of the data from the International Non-Hodgkin's Lymphoma Prognostic Factors Project, complete data on seven prognostic variables were available for 1760 patients, and there were 789 deaths in this group (Bernardo et al., 2000). Cox regression analyses showed that these seven prognostic factors were associated with shorter survival: an increasing number of extranodal sites of disease, advanced age, the presence of systemic symptoms, worsening ECOG performance status, an increasing concentration of the enzyme lactose dehydrogenase (LDH) above the upper limit of normal, a tumor that exceeds 10 cm in its largest dimension and worsening disease stage based on the Ann Arbor staging classification. In this dataset, only the presence of systemic symptoms and maximum tumor size were originally dichotomized. We retained the non-binary coding of the data for all analyses, except when the variable was the primary variable of interest. The primary variables were dichotomized as group 1 vs. group 2 as follows: extranodal disease site: none vs. at least one; age: < 60 vs. ≥ 60; performance status: ambulatory vs. non-ambulatory; disease stage: stage I and II vs. stage III and IV; LDH concentration: less than the upper limit of normal vs. greater than the upper limit of normal; systemic symptoms: absent vs. present; maximum tumor size: < 10 cm vs. ≥ 10 cm.

In this study, it was important to detect a log-hazard ratio (θ) between 0.18 and 0.22. The multiple correlation coefficient R^2, along with the proportion of patients belonging to group 1, ω_1 is also presented in Table 6.2. Table 6.2 shows the power of an unadjusted two-sample log-rank test and the power of a covariate adjusted score test using formula (6.4) for these two values of the log-hazard ratios for all seven variables, where the power of the unadjusted two-sample log-rank test is calculated by

$$power = \Phi\left(\sqrt{\omega_1\omega_2 D\theta_1^2} - z_{1-\alpha/2}\right),$$

and the power of the adjusted score test is calculated by

$$power = \Phi\left(\sqrt{\omega_1\omega_2 D\theta_1^2(1 - R^2)} - z_{1-\alpha/2}\right).$$

Each row in Table 6.2 presents a different example of a comparison of the

TABLE 6.1: A subset of multiple myeloma data (Krall et al., 1975)

time	status	Z_1	Z_2	Z_3	Z_4	Z_5	Z_6	Z_7	Z_8
1.25	1	2.2175	1	0	1	3.6628	1	12	2
1.25	1	1.9395	1	1	1	3.9868	1	20	1
2	1	1.5185	1	1	1	3.8751	1	2	1
2	1	1.7482	0	0	1	3.8062	1	0	2
2	1	1.3010	0	0	1	3.7243	1	3	1
3	1	1.5441	1	1	2	4.4757	0	12	2
5	1	2.2355	1	0	2	4.9542	1	4	1
5	1	1.6812	1	0	1	3.7324	0	5	2
6	1	1.3617	1	1	1	3.5441	0	1	2
6	1	2.1139	0	0	2	3.5441	1	1	2
6	1	1.1139	1	0	1	3.5185	1	0	2
6	1	1.4150	1	0	2	3.9294	1	0	2
7	1	1.9777	1	0	1	3.3617	1	5	2
7	1	1.0414	0	0	2	3.7324	1	1	2
7	1	1.1761	1	0	2	3.7243	1	1	1
9	1	1.7243	1	0	1	3.7993	1	0	2
11	1	1.1139	1	0	1	3.8808	1	0	2
11	1	1.2304	1	0	1	3.7709	1	1	1
11	1	1.3010	1	0	1	3.7993	1	1	2
11	1	1.5682	1	0	1	3.8865	0	0	2
11	1	1.0792	1	0	2	3.5051	1	0	2
13	1	0.7782	0	1	2	3.5798	1	2	2
14	1	1.3979	1	1	1	3.7243	1	2	1
15	1	1.6021	1	0	1	3.6902	1	0	2
16	1	1.3424	1	0	1	3.9345	1	0	2
16	1	1.3222	1	0	2	3.6990	1	17	2
17	1	1.2304	1	0	1	3.8808	1	4	2
17	1	1.5911	1	1	1	3.4314	0	1	2
18	1	1.4472	1	0	2	3.5682	0	7	2
19	1	1.0792	1	0	1	3.9191	1	6	2
19	1	1.2553	0	0	2	3.7924	1	5	1
24	1	1.3010	1	0	2	4.0899	1	0	2
25	1	1.0000	1	0	1	3.8195	1	0	2
26	1	1.2304	1	0	2	3.6021	1	27	1
32	1	1.3222	1	0	1	3.6990	1	1	2
35	1	1.1139	0	0	1	3.6532	1	4	1
37	1	1.6021	1	0	1	3.9542	0	7	1
41	1	1.0000	1	0	1	3.4771	1	6	1
41	1	1.1461	1	0	2	3.5185	1	0	2
51	1	1.5682	0	0	1	3.4150	1	4	1
52	1	1.0000	1	0	2	3.8573	1	4	1
54	1	1.2553	1	0	1	3.7243	1	2	1
58	1	1.2041	1	0	2	3.6990	1	22	1
66	1	1.4472	1	0	1	3.7853	1	0	2
67	1	1.3222	1	0	1	3.6435	1	1	1
88	1	1.1761	1	0	2	3.5563	0	21	1
89	1	1.3222	1	1	1	3.6532	1	1	1
92	1	1.4314	1	0	2	4.0755	1	4	1
4	0	1.9542	1	0	1	4.0453	0	12	1
4	0	1.9243	1	1	2	3.9590	0	0	2
7	0	1.1139	1	0	2	3.7993	0	0	2
7	0	1.5315	1	1	1	3.5911	0	0	2
8	0	1.0792	1	0	2	3.8325	1	0	2
12	0	1.1461	1	0	2	3.6435	0	0	2
11	0	1.6128	1	0	1	3.7324	1	3	1
12	0	1.3979	1	0	2	3.8388	1	0	2
13	0	1.6628	0	0	2	3.6435	0	0	2
16	0	1.1461	1	0	1	3.8573	0	0	2
19	0	1.3222	1	0	2	3.7709	1	1	2
19	0	1.3222	1	0	2	3.8808	1	0	2
28	0	1.2304	1	1	2	3.7482	1	0	2
41	0	1.7559	1	0	1	3.7243	1	1	1
53	0	1.1139	1	0	1	3.6128	1	1	2
57	0	1.2553	1	0	1	3.9685	0	0	2
77	0	1.0792	1	0	1	3.6812	0	0	2

Note: time: survival time from diagnosis to nearest month plus 1; status: 0 - alive, 1 - dead; Z_1: Log BUN at diagnosis; Z_2: Platelets at diagnosis 0 - abnormal, 1 - normal; Z_3: Infections at diagnosis 0 - none, 1 - present; Z_4: Sex 1 - Male, 2 - female; Z_5: Log WBC at diagnosis; Z_6: Fracture at diagnosis 0 - none, 1 - present; Z_7: Proteinuria at diagnosis; Z_8: Bence Jone protein in urine at diagnosis 1 - present, 2 - none.

TABLE 6.2: Power calculation based on the unadjusted two-sample log-rank test and the R^2 adjusted methods for a two-sided type I error of 0.05

Variable of interest	R^2	ω_1	θ	Power Unadjusted	R^2 adjusted
Extranodal disease sites	0.1968	0.68	0.18	0.65	0.56
			0.22	0.82	0.73
Age	0.0162	0.37	0.18	0.68	0.68
			0.22	0.85	0.84
Performance status	0.1746	0.24	0.18	0.58	0.50
			0.22	0.75	0.67
Disease stage	0.1538	0.65	0.18	0.67	0.60
			0.22	0.84	0.77
LDH	0.1563	0.55	0.18	0.71	0.64
			0.22	0.87	0.81
Systemic symptoms	0.1840	0.41	0.18	0.70	0.61
			0.22	0.86	0.78
Maximum tumor size	0.0532	0.29	0.18	0.63	0.61
			0.22	0.80	0.78

unadjusted and adjusted powers for one of the seven prognostic variables for a particular value of θ. Table 6.2 shows that when R^2 is relatively large, e.g., around 15% to 20%, the power based on the unadjusted log-rank test overestimates the true power by approximately 8% to 17%. However, when R^2 is close to 0, e.g., for age and maximum tumor size, the difference in power is small. We can see from the calculations in Table 6.2 that a failure to adjust for the presence of other covariates may lead us to believe that a particular comparison is adequately powered when in fact it is not. For example, in the comparison of extranodal disease sites when $\theta = 0.22$, the power based on the unadjusted log-rank test is found to be acceptable (82%), whereas the true power is only 73%, which is usually deemed unacceptable.

7

Complex Survival Trial Design

The sample size calculations presented thus far have been limited by some simplifying assumptions: that all patients in the trial are fully compliant with therapy and there is no noncompliance or drop-in. Here, noncompliance means that patients on active treatment discontinue their medication, and drop-in means that patients in the control group start taking medication on their own, i.e., they cross over to active treatment. Cancer survival trials are frequently complicated by noncompliance and drop-in, which can cause the hazard rate to vary during the trial. Thus, a proportional hazards assumption may be invalid. We illustrate this with a trial conducted by the Veterans Administration (VA) Lung Cancer Study Group (Prentice, 1973). In this trial, 137 patients with advanced lung cancer were randomized to one of two chemotherapeutic agents: the standard agent and the test agent. Figure 7.1 presents the overall survival Kaplan-Meier curves for the two groups. As the Kaplan-Meier curves cross each other, it is reasonable to suspect that the proportional hazards assumption is still valid. The reasons for this crossing can be complicated.

Another nonproportional hazards example, the Beta Blocker Heart Attack Trial (BHAT), is discussed by Lakatos (in Young and Chen, 2014). When the proportional hazards assumption is invalid, conventional methods such as the log-rank test perform poorly, and the sample size calculation discussed in the previous sections is inappropriate for trial design. Lachine (1981) discussed sample size calculation with allowance for nonuniform patient entry, loss to follow-up, noncompliance, and stratification, but this approach was limited to the exponential survival distribution. Fortunately, Lakatos (1988) derived a sample size calculation for the log-rank test in the general case that allows for any pattern of survival, noncompliance, drop-in, loss to follow-up, nonproportional hazards, or lag in the effectiveness of treatment during the course of a trial. The Lakatos method uses nonstationary Markov chains to model the trial process and adjust the sample size by specifying the state space, initial distributions, and transition probabilities between states according to various trial complications. Simulation results have shown that the Lakatos Markov approach outperforms two other popular methods: that of Rubinstein et al. (1980), under exponential models, and that of Freedman (1982), under proportional hazards models (Lakatos and Lan, 1992). The Lakatos method has been implemented in the SAS macro %SIZE (Shih, 1995). In this chapter, we will first extend the Freedman formula to the nonproportional hazards model.

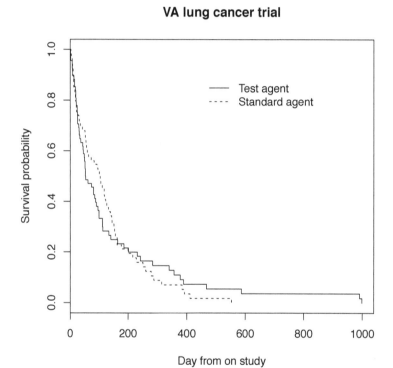

FIGURE 7.1: Overall survival Kaplan-Meier curves for the VA lung cancer data.

Then, we will discuss sample size calculation under a complicated survival model by using the Lakatos Markov chain approach.

7.1 Extension of the Freedman Formula

Let us assume that there are n patients who are allocated between the control and treatment groups, which are designated as group 1 and group 2, respectively. Assume the total number of deaths of two groups is d and all death times are distinct (no ties). Without a loss of generality, we assume that $k = 1, \ldots, d$ identify the patients who died. Let y_k be an indicator variable of the control group, that is, $y_k = 1$ if the kth subject belongs to the control group and $y_k = 0$ if the kth subject belongs to the treatment group. Let us define n_{1k} and n_{2k} to be the numbers at risk just before the kth death in the control and treatment groups, respectively. The weighted log-rank test statistic can then be expressed as

$$L_w = \sum_{k=1}^{d} w_k \left(y_k - \frac{n_{1k}}{n_{1k} + n_{2k}} \right) / \left[\sum_{k=1}^{d} w_k^2 \frac{n_{1k} n_{2k}}{(n_{1k} + n_{2k})^2} \right]^{1/2},$$

where the sum is over the total number of deaths d, $\{w_k\}$ are the weights. Conditional on n_{1k} and n_{2k}, the $\{y_k\}$ are a sequence of uncorrelated Bernoulli random variables with means

$$\mu_k = \frac{n_{1k} \lambda_{1k}}{n_{1k} \lambda_{1k} + n_{2k} \lambda_{2k}}$$

and variances $\mu_k(1 - \mu_k)$, where λ_{1k} and λ_{2k} are the hazards just before the kth death in the control and treatment groups, respectively. To obtain the asymptotic distribution of L_w, we assume a contiguous alternative $\log(\lambda_{1k}/\lambda_{2k}) = O(n^{-1/2})$; then, as shown in section 5.6 of Chapter 5, we have

$$L_w = \sum_{k=1}^{d} w_k (y_k - \mu_k) / \left[\sum_{k=1}^{d} w_k^2 \mu_k (1 - \mu_k) \right]^{1/2} + E + O_p(n^{-1/2}),$$

where

$$E = \sum_{k=1}^{d} w_k \left(\mu_k - \frac{n_{1k}}{n_{1k} + n_{2k}} \right) / \left[\sum_{k=1}^{d} w_k^2 \frac{n_{1k} n_{2k}}{(n_{1k} + n_{2k})^2} \right]^{1/2}.$$

Thus, L_w is approximately normal distributed with unit variance, and the mean E given by

$$E = \sum_{k=1}^{d} w_k \left(\frac{\phi_k \theta_k}{1 + \phi_k \theta_k} - \frac{\phi_k}{1 + \phi_k} \right) / \left[\sum_{k=1}^{d} w_k^2 \frac{\phi_k}{(1 + \phi_k)^2} \right]^{1/2},$$

where $\phi_k = n_{1k}/n_{2k}$ and $\theta_k = \lambda_{1k}/\lambda_{2k}$. Now let us partition the study period $[0, \tau]$ into N subintervals with equal length $\{t_0 = 0, t_1, t_2, \ldots, t_N = \tau\}$, where $N = [\tau b]^-$, b is the number of subintervals per time unit, and $[x]^-$ is defined as the largest integer not greater than x. Let there be d_i deaths in the ith subinterval $(t_{i-1}, t_i], i = 1, \ldots, N$; then, the mean of L_w can be expressed as

$$E = \sum_{i=1}^{N} \sum_{k=1}^{d_i} w_{i_k} \left(\frac{\phi_{i_k} \theta_{i_k}}{1 + \phi_{i_k} \theta_{i_k}} - \frac{\phi_{i_k}}{1 + \phi_{i_k}} \right) \Big/ \left[\sum_{i=1}^{N} \sum_{k=1}^{d_i} w_{i_k}^2 \frac{\phi_{i_k}}{(1 + \phi_{i_k})^2} \right]^{1/2},$$

where $\phi_{i_k} = n_{1i_k}/n_{2i_k}$ is the ratio of patients in the two groups at risk up to the kth death in the ith subinterval and $\theta_{i_k} = \lambda_{1i_k}/\lambda_{2i_k}$ is the ratio of the hazards of dying in the two groups just before the kth death in the ith subinterval. If we assume that $\phi_{i_k} = \phi_i$, $\theta_{i_k} = \theta_i$, and $w_{i_k} = w_i$ are constants for all k in the ith subinterval, then E can be written as

$$E = \frac{\sum_{i=1}^{N} w_i d_i \gamma_i}{(\sum_{i=1}^{N} w_i^2 d_i \eta_i)^{1/2}},$$

where

$$\gamma_i = \frac{\phi_i \theta_i}{1 + \phi_i \theta_i} - \frac{\phi_i}{1 + \phi_i} \quad \text{and} \quad \eta_i = \frac{\phi_i}{(1 + \phi_i)^2}.$$

Let ω_j be the proportion assigned to group j and n be the total sample size; then the number of subjects at risk just before i^{th} subinterval $(t_{i-1}, t_i](i = 1, \ldots, N)$ in group j can be calculated as follows:

$$\begin{aligned} N_j(1) &= n\omega_j \\ N_j(i) &= N_j(i-1)[1 - \lambda_j(t_{i-1})\epsilon - h(t_{i-1})\epsilon], \ i > 1, \end{aligned}$$

where $\epsilon = b^{-1}$ is the length of each subinterval, $\lambda_j(t)$ is the hazard function of the failure time for group j, and $h(t)$ is the hazard function of the censoring time. Then, the expected number of events for each subinterval $(t_{i-1}, t_i]$ is calculated by

$$D_i = [\lambda_1(t_i)N_1(i) + \lambda_2(t_i)N_2(i)]\epsilon.$$

Substituting d_i by D_i, we obtain

$$E = \sqrt{n}E^* = \frac{\sum_{i=1}^{N} w_i D_i^* \gamma_i}{(\sum_{i=1}^{N} w_i^2 D_i^* \eta_i)^{1/2}},$$

where

$$\begin{aligned} \theta_i &= \lambda_1(t_i)/\lambda_2(t_i) \\ \phi_i &= N_1^*(i)/N_2^*(i) \\ D_i^* &= [\lambda_1(t_i)N_1^*(i) + \lambda_2(t_i)N_2^*(i)]\epsilon \\ N_j^*(1) &= \omega_j \\ N_j^*(i) &= N_j^*(i-1)[1 - \lambda_j(t_{i-1})\epsilon - h(t_{i-1})\epsilon]. \end{aligned}$$

Given a two-sided type I error of α, the study power of $1 - \beta$ satisfies the following:

$$
\begin{aligned}
1 - \beta &= P(|L_w| > z_{1-\alpha/2}|H_1) \\
&\simeq P(L_w - E > z_{1-\alpha/2} - E|H_1) \\
&= \Phi(E - z_{1-\alpha/2}).
\end{aligned}
$$

It follows that

$$
E = z_{1-\alpha/2} + z_{1-\beta}.
$$

Thus, solving for n, the required total sample size for the trial is given by

$$
n = \frac{(z_{1-\alpha/2} + z_{1-\beta})^2 (\sum_{i=1}^{N} w_i^2 D_i^* \eta_i)}{(\sum_{i=1}^{N} w_i D_i^* \gamma_i)^2}, \tag{7.1}
$$

and the total number of events is given by

$$
D = n \sum_{i=1}^{N} D_i^*. \tag{7.2}
$$

Remark 1: Cantor (1998) and Hasegawa (2014) developed a similar approach; however, formula (7.1) is slightly different from the version given by Hasegawa (2014). Here we use the log-rank score $U = O_1 - E_1$, whereas Hasegawa uses $U = O_2 - E_2$, resulting in a different calculation for ϕ_i and θ_i.

7.1.1 Example and R code

Example 7.1 *Cancer Vaccine Trial*

Kantoff et al. (2010) conducted a double-blind, placebo-controlled immunotherapy trial for castration-resistant prostate cancer, in which patients were randomly assigned in a 2:1 ratio to receive either sipuleucel-T or placebo. The primary endpoint was overall survival. The median survival was 25.8 months in the sipuleucel-T group and 21.7 months in the placebo group. Visual separation of the overall survival Kaplan-Meier curves (Kantoff et al., 2010) occurred approximately 6 months after the randomization. This implies that the proportional hazard assumption no longer holds, and the conventional sample size and power calculation methods based on the standard log-rank test would lead to a loss of power. Hasegawa (2014) proposed a sample size calculation for the weighted log-rank test with the Fleming-Harrington $\mathcal{G}^{\rho,\nu}$ class of weights for use in cancer vaccine studies. For the delayed treatment-effect model, formula (7.1) can be used for the sample size calculation because it assumes only that the hazard ratio is constant within each subinterval and there is no need to satisfy the PH assumption. We illustrate the sample size calculation by using the cancer vaccine trial of Kantoff as an example.

Here, we illustrate sample size calculation using the proposed method for a potential new trial to detect the difference in overall survival between the sipuleucel-T group and the placebo group by using the weighted log-rank test with Fleming-Harrington $\mathcal{G}^{\rho,\nu}$ class of weights. We assume that the overall survival times for patients receiving placebo follow an exponential distribution, whereas the overall survival times for patients receiving sipuleucel-T follow a piecewise exponential distribution with a delayed onset time of $t_0 = 6$ months as follows:

$$S_1(t) = e^{-\lambda t}$$

$$S_2(t) = \begin{cases} e^{-\lambda t} & 0 \le t < t_0 \\ ce^{-\delta\lambda t} & t \ge t_0 \end{cases} \quad,$$

where $c = e^{-t_0\lambda(1-\delta)}$ is a normalizing constant, λ is the hazard of the placebo group and of the cancer vaccine group before time t_0 (months), and $\delta\lambda$ is the hazard of the cancer vaccine group after time t_0 (Figure 7.2). Thus, the hazard ratio can be expressed as

$$\frac{\lambda_2(t)}{\lambda_1(t)} = \begin{cases} 1 & 0 \le t < t_0 \\ \delta & t \ge t_0 \end{cases} \quad.$$

Based on the results of the trial conducted by Kantoff et al., the hazard rate λ and hazard ratio δ after the delayed onset time are 0.032 and 0.79, respectively. We further assume that patients are accrued to the trial for $t_a = 48$ months at a constant rate (uniform accrual) and are followed for $t_f = 18$ months. The hazard function of the censoring time (administrative censoring) is given by

$$h(t) = \begin{cases} \frac{1}{t_a+t_f-t} & t_f < t \le \tau \\ 0 & otherwise \end{cases} \quad,$$

where $\tau = t_a + t_f$ is the study duration. Assume the treatment to control allocation ratio is 2:1; that is, $\omega_1 = 1/3$ and $\omega_2 = 2/3$. The sample size calculation is based on the weighted log-rank test with the Fleming-Harrington weight function $W(t) = \{\hat{S}(t^-)\}^\rho\{1 - \hat{S}(t^-)\}^\nu$ for $\rho = 0$ and $\nu = 1$, where $\hat{S}(t^-)$ is the left-continuous version of the Kaplan-Meier estimate computed from the pooled sample of the two groups. Then, the total numbers of deaths and subjects required to achieve the desired power of 90% with a two-sided significance level of 5% are 1279 and 1912 using the $\mathcal{G}^{0,1}$ weighted log-rank test, respectively. The total required number of deaths and subjects for the standard log-rank test are 1508 and 2254, respectively. The R function 'SizeFH' is given below for the sample size calculation by using the Fleming-Harrington weighted log-rank test.

Remark 2: Recently, Xu et al. (2016) showed that the piecewise weighted log-rank test was optimal for cases of delayed onset of treatment effect and derived sample size and power calculations using this test under the exponential delayed treatment effect model.

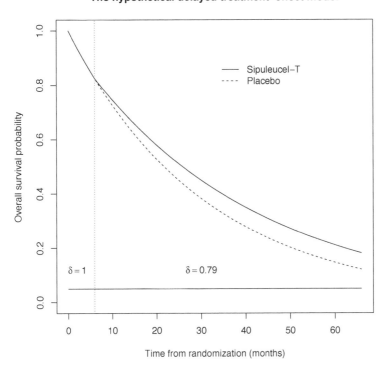

FIGURE 7.2: Hypothetical piecewise exponential survival curve for the sipuleucel-T group and exponential survival curve for the placebo group.

```
############################## Input parameters ##############################
###   lambda is the hazard rate for control;  psi is the hazard ratio;      ###
###   ta and tf are the accrual time and follow-up time;                    ###
###   epsilon is the delayed onset time; b the number of subintervals;      ###
###   alpha and beta are the type I and II error; power=1-beta;             ###
###   omega1 is the sample size allocation ratio of the control;            ###
###   rho and nu are the parameters of Fleming-Harrington weight function.  ###
##############################################################################
SizeFH=function(lambda, psi, ta, tf, t0, omega1, b, rho, nu, alpha, beta)
{tau=ta+tf; M=tau*b
 t=seq(0, tau, length=M)[-1]
 c=exp(-t0*psi*lambda*(1/psi-1))
 I=function(t){ if (t<=tf) {ans=0}
     else {ans=1}; return(ans) }
 h1=function(t){ lambda}
 h2=function(t){ if (t<t0) {ans=lambda}
     else {ans=psi*lambda}; return(ans) }
 S1=function(t){exp(-lambda*t)}
 S2=function(t){ if (t<t0) {ans=exp(-lambda*t)}
     else {ans=c*exp(-psi*lambda*t)} ; return(ans)}
 W=function(t){ S=omega1*S1(t)+(1-omega1)*S2(t)
     ans=S^rho*(1-S)^nu; return(ans) }
 D=N1=N2=rr=theta=phi=rep(0,M)
 N1[1]=omega1; N2[1]=1-omega1
 for (i in 2:(M-1))
 {N1[i]=N1[i-1]*(1-h1(t[i-1])/b-I(t[i-1])/(b*(tau-t[i-1])))
  N2[i]=N2[i-1]*(1-h2(t[i-1])/b-I(t[i-1])/(b*(tau-t[i-1])))}
 for (i in 1:(M-1))
 {D[i]=(h1(t[i])*N1[i]+h2(t[i])*N2[i])/b
  rr[i]=W(t[i])
  theta[i]=h1(t[i])/h2(t[i])
  phi[i]=N1[i]/N2[i]}
 num=dem=NULL
 for (i in 1:(M-1))
 {num[i]=D[i]*rr[i]*(phi[i]*theta[i]/(1+phi[i]*theta[i])-phi[i]/(1+phi[i]))
  dem[i]=D[i]*(rr[i]^2)*phi[i]/(1+phi[i])^2}
 e=sum(num)/sqrt(sum(dem))
 z0=qnorm(1-alpha/2)
 z1=qnorm(1-beta)
 n=ceiling((z0+z1)^2/e^2)
 d=ceiling(n*sum(D))
 return(c(d=d,n=n))}
SizeFH(lambda=0.032,psi=0.79,ta=48,tf=18,t0=6,omega1=1/3,b=100,rho=0,
     nu=1,alpha=0.05,beta=0.1)
    d    n #d is the number of events; n is the sample size #
1279 1912 #sample size calculated using the weighted log-rank test#

SizeFH(lambda=0.032,psi=0.79,ta=48,tf=18,t0=6,omega1=1/3,b=100,rho=0,
     nu=0,alpha=0.05,beta=0.1)
    d    n
1508 2254 #sample size calculated using the standard log-rank test#
```

7.2   Lakatos Formula

Lakatos developed a more sophisticated method by using a Markov chain approach to handle complicated survival trial design that allows for loss to follow-up, noncompliance, drop-in, and a nonproportional hazards model. We will discuss the sample size formula, computation method, and R code for the Lakatos Markov chain approach in detail and illustrate it by several examples.

Using the same notation as in the previous section, the weighted log-rank test statistic can be expressed as

$$L_w = \sum_{k=1}^{d} w_k \left(y_k - \frac{n_{1k}}{n_{1k} + n_{2k}} \right) / \left[\sum_{k=1}^{d} w_k^2 \frac{n_{1k} n_{2k}}{(n_{1k} + n_{2k})^2} \right]^{1/2},$$

where the sum is over the total number of deaths d, $\{w_k\}$ are the weights, y_k is the indicator variable of the control group, and n_{1k} and n_{2k} are the numbers at risk just before the kth death in the control and treatment groups, respectively. As we have shown, the weighted log-rank test L_w is approximately normal distributed with unit variance and mean E given by

$$E = \sum_{k=1}^{d} w_k \left(\frac{\phi_k \theta_k}{1 + \phi_k \theta_k} - \frac{\phi_k}{1 + \phi_k} \right) / \left[\sum_{k=1}^{d} w_k^2 \frac{\phi_k}{(1 + \phi_k)^2} \right]^{1/2},$$

where $\phi_k = n_{1k}/n_{2k}$ and $\theta_k = \lambda_{1k}/\lambda_{2k}$. To use the Markov chain model, we partition the study duration into N equal subintervals, and assume there will be d_i deaths in the ith interval. Then, the mean can be expressed as

$$E = \sum_{i=1}^{N} \sum_{k=1}^{d_i} w_{i_k} \left(\frac{\phi_{i_k} \theta_{i_k}}{1 + \phi_{i_k} \theta_{i_k}} - \frac{\phi_{i_k}}{1 + \phi_{i_k}} \right) / \left[\sum_{i=1}^{N} \sum_{k=1}^{d_i} w_{i_k}^2 \frac{\phi_{i_k}}{(1 + \phi_{i_k})^2} \right]^{1/2}.$$

If we assume that $\phi_{i_k} = \phi_i$, $\theta_{i_k} = \theta_i$, and $w_{i_k} = w_i$ are constants for all k in the ith interval and let $\rho_i = d_i/d$, where $d = \sum_{i=1}^{N} d_i$, then E can be written as

$$E = e(D)\sqrt{d},$$

where

$$e(D) = \frac{\sum_{i=1}^{N} w_i \rho_i \gamma_i}{(\sum_{i=1}^{N} w_i^2 \rho_i \eta_i)^{1/2}}$$

and

$$\gamma_i = \frac{\phi_i \theta_i}{1 + \phi_i \theta_i} - \frac{\phi_i}{1 + \phi_i} \quad \text{and} \quad \eta_i = \frac{\phi_i}{(1 + \phi_i)^2}.$$

Thus, given a two-sided type I error of α, the study power of $1 - \beta$ satisfies the following:

$$1 - \beta = P(|L_w| > z_{1-\alpha/2}|H_1)$$
$$\simeq P(L_w - E > z_{1-\alpha/2} - E|H_1)$$
$$\simeq \Phi(E - z_{1-\alpha/2}).$$

It follows that

$$E = z_{1-\alpha/2} + z_{1-\beta}.$$

Thus, solving for d, the required number of events for the trial is given by

$$d = \frac{(z_{1-\alpha/2} + z_{1-\beta})^2 (\sum_{i=1}^{N} w_i^2 \rho_i \eta_i)}{(\sum_{i=1}^{N} w_i \rho_i \gamma_i)^2}. \tag{7.3}$$

The quantities ϕ_i, θ_i, ρ_i, η_i, and γ_i can be determined using the Markov chain model as discussed in the next section. If we assume that the proportions of allocation to the control and treatment groups are w_1 and w_2 ($w_1 + w_2 = 1$), respectively, and let P_C and P_E be the probabilities of failure for the control and treatment groups, respectively, then the total sample size of the two groups is given by

$$n = \frac{d}{w_1 P_C + w_2 P_E}. \tag{7.4}$$

7.3   Markov Chain Model with Simultaneous Entry

The Lakatos method uses nonstationary Markov chains to model the trial process and adjust the sample size by specifying the state space, initial distributions, and transition probabilities between states according to various trial complications including loss to follow-up, noncompliance and drop-in. We will briefly introduce the Lakatos method as follows. Consider a randomized trial that compares two groups: the control group and the treatment group. Assume that all patients enter simultaneously at time $t = 0$ and there is no time lag in the effectiveness of the treatments; then, patients initially randomized to the treatment (control) group occupy the state A_E (A_C), which designates the patient to be at risk at the treatment (control) rate. During the trial, patients can remain in state A_E (A_C) or transition to one of three other states: state A_C (A_E) for those patients who are no longer compliant with their treatment (control) regimen and are at risk at the control (treatment) rate; state E for patients who experience the event of interest; or state L for patients who are lost to follow-up or for patients whose time-to-event is censored because they are still at risk for the event of interest. Thus, a patient's status follows a Markov chain with four possible states: lost to follow-up (L), experienced an event (E), active on treatment (A_E), and active on control

(A_C), where L and E are absorbing states. Hence, at any time t, a patient is in one of these four states, corresponding to a vector of occupancy probabilities $D_t = (P_L(t), P_E(t), P_{A_E}(t), P_{A_C}(t))'$. Let the transition matrix at time t be $T_t = \{p_t(j,l)\}$, where $p_t(j,l)$ is the probability of going from state l to state j during the period $[0,t]$ and $j,l = L, E, A_E, A_C$. The initial distribution for the treatment group is $D_{t_0} = (0,0,1,0)'$, and that for the control group is $D_{t_0} = (0,0,0,1)'$, where $t_0 = 0$. Thus, the occupancy probability distribution of states at time t is given by

$$D_t = T_t * D_{t_0},$$

where " $*$ " indicates matrix multiplication. For computation purposes, we can approximate the continuous process by a discrete process as follows. The study duration is partitioned into N subintervals of equal length $[t_{i-1}, t_i], i = 1, \ldots, N$, then the 4×4 transition matrices $T_{i-1,i} = \{p_{i-1,i}(j,l)\}$ are constructed so that $p_{i-1,i}(j,l)$ is the conditional probability of transferring from the previous state l to the current state j during the time interval $[t_{i-1}, t_i]$, which is given by

$$T_{i-1,i} = \begin{pmatrix} & L & E & A_E & A_C \\ L & 1 & 0 & p_{loss_E,i} & p_{loss_C,i} \\ E & 0 & 1 & p_{event_E,i} & p_{event_C,i} \\ A_E & 0 & 0 & 1 - \Sigma_1 & p_{dropin,i} \\ A_C & 0 & 0 & p_{noncmpl,i} & 1 - \Sigma_2 \end{pmatrix}.$$

Here, the first column and row are used to identify the states and are not part of the matrix, and Σ_i represents the sum of the three other entries in the same column. In the transition matrix, $p_{loss_E,i}(p_{loss_C,i})$ is the probability of a patient transferring from state $A_E(A_C)$ to the lost to follow-up state L in the ith interval; $p_{event_E,i}(p_{event_C,i})$ is the probability of a patient transferring from state $A_E(A_C)$ to event state E in the ith interval; $p_{noncmpl,i}$ is the probability of a patient transferring from state A_E to state A_C, which indicates noncompliance in the ith interval; and $p_{dropin,i}$ is the probability of a patient transferring from state A_C to state A_E, which indicates drop-in in the ith interval. These transition probabilities of the transition matrix $T_{i-1,i}$ can be obtained from the assumptions about the trial. With this model, patients can transfer to states at time $t_i(i = 1, \ldots, N)$. In the real setting, transitions can take place at any time.

This Markov chain model creates a sequence of occupancy probability distribution $\{D_{t_i}, i = 1, \ldots, N\}$ for each group, where

$$D_{t_i} = T_{i-1,i} * D_{t_{i-1}}. \tag{7.5}$$

Then, the parameters ϕ_i, θ_i, ρ_i, η_i, and γ_i in sample size formula (7.4) can readily be determined by using the probability distribution $\{D_{t_i}, i = 1, \ldots, N\}$ obtained from the Markov chain model. The computation formulae of these parameters are given in the following section.

7.4   Computation Formulae

To use the Markov chain model for sample size calculation, we have to calculate the parameters $\phi_i, \theta_i, \rho_i\, \eta_i$, and γ_i for each time point t_i, $i = 1, \ldots, N$, where N is the total number of subintervals for the trial duration. Let $D_{1,i} = (p_{1,i,1}, p_{1,i,2}, p_{1,i,3}, p_{1,i,4})'$ and $D_{2,i} = (p_{2,i,1}, p_{2,i,2}, p_{2,i,3}, p_{2,i,4})'$ be the occupancy probabilities at time point t_i for the control and treatment groups, respectively, and assume that the allocation ratio of control to treatment is $r_1 : r_2$; then, the probability of having an event for the control and treatment groups at the interval $[t_{i-1}, t_i]$ can be calculated by

$$
\begin{aligned}
d_{1,i} &= p_{1,i,2} - p_{1,i-1,2}, \\
d_{2,i} &= p_{2,i,2} - p_{2,i-1,2},
\end{aligned}
$$

and the probability of being at risk for the control and treatment groups at the interval $[t_{i-1}, t_i]$ can be calculated by

$$
\begin{aligned}
a_{1,i} &= p_{1,i-1,3} + p_{1,i-1,4}, \\
a_{2,i} &= p_{2,i-1,3} + p_{2,i-1,4},
\end{aligned}
$$

where $p_{1,0,j} = p_{2,0,j} = 0$ for $j = 2, 3, 4$. Thus, the parameters $\phi_i, \theta_i, \rho_i\, \eta_i$ and γ_i for each time point t_i can be calculated as follows

$$
\begin{aligned}
\rho_i &= d_i/(r_1 p_{1,N,2} + r_2 p_{2,N,2}), \quad \text{where } d_i = r_1 d_{1,i} + r_2 d_{2,i}, \\
\phi_i &= r_1 a_{1,i}/(r_2 a_{2,i}), \\
\theta_i &= \log(1 - d_{1,i}/a_{1,i})/\log(1 - d_{2,i}/a_{2,i}), \\
\eta_i &= \frac{\phi_i}{(1 + \phi_i)^2}, \\
\gamma_i &= \frac{\phi_i \theta_i}{1 + \phi_i \theta_i} - \frac{\phi_i}{1 + \phi_i},
\end{aligned}
$$

where $p_{1,N,2}$ and $p_{2,N,2}$ are the probabilities of an event at the end of the trial for the control group (group 1) and the treatment group (group 2), respectively.

The following example illustrates how to set up transition matrix and calculate the occupancy probability of the distribution $\{D_{t_i}, i = 1, \ldots, N\}$.

Example 7.2 *Cardiovascular trial*

Consider a two-year cardiovascular trial (Lakatos, 1988). It is assumed that the yearly hazard rates are 1 and 0.5 for the control and treatment groups, respectively. Hence, under the exponential model, the yearly event rates are $1 - e^{-1} = 0.6321$ and $1 - e^{-0.5} = 0.3935$ for the control and treatment groups, respectively. It is also assumed that the yearly loss to follow-up rate is 3% for both the control and treatment groups, the yearly noncompliance rate is 4%, and the drop-in rate (e.g., the rate at which patients assigned to the control group begin taking a medication similar to the treatment) is 5%. Then the unit time (year) transition matrix for both the first year and second year is given by

$$
T = \begin{pmatrix}
1 & 0 & 0.03 & 0.03 \\
0 & 1 & 0.3935 & 0.6321 \\
0 & 0 & 1 - \Sigma_1 & 0.05 \\
0 & 0 & 0.04 & 1 - \Sigma_2
\end{pmatrix},
$$

where $1 - \Sigma_1 = 1 - (0.03 + 0.3935 + 0.04) = 0.5365$ and $1 - \Sigma_2 = 1 - (0.03 + 0.6321 + 0.05) = 0.2879$. For illustration purposes, let us assume that each unit time (year) has been divided into $K = 10$ equal-length intervals, with a total of $N = 20$ subintervals in a 2-year study period. When only year rates are given and a constant hazard rate within each year is assumed, the transition matrix within each subinterval can be obtained by replacing each off-diagonal entry x in T (per year transition matrix) by $1 - (1 - x)^{1/K}$, and the resulting transition matrix for each interval is $T_{i-1,i} = T_{1/K}$, which is given by

$$
T_{1/K} = \begin{pmatrix}
1 & 0 & 0.003 & 0.003 \\
0 & 1 & 0.0488 & 0.0951 \\
0 & 0 & 1 - \Sigma_1 & 0.0051 \\
0 & 0 & 0.0041 & 1 - \Sigma_2
\end{pmatrix},
$$

where Σ_1 and Σ_2 represent the sum of the remainder of the corresponding column, that is, $1 - \Sigma_1 = 0.9441$ and $1 - \Sigma_2 = 0.8968$. Then, we can use $T_{i-1,i} = T_{1/K}$ approximately to calculate distribution D_{t_i} recursively by using equation (7.5). Under equal allocation ($r_1 : r_2 = 1 : 1$), the resulting sequence distributions $\{D_{t_i}, i = 1, \ldots, 20\}$ and parameters $\rho_i, \phi_i, \theta_i, \eta_i$ and γ_i are given in Table 7.1. For example, at the end of the 2-year trial, in the control group, 2.7% have been lost to follow-up, 83.7% have had events, 11.4% are complying with the control, and 2.2% are drop-ins. For treatment group, 3.8% have been lost to follow-up, 62.7% have had events, 31.8% are complying with the treatment, and 1.8% are drop-ins.

For illustration purposes, the calculations for $t_i = 0.2$ are given as follows. Patients at risk just before $t_i = 0.2$ are the patients still active ($A_E + A_C$) at time $t_i = 0.1$; thus, $a_{1,i} = (0.897 + 0.005) = 0.902$ for the control group and $a_{2,i} = (0.944 + 0.004) = 0.948$ for the treatment group. Hence, $\phi_i = a_{1,i}/a_{2,i} = 0.902/0.948 = 0.951$ and $\eta_i = 0.951/(1 + 0.951)^2 = 0.025$. Next, we calculate θ_i, which is the hazard ratio within this interval. When $t_i = 0.2$, the event rates are $d_{1,i} = 0.181 - 0.095 = 0.086$ for the control group and $d_{2,i} = 0.095 - 0.049 = 0.046$ for the treatment group; thus, $\theta_i = \log(1 - 0.08557/0.9018)/\log(1 - 0.04644/0.94818) = 1.986$ (note: to be more accurate, we use more decimal places for the calculation). Finally, we calculate ρ_i and γ_i. The sum of the event rates for the two groups is $a_{1,i} + a_{2,i} = 0.086 + 0.046 = 0.132$, and the sum of the total event rates is $p_{1,N,2} + p_{2,N,2} = (0.837 + 0.627) = 1.464$.

Thus, $\rho_i = 0.132/1.464 = 0.090$ and $\gamma_i = 0.951 \times 1.986/(1 + 0.951 \times 1.986) - 0.951/(1+0.951) = 0.166$. The values of these parameters at other time points can be obtained similarly.

Once all the derived parameters are obtained, we can calculate the required number of events for the standard log-rank test by using formula (7.3). From Table 7.1, we have $\sum_{i=1}^{N} \rho_i \eta_i = 0.2399$ and $\sum_{i=1}^{N} \rho_i \gamma_i = 0.1574$; thus, given a two-sided type I error $\alpha = 0.05$ and power of 90%, the required total number of events is

$$d = \frac{(1.96 + 1.28)^2 \times 0.2399}{(0.1574)^2} = 101.7 \simeq 102.$$

On the other hand, the overall event rate for the control group is $P_C = p_{1,N,2} = 0.837$, and for the treatment group it is $P_E = p_{2,N,2} = 0.627$. Hence, the total sample size for a balanced design ($r_1 : r_2 = 1 : 1$) is given by

$$n = \frac{2d}{P_E + P_C} = \frac{2 \times 102}{0.837 + 0.627} = 138.9 \simeq 139.$$

Remark 3: The algorithm requires that each unit time be partitioned into a number of equal-width subintervals. All parameters such as the hazard ratio, loss to follow-up rate, drop-in rate, and noncompliance rate are assumed to be constant for each subinterval within a unit time.

Remark 4: Lakatos did not discuss how many subintervals should be chosen for the sample size calculation. The user specifies how finely each unit time will be subdivided in the application. From our experience, 20 to 200 subintervals for each unit time should be adequate (see section 7.8).

7.5 Markov Chain Model with Staggered Entry

In a cancer clinical trial, patients enter in a staggered fashion. To preserve the Markov property, we will continue to assume that all patients enter simultaneously, and we will account for staggered entry by "administratively censoring" patients in accordance with their accrual pattern. The study duration is divided into N equal-length intervals. Let p_i ($\sum_{i=1}^{N} p_i = 1$) be the probability of a patient entering during the ith interval; then, conditional on the patient being in an active state during the $(N - k + 1)^{th}$ interval, the probability of their being administratively censored during the $(N - k + 1)^{th}$ interval is given by

$$a_k = \frac{p_k}{\sum_{i=1}^{k} p_i}.$$

For example, in the last (N^{th}) interval, $k = 1$ and $a_1 = p_1/p_1 = 1$; in the $(N - 1)^{th}$ interval, $k = 2$ and $a_2 = p_2/(p_1+p_2)$; and in the $(N - 2)^{th}$ interval,

TABLE 7.1: The sequence distributions $\{D_{t_i}\}$ for the example with simultaneous entry

t_i	Control				Treatment				Parameters				
	L	E	A_E	A_C	L	E	A_E	A_C	γ	η	ρ	θ	ϕ
.1	0.003	0.095	0.005	0.897	0.003	0.049	0.944	0.004	0.167	0.250	0.098	2.000	1.000
.2	0.006	0.181	0.009	0.804	0.006	0.095	0.891	0.008	0.166	0.250	0.090	1.986	0.951
.3	0.008	0.258	0.013	0.721	0.009	0.139	0.842	0.010	0.166	0.249	0.083	1.972	0.905
.4	0.010	0.327	0.016	0.647	0.011	0.181	0.795	0.013	0.165	0.249	0.076	1.959	0.862
.5	0.012	0.389	0.018	0.580	0.014	0.221	0.750	0.015	0.164	0.248	0.070	1.945	0.821
.6	0.014	0.445	0.020	0.520	0.016	0.259	0.708	0.016	0.163	0.246	0.064	1.932	0.782
.7	0.016	0.496	0.022	0.467	0.018	0.296	0.669	0.018	0.162	0.245	0.059	1.920	0.746
.8	0.017	0.541	0.023	0.419	0.020	0.330	0.632	0.018	0.160	0.243	0.054	1.907	0.712
.9	0.019	0.582	0.024	0.376	0.022	0.362	0.596	0.019	0.158	0.241	0.050	1.894	0.679
1.0	0.020	0.619	0.024	0.337	0.024	0.393	0.563	0.020	0.156	0.239	0.046	1.882	0.649
1.1	0.021	0.652	0.025	0.302	0.026	0.423	0.532	0.020	0.154	0.236	0.043	1.870	0.620
1.2	0.022	0.682	0.025	0.271	0.027	0.450	0.502	0.020	0.152	0.234	0.039	1.857	0.593
1.3	0.023	0.709	0.025	0.243	0.029	0.477	0.474	0.020	0.149	0.231	0.036	1.845	0.567
1.4	0.024	0.733	0.025	0.218	0.030	0.502	0.448	0.020	0.147	0.228	0.034	1.833	0.543
1.5	0.024	0.755	0.024	0.196	0.032	0.526	0.423	0.020	0.144	0.225	0.031	1.820	0.520
1.6	0.025	0.775	0.024	0.176	0.033	0.548	0.399	0.019	0.141	0.222	0.029	1.808	0.498
1.7	0.025	0.793	0.024	0.158	0.034	0.569	0.377	0.019	0.138	0.219	0.027	1.796	0.477
1.8	0.026	0.809	0.023	0.142	0.035	0.590	0.356	0.019	0.135	0.215	0.025	1.783	0.458
1.9	0.027	0.824	0.023	0.127	0.037	0.609	0.336	0.018	0.132	0.212	0.023	1.771	0.439
2.0	0.027	0.837	0.022	0.114	0.038	0.627	0.318	0.018	0.129	0.209	0.021	1.758	0.422

Note: In the original Table 1 of Lakatos, the values of η were recorded in error, and A_C and A_E for the control and treatment groups were switched. These errors have been corrected in Table 7.1.

$k = 3$ and $a_3 = p_3/(p_1 + p_2 + p_3)$, and so on, where p_i can be determined by the accrual pattern specifying the accrual ratio in each accrual period. For example, suppose a trial has a 2-year duration with 1-year accrual and 1-year follow-up, and the accrual pattern is divided into two periods 0.5 years and 1 year, with an accrual ratio of 1:2 for these two periods. Assume each year is divided into 4 intervals. Then, the accrual pattern in each interval for a total of $N = 8$ intervals is $(1, 1, 2, 2, 0, 0, 0, 0)$; thus, the probabilities of being administratively censored for $N = 8$ intervals are given by $(0, 0, 0, 0, 0.3333, 0.5, 0.5, 1)$. Hence, we can model staggered entry by assuming additional transitions of active patients (in state A_E or A_C) to a lost to follow-up state (L) with these probabilities. To accomplish this, we define the administrative censoring transition matrix A_i for the ith interval by

$$A_i = \begin{pmatrix} 1 & 0 & a_i & a_i \\ 0 & 1 & 0 & 0 \\ 0 & 0 & 1 - a_i & 0 \\ 0 & 0 & 0 & 1 - a_i \end{pmatrix}.$$

Then, the Markov model for staggered entry is given by

$$D_{t_i} = (A_i * T_{i-1,i}) * D_{t_{i-1}}.$$

Remark 5: Lakatos (1992) used the equation $D_{t_i} = (T_{i-1,i} * A_i) * D_{t_{i-1}}$ which contains a typographic error by switching the matrix multiplication $A_i * T_{i-1,i}$ to $T_{i-1,i} * A_i$.

Remark 6: The weighted log-rank test statistic L in Lakatos's 1988 paper was given by

$$L_w = \sum_{k=1}^{d} w_k \left(X_k - \frac{m_k}{m_k + n_k} \right) \bigg/ \left[\sum_{k=1}^{d} w_k^2 \frac{m_k n_k}{(m_k + n_k)^2} \right]^{1/2}$$

(using Lakatos' notations), where X_k is the indicator of the control group instead of the experimental group, and m_k and n_k are the numbers at risk, just before the kth death, in the experimental and control groups, respectively. This was an error, because X_k is the indicator of the control group; thus, the correct version of the weighted log-rank test is

$$L_w = \sum_{k=1}^{d} w_k \left(X_k - \frac{n_k}{m_k + n_k} \right) \bigg/ \left[\sum_{k=1}^{d} w_k^2 \frac{m_k n_k}{(m_k + n_k)^2} \right]^{1/2}$$

Remark 7: The SAS code of Lakatos (1988, Appendix) for the calculation of $\theta = (d_{1,i}/a_{1,i})/(d_{2,i}/a_{2,i})$ was in error. It has been corrected as $\theta_i = \log(1 - d_{1,i}/a_{1,i})/\log(1 - d_{2,i}/a_{2,i})$ in our computation formula (section 7.6) and it has also been corrected in Shih's SAS code '%SIZE' (personal communication).

7.6   Examples and R code

To implement the Lakatos method, a simple R function 'SizeLak' has been developed to design complex survival trials (see Appendix D). We will illustrate trial design using the R function 'SizeLak' in a step by step manner via examples.

```
SizeLak(ploss,    # vector of probability of loss to follow-up for both groups#
        pc,       # vector of probability of having an event in control group #
        k,        # vector of hazard ratio #
        pnoncmpl, # vector of probability of noncompliance #
        pdropin,  # vector of probability of drop-in #
        rectime,  # vector of accrual times (in unit time); default if simul=1#
        recratio, # vector of accrual rates; default if simul=1#
        logr,     # vector of weight of the log-rank test #
        ratio,    # vector of randomization allocation ratio #
        simul,    # staggered entry (0) or simultaneously entry (1) #
        sbdv,     # number of intervals to be divided for each unit time #
        alpha,    # type I error for a two-sided test #
        beta)     # type II error #

## parameter input 1: Cardiovascular trial example ##
 ploss=rep(0.03,2) # 3% yearly loss to follow-up with two years study period #
 pnoncmpl=rep(0.04,2) # 4% yearly noncompliance rate #
 pdropin=rep(0.05,2)  # 5% yearly drop-in rate #
 pc=rep(0.6321,2)  # 1-e^(-1)=0.6321 #
 k=rep(0.5,2)      # hazard ratio=0.5/1=0.5 #
 logr=rep(1,2)     # standard log-rank test #
 ratio=1           # equal allocation #
 sbdv=20           # 20 subintervals #
 simul=1           # simultaneously entry #
 alpha=0.05        # 5% type I error #
 beta=0.1          # 90% power #
 SizeLak(ploss,pc,k,pnoncmpl,pdropin,rectime,recratio,
         logr,ratio,simul,sbdv,alpha,beta)
## output ##
d_LR      n_LR      p_e     p_c
101.4268  138.5736  0.6265  0.8373
```

1. Number of subintervals

One concern of the Lakatos approach is the convergence of the discrete Markov chains. To investigate this issue further, we will look at the effect of the number of subintervals on the sample size calculation. Using the same parameters as input 1, where the yearly hazard rate of control is set to $\lambda = 1$, and the number of subintervals sbdv is taken to be 20, 50, 75, 100, 150 or 200, the calculated sample sizes are 138.57, 138.35, 138.29, 138.27, 138.24, and 138.23, respectively. If the yearly hazard rate of control increases to $\lambda = 5$, the calculated sample sizes are 100.47, 99.83, 99.69, 99.62, 99.56, and 99.52 for the number of subintervals 20, 50, 75, 100, 150 and 200 intervals, respectively;

and if the yearly hazard rate of control increases to $\lambda = 15$, the calculated sample sizes are 97.62, 96.39, 96.15, 96.03, 95.92, and 95.87 for the number of subintervals 20, 50, 75, 100, 150 and 200 intervals, respectively. Thus, the results are very stable for numbers of subintervals ranging from 20 to 200.

2. Parameter specification for the R function 'SizeLak'

Let us assume that the duration of a trial is expressed as τ unit time, where τ is an integer in unit time, e.g., day, month, year, etc. In using the Markov model approach to calculate the sample size by the function 'SizeLak,' we assume each unit time to be partitioned into a number of equal-width intervals. All parameters such as probability of failure, loss to follow-up, drop-in, non-compliance, and hazard ratio are assumed to be constant for each subinterval within a unit time, but they can be different for other time intervals.

2.1. Probability of failure

The parameter *pc* specifies a vector of conditional probability of failure for the control group, with length τ. Each element of *pc* is the conditional probability of failure in that unit time interval. If $S(t)$ is the survival distribution, e.g., an exponential distribution or Kaplan-Meier curve of the control group, then the conditional transition probability in the unit time interval $[t_{i-1}, t_i]$ can be calculated by $S(t_i|t_{i-1}) = 1 - S(t_i)/S(t_{i-1})$ for the control group. For example, for a two-year trial ($\tau = 2$), the yearly hazard rate is 1 for the control group. Then, under the exponential distribution $S(t) = e^{-t}$, the conditional probabilities of failure in the first year and second year are $S(1) = 1 - e^{-1} = 0.6321$ and $S(2|1) = 1 - S(2)/S(1) = 1 - e^{-(2-1)} = 0.6321$, respectively. Thus, *pc* is set to be the vector of $c(0.6321, 0.6321)$.

2.2. Loss to follow-up and noncompliance

The parameter *ploss* specifies a vector of conditional probability of loss to follow-up, with length τ. If the survival distribution of the loss to follow-up can be specified during the design stage, then *ploss* can be calculated using the same method for calculating *pc*; otherwise, it is usually specified by a constant loss to follow-up rate at each unit time interval according to the historical data. A similar approach is used to set up the parameters *pnoncmpl* and *pdropin*, which are vectors of conditional probability of noncompliance and drop-in, respectively. For example, for a two-year trial, it is assumed that the yearly loss to follow-up rate is 3% for both the control and treatment groups, the yearly noncompliance rate is 4%, and the drop-in rate is 5%. Thus, *ploss*=c(0.03, 0.03), *pnoncmpl*=c(0.04, 0.04) and *pdropin*=c(0.05,0.05).

Remark 8: In the R function 'SizeLak', we have set *ploss* to be the same for the control and treatment groups but this is unnecessary: One can set different loss to follow-up probabilities for the control and treatment groups, and the R code can be easily modified to accommodate this change.

2.3. Staggered entry and accrual distribution

The parameter *simul* is a 0/1 indicator variable. If *simul*= 1, then patients enter the trial simultaneously. If *simul*= 0, then patients enter the trial according to the accrual distribution specified by the parameters *rectime* and *recratio*. The parameter *rectime* specifies a vector of accrual time in terms of unit time or a fraction of unit time. In each subinterval of *rectime*, the accrual rate is assumed to be constant. The parameter *recratio* is a vector of the relative accrual rates over the accrual times. The length of *recratio* and the length of *rectime* must be equal. For a uniform accrual with an accrual period of 2 years, one can set *rectime* to 2 and *recratio* to 1.

2.4. Treatment allocation

The parameter *ratio* specifies the equal or unequal treatment allocation for the trial, which is a vector with a length of 2, referring to the ratio of the sample size in the control group to that in the treatment group. For example, if the allocation *ratio* is 2:1, then *ratio*= $c(2, 1)$.

2.5. Hazard ratio

The parameter k specifies a vector of the hazard ratio, with length τ. A constant hazard ratio vector k specifies a proportional hazards model; otherwise, it specifies a nonproportional hazards model. For a nonproportional hazards model, the hazard ratio in each unit time interval is assumed to be constant. For example, if a 2-year (where the unit time is a year) trial is to detect a hazard ratio of 0.583 under a proportional hazards model, then k=c(0.583, 0.583).

2.6. Weights for the log-rank test

For the nonproportional hazards model, the weighted log-rank test may be more efficient than the standard log-rank test. The parameter *logr* specifies a vector of weights, with length τ. For the standard log-rank test, the *logr* is set to a unit vector of length τ.

2.7. Other parameters

The parameter *sbdv* specifies the number of subintervals into which each unit time interval is to be divided. The parameters *alpha* and *beta* specify the type I error (two-sided) and type II error of the trial, respectively.

Remark 9: The R code 'SizeLak' is less comprehensive than the SAS code '%SIZE' developed by Shih but it is much simpler and easy to use and includes most of the same features as the Lakatos Markov approach. The computation for the occupancy probability distribution in R code is slightly different to that in '%SIZE'. Thus, the sample size calculated by the R code 'SizeLak' may not be identical to that calculated by the SAS code '%SIZE'. However, our simulation results showed that the results with the R code 'SizeLak' are very reliable.

Example 7.3 *The SHEP Trial*

Lakatos (1996) considers the sample size calculation for the Systolic Hypertension in the Elderly (SHEP) trial. In this trial, patients are randomized to hypertension medication or a control. The primary outcome is fatal or nonfatal stroke. Those participants who die of nonstroke causes can no longer be followed for the outcome. The rate of loss to follow-up for both the control and treatment groups is estimated to be 3% in the first year and is expected to increase uniformly to 4% over the next 6 years. The parameter specification is given in Table 7.2, where the drop-in rates and noncompliance rates are derived from experience in several clinical trials. The event (stroke) rate of patients in the control group is assumed to be 1.6% per year. Assuming a proportional hazards model, the study is designed to detect a hazard ratio of $k = 0.5981$ for the treatment group versus the control group. The unit time (year) transition matrix is given by

$$T = \begin{pmatrix} 1 & 0 & 0.03 & 0.03 \\ 0 & 1 & 0.0096 & 0.016 \\ 0 & 0 & 1-\Sigma_1 & 0.09 \\ 0 & 0 & 0.07 & 1-\Sigma_2 \end{pmatrix},$$

where $\Sigma_1 = 0.03+0.0096+0.07 = 0.1096$ and $\Sigma_2 = 0.03+0.016+0.09 = 0.136$.

Suppose that the SHEP trial is designed with a 2-year recruitment phase and 4-year follow-up, so that the study duration is 6 years. Lakatos and Shih consider the accrual ratio to be 2:4:5 for the first quarter, the second quarter, and the last 18 months, respectively; that is, the accrual period is $(0.25, 0.5, 2)$ in terms of unit time (year). If we assume equal allocation $(r_1 : r_2 = 1 : 1)$, each unit time (year) is divided into $K = 100$ equal-length intervals, and the probability of an event is constant across intervals within a given year, then we have $\sum_{i=1}^{N} \rho_i \eta_i = 0.249987$ and $\sum_{i=1}^{N} \rho_i \gamma_i = 0.097306$, where $N = 6 \times 100 = 600$. Thus, given a two-sided type I error of $\alpha = 0.05$ and power of 90%, the required total number of events is

$$d = \frac{(1.959964 + 1.281552)^2 \times 0.249987}{(0.097306)^2} = 277.4 \simeq 278.$$

The probabilities of an event by the end of the trial are $P_E = 0.0454997$ and $P_C = 0.066608$ for the control and treatment groups, respectively; therefore, the total sample size is $n = 2d/(P_E + P_C) = 4949.1 \simeq 4950$.

```
### parameter input 2: SHEP trial with non-uniform accrual ###
ploss=c(0.03, 0.032, 0.034, 0.036, 0.038, 0.040)
```

TABLE 7.2: Yearly rates of loss to follow-up, noncompliance, and drop-in for the SHEP trial

State	Year 1	Year 2	Year 3	Year 4	Year 5	Year 6
Lost to follow-up	0.030	0.032	0.034	0.036	0.038	0.040
Event (*pc*)	0.016	0.016	0.016	0.016	0.016	0.016
Noncompliance	0.070	0.035	0.035	0.035	0.035	0.035
Drop-in	0.090	0.045	0.050	0.055	0.060	0.065

```
pnoncmpl=c(0.07, 0.035, 0.035, 0.035, 0.035, 0.035)
pdropin=c(0.09, 0.045, 0.050, 0.055, 0.060, 0.065)
pc=rep(0.016, 6)
k=rep(0.5981, 6)
rectime=c(0.25, 0.50, 2)  # vector of accrual times (in unit time - year)  #
recratio=c(2, 4, 5)  # vector of accrual ratios over accrual times in rectime#
sbdv=100
simul=0
ratio=1
logr=rep(1,6)
alpha=0.05
beta=0.1
### output ###
d_LR     n_LR      p_e     p_c
277.4197 4949.1473 0.0455  0.0666
```

Example 7.4 *The PBC Trial*

1. Trial design under the parametric Weibull model

   The survival distribution of the DPCA arm of the PBC trial can be fitted by the Weibull distribution

$$S(t) = e^{-\log(2)(\frac{t}{m_1})^{\kappa}},$$

where the median $m_1 = 9$ and $\kappa = 1.22$. The trial was designed to detect a hazard ratio of $k = 0.5834$ with power of 90% and type I error of 5% for a two-sided test. We assume a uniform accrual with accrual duration $t_a = 6$ (years) and follow-up time $t_f = 3$ (years), equal allocation, no loss to follow-up, no drop-in, and no noncompliance. To use the Lakatos method, we calculate the conditional failure rate for each year of the 9-year study as shown in Table 7.3.

   Thus, we can set up the following parameter input 3 for the Lakatos method. The calculated total number of events is 149, and the total sample size is 532.

```
### parameter input 3: PBC trial design under the Weibull model ###
ploss=rep(0,9)
```

TABLE 7.3: Conditional failure rate for each year of a 9-year study based on the Weibull distribution

t_i (year)	$S(t_i)$	$1 - S(t_i)/S(t_{i-1})$
1	0.95362	0.04638
2	0.89526	0.06119
3	0.83407	0.06835
4	0.77280	0.07345
5	0.71293	0.07748
6	0.65530	0.08084
7	0.60043	0.08374
8	0.54861	0.08630
9	0.50000	0.08860

```
pnoncmpl=rep(0,9)
pdropin=rep(0,9)
pc=c(0.04638,0.06119,0.06836,0.07345,0.07748,0.08084,0.08374,0.08630,0.08860)
k=rep(0.5834,9)
rectime=c(1,2,3,4,5,6)
recratio=rep(1,6)
sbdv=100
simul=0
ratio=1
logr=rep(1,9)
alpha=0.05
beta=0.1
### output ###
d_LR        n_LR        p_e        p_c
148.63      531.48      0.2181     0.3412
```

2. Trial design based on the Kaplan-Meier curve

To avoid an assumption of the parametric Weibull distribution, we use the Kaplan-Meier estimate given in Table 7.4 for the sample size calculation. Based on the Kaplan-Meier estimate, we calculate the conditional failure rate for each year of the 9-year study as shown in Table 7.5. Thus, we set up parameter input 4; the calculated total number of events is 149, and the total sample size is 519, which are close to those calculated under the Weibull model.

3. Trial design under nonuniform accrual and unbalanced allocation

To give an example of how to set up nonuniform accrual and unequal allocation, let us assume that the ratio of the accrual rates for a 6-year accrual period is 1:1:1:2:2:2 and the sample size allocation ratio is $r_1 : r_2 = 1 : 2$. Furthermore, let us assume that the yearly rates of loss to follow-up, noncompliance, and drop-in are 3%, 5%, and 4%, respectively. We then set up

TABLE 7.4: Kaplan-Meier estimate of PBC data

Time	Risk	Fail	Censor	$\hat{S}(t)$	SE
0	158	0	0	1.000	0.000
1	158	9	0	0.943	0.018
2	149	5	1	0.911	0.023
3	143	13	6	0.826	0.031
4	124	9	14	0.764	0.037
5	101	7	12	0.708	0.042
6	82	5	12	0.661	0.047
7	65	7	12	0.584	0.055
8	46	3	9	0.542	0.062
9	34	3	10	0.478	0.074
10	21	2	3	0.425	0.078
11	16	0	6	0.425	0.097
12	10	2	4	0.319	0.118
13	4	0	4	0.319	0.263

parameter input 5; the calculated total number of events is 256, and the total sample size is 1126.

```
## parameter input 4: PBC trial design based on the Kaplan-Meier curve ##
ploss=rep(0,9)
pnoncmpl=rep(0,9)
pdropin=rep(0,9)
pc=c(0.057,0.03393,0.09330,0.07506,0.07330,0.06638,0.11649,0.07192,0.11808)
k=rep(0.5834,9)
rectime=c(1,2,3,4,5,6)
recratio=rep(1,6)
sbdv=100
simul=0
ratio=1
logr=rep(1,9)
alpha=0.05
beta=0.1
### output ###
d_LR      n_LR       p_e     p_c
148.5802  518.9503   0.2237  0.3489

### parameter input 5: PBC trial design adjusted for loss follow-up ##
###   noncompliance, drop-in and non-uniform accrual ###
ploss=rep(0.03,9)
pnoncmpl=rep(0.05,9)
pdropin=rep(0.04,9)
pc=c(0.057,0.03393,0.09330,0.07506,0.07330,0.06638,0.11649,0.07192,0.11808)
k=rep(0.5834,9)
rectime=c(1,2,3,4,5,6)
recratio=c(1,1,1,2,2,2)
sbdv=100
simul=0
```

TABLE 7.5: Conditional failure rate for each year of the 9-year study based on the Kaplan-Meier survival curve

t_i (year)	$\hat{S}(t_i)$	$1 - \hat{S}(t_i)/\hat{S}(t_{i-1})$
1	0.943	0.05700
2	0.911	0.03393
3	0.826	0.09330
4	0.764	0.07506
5	0.708	0.07330
6	0.661	0.06638
7	0.584	0.11649
8	0.542	0.07192
9	0.478	0.11808

```
ratio=c(1,2)
logr=rep(1,9)
alpha=0.05
beta=0.1
### output ###
d_LR       n_LR      p_e     p_c
255.2042  1125.851  0.1996  0.2809
```

Example 7.5 *Nonproportional Hazards Model*

Yang and Prentice (2005) developed a semiparametric model that can accommodate different short-term and long-term hazard ratios. In the two-sample case, the model has the following form:

$$\frac{\lambda_2(t)}{\lambda_1(t)} = \frac{\gamma_1\gamma_2}{\gamma_1 + (\gamma_2 - \gamma_1)S_1(t)}. \tag{7.6}$$

The hazard ratio in (7.6) is a function of the two positive parameters, γ_1 and γ_2, and the baseline survival function $S_1(t)$. This is a monotone function in t for fixed values of γ_1 and γ_2. Notice that $\gamma_1 = \lim_{t \to 0} \lambda_1(t)/\lambda_2(t)$ and $\gamma_2 = \lim_{t \to \infty} \lambda_1(t)/\lambda_2(t)$; therefore, γ_1 can be interpreted as the short-term hazard ratio and γ_2 as the long-term hazard ratio. The model reduces to the Cox proportional hazards model when $\gamma_1 = \gamma_2$. When $\gamma_2 = 1$, the model becomes the proportional odds model. The proportional odds model has a nonconstant hazard ratio, and the corresponding hazard functions are not proportional. The treatment effect would fade away over time for the proportional odds model. A case of special interest is what we call the long-term effect model, in which $\gamma_1 = 1$. This means that there is no treatment effect at the beginning of the trial but the effect shows up later on. The long-term effect model has a nonconstant hazard ratio, and the corresponding hazard functions are nonproportional (Wang, 2013).

Proportional odds model

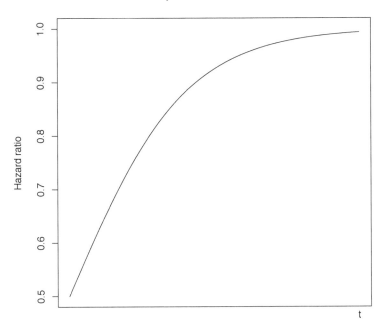

FIGURE 7.3: Hazard ratio curve of the proportional odds model with $\gamma_1 = 0.5$, $\gamma_2 = 1$, and the baseline survival distribution $S_1(t) = e^{-0.5t}$.

To calculate the sample size under the proportional odds model, the parameters are set for the sample size calculation as given by $\gamma_1 = 0.5$, $\gamma_2 = 1$, and the baseline survival distribution $S_1(t) = e^{-0.5t}$.

The hazard ratio for each year can be calculated as given in parameter input 6. Thus, with equal allocation, 5-year uniform accrual, 3-year follow-up, a two-sided type I error of $\alpha = 0.05$, and power of 90% for testing the hypothesis

$$H_0 : \gamma_1 = 0 \quad vs. \quad H_1 : \gamma_1 = 0.5,$$

where $\gamma_2 = 1$ is fixed, the total number of events and the sample size are $d = 435$ and $n = 487$, respectively.

```
#parameter input 6: Sample size calculation under the proportional odds model#
ploss=rep(0, 8)
pnoncmpl=rep(0, 8)
pdropin=rep(0, 8)
pc=rep(0.39347, 8)     ## 1-exp(-0.5)= 0.39347 #
k=c(0.6225, 0.7311, 0.8176, 0.8808, 0.9241, 0.9526, 0.9707, 0.9820)
```

Long–term effect model

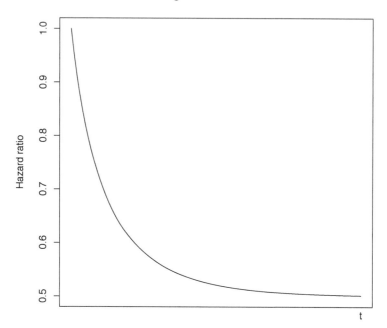

FIGURE 7.4: Hazard ratio curve of the long-term effect model with $\gamma_1 = 1$, $\gamma_2 = 0.5$, and the baseline survival distribution $S_1(t) = e^{-0.5t}$.

```
rectime=c(1,5)
recratio=c(1,1,1,1,1)
logr=rep(1, 8)
ratio=1
simul=0
alpha=0.05
beta=0.1
sbdv=100
```

For the long-term effect model, the parameters are set for the sample size calculation as given by $\gamma_1 = 1$, $\gamma_2 = 0.5$, and the baseline survival distribution $S_1(t) = e^{-0.5t}$.

The hazard ratio for each year can be calculated as given in parameter input 7. Thus, with equal allocation, 5-year uniform accrual, 3-year follow-up, a two-sided type I error of $\alpha = 0.05$, and power of 90% for testing the hypothesis

$$H_0 : \gamma_2 = 0 \quad vs. \quad H_1 : \gamma_2 = 0.5,$$

where $\gamma_1 = 1$ *is fixed, the total number of events and the sample size are* $d = 196$ *and* $n = 230$, *respectively.*

```
#parameter input 7: Sample size calculation under the long-term effect model#
 ploss=rep(0, 8)
 pnoncmpl=rep(0, 8)
 pdropin=rep(0, 8)
 pc=rep(0.39347, 8)     ## 1-exp(-0.5)= 0.39347 #
 k=c(0.7176, 0.6127, 0.5628, 0.5363, 0.5214, 0.5128, 0.5077, 0.5046)
 rectime=c(1,5)
 recratio=c(1,1,1,1,1)
 logr=rep(1, 8)
 ratio=1
 simul=0
 alpha=0.05
 beta=0.1
 sbdv=100
```

Example 7.6 *Piecewise proportional hazards adjusted for loss to follow-up, drop-in, and noncompliance*

Consider the sample size calculation for a piecewise proportional hazards model with loss to follow-up, drop-in, and noncompliance as given in Table V of Barthel et al. (2006). Assume a randomized trial has a 2-year accrual, 2-year follow-up, equal allocation, uniform accrual, exponential survival distribution, and 1-year median survival in the control group ($m_1 = 1$). The sample sizes are calculated for 90% power with a two-sided type I error of 5%. Other design parameters are given in Table 7.6. In this piecewise proportional hazards model, we assumed that the hazard in the experimental group was changed for each patient after they had survived for 2 years in the trial, which resulted in a change in the overall hazard ratio from HR1 for the first 2 years to HR2 after 2 years. In addition, Π_1^L and Π_2^L are the proportions lost to follow-up in the control and experimental groups, respectively, by the end of the trial, and Π_1^C and Π_2^C are the proportions of drop-in and noncompliance, respectively, by the end of trial. The input parameters for the sample size calculation using 'SizeLak' for the first case are given as follows in parameter input 8. The sample sizes N_L (by the Lakatos method) and N_B (by the method of Barthel et al.) calculated for cases 1 to 8 are identical to those obtained by Barthel et al. (Table V). For cases 9 to 11, the sample sizes calculated using the Lakatos method are slightly different to those obtained by Barthel et al.(2006) (Table V). This is because of the different assumptions underlying the sample size calculations: with the calculation method of Barthel et al., patients crossing over to the other treatment group are not allowed to return to their original treatment, whereas the Lakatos Markov approach allows patients to change treatment groups more than once over the course of trial.

```
### parameter input 8: Example 7.6 case 1 ###
 ploss=rep(0.08530878, 4)       ### 1-(1-0.3)^(1/4)=0.08530878 ##
 pnoncmpl=rep(0.05425839, 4)    ### 1-(1-0.2)^(1/4)=0.05425839 ##
 pdropin=rep(0, 4)
```

TABLE 7.6: Sample sizes for the piecewise proportional hazards model adjusted for loss to follow-up, drop-in, and noncompliance

Case	HR1	HR2	$\Pi_1^L(\%)$	$\Pi_2^L(\%)$	$\Pi_1^C(\%)$	$\Pi_2^C(\%)$	N_L	N_B
1	0.6	0.7	30	30	0	20	274	274
2	0.6	0.7	30	30	0	30	291	291
3	0.6	0.8	30	30	0	20	296	296
4	0.6	0.8	30	30	0	30	313	313
5	0.6	0.9	30	30	0	20	319	319
6	0.6	0.9	30	30	0	30	337	337
7	0.8	0.6	30	30	0	20	963	964
8	0.8	0.6	30	30	0	30	1036	1036
9	0.6	0.8	20	20	10	10	288	292
10	0.6	0.8	20	20	10	20	303	308
11	0.6	0.8	20	20	20	20	321	331

Note: HR1, hazard ratio in favor of the experimental group for the first 2 years of the trial; HR2, hazard ratio after the first 2 years; Π_1^L, proportion lost to follow-up in the control group by the end of the trial; Π_2^L, proportion crossing over to different treatment regimens from the control group by the end of the trial; N_L, sample size calculated by the Lakatos Markov method; N_B, sample size calculated by the method proposed by Barthel et al.

```
pc=rep(0.5, 4)                    ### 1-exp(-log(2)/m1)=0.5 (m1=1) ##
k=c(0.6, 0.6, 0.7, 0.7)
rectime=c(1,2)
recratio=c(1,1)                   ### 2-year uniform accrual  ##
logr=rep(1, 4)
ratio=1
simul=0
alpha=0.05
beta=0.1
sbdv=100
```

Example 7.7 *Comparison of sample size calculations*

First, we will compare the sample size calculations by the method proposed by Barthel et al. (2006) and by the Lakatos Markov approach by using the R code 'SizeLak' and the SAS code '%SIZE' under both the PH model and the piecewise proportional hazards model. The study designs given in Table 7.7, which are the same as those given in Tables II and III in the paper by Barthel et al., assume a randomized trial with 2-year accrual, 2-year follow-up, equal allocation, uniform accrual, exponential survival distribution and 1-year median survival in the control group $(m_1 = 1)$. Sample sizes are calculated for 90% power with a two-sided type I error of 5%. The parameter inputs for the sample size calculations using 'SizeLak' are given in parameter inputs 9 (case 3) and 10 (case 11). The results in Table 7.7 show that the sample sizes calculated by the Lakatos method using R code 'SizeLak' and by the method of Barthel et al. are almost identical for 16 cases and that the sample sizes calculated by the Lakatos method using SAS code %SIZE are slightly larger. Based on their power simulations, Barthel et al. concluded that the '%SIZE' code can lead to slightly overpowered designs.

We have presented two more sample size formulae in this chapter, including extensions of the Freedman formula and Lakatos formula. Even though these formulae were developed for sample size calculation under the nonproportional hazards model, it is interesting how accurate they are when compared to the five formulae developed under the PH model in Chapter 4. To investigate this further, we calculated the sample sizes by the extension of the Freedman formula and the Lakatos formula for the same scenarios as in Example 5.4, and the results are recorded in the last two columns of Table 7.8. The results are almost identical to the sample sizes calculated from the precise formula and are more accurate than those obtained with the widely used Schoenfeld, Rubinstein, and Freedman formulae.

```
### parameter input 9: Example 7.7 case3 ###
 ploss=rep(0.01274, 4)              ### 1-(1-0.05)^(1/4)=0.01274##
 pnoncmpl=rep(0, 4)
 pdropin=rep(0, 4)
 pc=rep(0.5, 4)                     ### 1-exp(-log(2)/m1)=0.5 (m1=1)##
 k=c(0.7, 0.7, 0.7, 0.7)
 rectime=c(1,2)
 recratio=c(1,1)                    ### 2-year uniform accrual  ##
 logr=rep(1, 4)
 ratio=1
 simul=0
 alpha=0.05
 beta=0.1
 sbdv=100


### parameter input 10: Example 7.7 case 11 ###
 ploss=rep(0, 4)
 pnoncmpl=rep(0, 4)
 pdropin=rep(0, 4)
 pc=rep(0.5, 4)                     ### 1-exp(-log(2)/m1)=0.5 (m1=1)##
 k=c(0.6, 0.6, 0.9, 0.9)
 rectime=c(1,2)
 recratio=c(1,1)                    ### 2-year uniform accrual  ##
 logr=rep(1, 4)
 ratio=1
 simul=0
 alpha=0.05
 beta=0.1
 sbdv=100
```

TABLE 7.7: Comparison of sample size calculations by the method proposed by Barthel et al. (2006) and by the Lakatos Markov approach using the R code 'SizeLak' and the SAS code '%SIZE' under the PH model and the piecewise proportional hazards model

			Design		Sample size		
Case	HR1	HR2	$\Pi_1^L(\%)$	$\Pi_2^L(\%)$	Barthel	SizeLak	%SIZE
1	0.7	0.7	0	0	408	408	415
2	0.8	0.8	0	0	1029*	1014	1029
3	0.7	0.7	5	5	414	414	423
4	0.7	0.7	20	20	433	433	447
5	0.7	0.7	30	30	448	448	466
6	0.7	0.7	40	40	466	466	489
7	0.7	0.7	50	50	487	487	516
8	0.8	0.8	30	30	1112	1111	1154
9	0.8	0.8	40	40	1155	1154	1209
10	0.8	0.8	50	50	1206	1206	1276
11	0.6	0.9	0	0	274	275	281
12	0.6	0.8	0	0	249	249	255
13	0.6	0.7	0	0	227	227	232
14	0.7	0.8	0	0	458	458	466
15	0.8	0.7	0	0	869	868	882
16	0.8	0.6	0	0	749	748	761

Note: HR1, hazard ratio in favor of experimental group for the first 2 years of the trial; HR2, hazard ratio after the first 2 years; Π_1^L, proportion lost to follow-up in the control group by the end of the trial; Π_2^L, proportion crossing over to different treatment regimens from the control group by the end of the trial. *, The sample size 1029 recorded in Table II in the paper by Barthel et al. could be a typographic error.

TABLE 7.8: Comparison of the calculated sample size and empirical power for seven sample size formulae

Design	x	t_a	t_f	Schoenfeld	Rubinstein	Freedman	Precise	Exact	Extension*	Lakatos
$S_1(x) = 20\%$	12	24	12	547(.898)	547(.902)	554(.904)	549(.903)	551(.901)	549	548
$S_2(x) = 30\%$	24	24	24	579(.901)	580(.900)	587(.904)	579(.902)	581(.901)	579	579
$\delta = .748$	12	36	12	532(.899)	532(.899)	539(.903)	535(.900)	538(.900)	535	535
	24	36	24	559(.900)	560(.899)	567(.902)	561(.902)	563(.902)	561	560
$S_1(x) = 40\%$	12	24	12	171(.899)	174(.904)	181(.915)	172(.900)	173(.903)	172	172
$S_2(x) = 60\%$	24	24	24	195(.903)	200(.907)	206(.915)	196(.902)	195(.902)	196	196
$\delta = .557$	12	36	12	159(.900)	160(.901)	161(.902)	160(.900)	161(.904)	160	159
	24	36	24	181(.902)	185(.907)	191(.917)	182(.900)	182(.903)	182	182
$S_1(x) = 70\%$	12	24	12	83(.882)	104(.939)	104(.938)	93(.915)	85(.889)	93	92
$S_2(x) = 90\%$	24	24	24	102(.871)	132(.942)	128(.935)	117(.915)	107(.892)	117	117
$\delta = .295$	12	36	12	71(.885)	87(.938)	89(.941)	78(.906)	73(.891)	78	78
	24	36	24	91(.872)	116(.940)	114(.936)	103(.915)	94(.884)	103	103

Notes: *, Extension of Freedman's formula. The sample sizes are calculated under the exponential model with a uniform accrual, two-sided type I error of 5%, and power of 90%. The empirical powers were estimated based on 100,000 simulation runs.

8

Survival Trial Design under the Mixture Cure Model

8.1 Introduction

The treatment of cancer has progressed dramatically in recent decades, such that it is no longer uncommon to see a cure or long-term survival in a significant proportion of patients with various types of cancer, e.g., breast cancer, non-Hodgkin lymphoma, leukemia, prostate cancer, melanoma, or head and neck cancer (Ewell and Ibrahim, 1997).

To adequately account for cured (non-susceptible) patients in survival data from clinical trials, cure models are increasingly useful. Various parametric and semiparametric cure models have been proposed by Farewell (1982), Peng et al. (1998), and Kuk and Chen (1992), among others, and a maximum-likelihood EM algorithm for parametric and semiparametric mixture cure models has been proposed by Peng and Dear (2000) and Sy and Taylor (2000). A SAS macro, 'PSPMCM', developed by Corbière and Joly (2007), is available to fit both parametric and semiparametric mixture cure models. We will illustrate the cure models by using data from the Eastern Cooperative Oncology Group (ECOG) trial e1684. This trial tested the ability of interferon alpha-2b administered at the maximum tolerated doses for 1 year to prevent relapse and death in patients at high risk after curative surgery for melanoma. This randomized controlled trial accrued patients between 1984 and 1990 and remained blinded under analysis until 1993. The primary objective was to compare the relapse-free survival (RFS) in a high-dose interferon alpha-2b arm with that in an observation arm. Figure 8.1 shows Kaplan-Meier RFS curves for the two arms. The long and stable plateau of the Kaplan-Meier curve for the treatment group shows that a significant proportion of patients were cured.

The traditional methods for designing survival trials may not be appropriate when there are non-susceptible patients in the survival data. Sample size calculations have recently been developed for clinical trial design under mixture cure models. For example, Halpern and Brown (1987) developed a computer program to calculate the power and sample size for exponential mixture cure models based on Monte Carlo simulation. Ewell and Ibrahim (1997) provided a power formula for exponential mixture cure models by con-

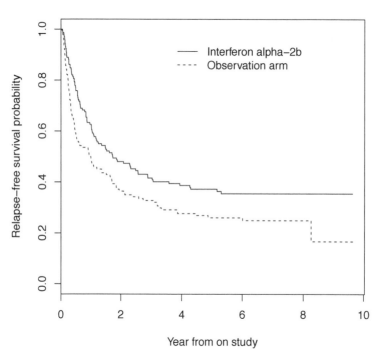

FIGURE 8.1: Kaplan-Meier relapse-free survival curves for the ECOG e1684 data. The solid line is the interferon alpha-2b arm and the dash line is the observation arm.

sidering a general alternative that allows for the effects of treatment on both short- and long-term survival. Recently, Wang et al. (2012) considered a proportional hazards mixture cure model, a special case of the general alternative proposed by Ewell and Ibrahim, and derived a sample size formula for the log-rank test under the local alternative. However, the formula derived by Wang et al. does not provide adequate sample size or power for clinical trial design (Wu, 2015).

In this chapter, we will first derive a sample size calculation for testing the difference between cure rates as proposed by Gray and Tsiatis (1989). Then, we will derive the sample size formula for the weighted log-rank test for testing differences in short- and long-term survival as proposed by Ewell and Ibrahim (1997).

8.2 Testing Differences in Cure Rates

In a cancer clinical trial in which a portion of the patients experience long-term survival, the main interest is usually in the differences between the cure rates. Examples from Children's Cancer Group trials are given by Lee and Sather (1995). To develop an appropriate test for the differences between cure rates, Gray and Tsiatis (1989) proposed a family of cure models with a proportional distributions alternative. The optimal log-rank test was discussed under the proportional distributions alternative, which has the form of a Harrington and Fleming $\mathcal{G}^\rho$ test where $\rho = -1$ (Harrington and Fleming, 1982), and its efficacy relative to that of the standard log-rank test was also investigated. Ewell and Ibrahim (1997) extended the work of Gray and Tsiatis by deriving the large sample distribution of the weighted log-rank test under a more general sequence of local alternatives that allows for the effects of treatment on both short- and long-term survival.

In this section, we focus on the situation in which the main interest is in the differences between the cure rates for two groups. Following the work of Ewell and Ibrahim, sample size formulae are derived for both the standard log-rank test and the optimal weighted log-rank test. The relative efficacy of the two tests is also discussed (Wu, 2016).

8.2.1 Mixture Cure Model

When the study population consists of both susceptible and non-susceptible patients, the failure time, T^*, takes the form of $vT + (1 - v)\infty$, where v is an indicator of whether a subject will eventually ($v = 1$) or never ($v = 0$) experience treatment failure, and T denotes the failure time of a susceptible subject, with a survival distribution $S(t)$, which is the conditional distribution for patients who will experience treatment failure and is usually called the latency distribution. Thus, the unconditional survival distribution of T^* is a mixture model with a cure rate of $\pi = P(v = 0)$ and a latency distribution $S(t)$ given by

$$S^*(t) = \pi + (1 - \pi)S(t),$$

which is often referred to as a mixture cure model. Let $\lambda^*(t)$ and $\lambda(t)$ be the hazard functions of T^* and T, respectively. We then have the following relation between the two hazard functions:

$$\lambda^*(t) = \frac{(1 - \pi)S(t)}{\pi + (1 - \pi)S(t)}\lambda(t).$$

For a two-arm randomized survival trial, let T_{ij}^* and C_{ij} denote the survival and censoring times, respectively, of patient i in the jth group, where $j = 1, 2$ (1 for the control group and 2 for the treatment group). The observed data then consist of $\{X_{ij}; \Delta_{ij}; i = 1, \cdots, n_j, j = 1, 2\}$, where $X_{ij} = T_{ij}^* \wedge C_{ij}$ and $\Delta_{ij} = I(T_{ij}^* \leq C_{ij})$. It is commonly assumed that $\{T_{ij}^*, C_{ij}, i = 1, \cdots, n_j\}$ are independent and identically distributed samples of (T_j^*, C_j) for the control $(j = 1)$ and treatment $(j = 2)$ groups and that T_{ij}^* is independent of C_{ij}. Let $S_j^*(t)$ denote the unconditional survival distribution, and let $\lambda_j^*(t)$ denote its hazard function for the jth group. When the main interest is in testing for differences between cure rates, it is reasonable to assume that the latency distributions are the same for the two groups and can be denoted by $S(t)$, with the hazard function and cumulative hazard function being denoted by $\lambda(t)$ and $\Lambda(t)$, respectively. The cure rate for the jth group is defined by π_j, where $0 \leq \pi_j < 1$. Then, the survival distribution of the mixture cure model for the jth group is given by

$$S_j^*(t) = \pi_j + (1 - \pi_j)S(t), \tag{8.1}$$

and the hazard function for the jth group is given by

$$\lambda_j^*(t) = \frac{(1 - \pi_j)S(t)}{\pi_j + (1 - \pi_j)S(t)}\lambda(t).$$

We are interested in testing the following hypothesis:

$$H_0 : \pi_1 = \pi_2 \quad vs. \quad H_1 : \pi_1 \neq \pi_2. \tag{8.2}$$

We define the parameters γ and π_0 as follows:

$$\gamma = \frac{1}{2}\log\frac{1 - \pi_2}{1 - \pi_1},$$

$$\pi_0 = 1 - [(1 - \pi_1)(1 - \pi_2)]^{1/2},$$

where γ is the half-log ratio of the failure rates, and π_0 is the proportion of cured patients under the null hypothesis. Then, hypothesis (8.2) is equivalent to the following hypothesis:

$$H_0 : \gamma = 0 \quad vs. \quad H_1 : \gamma \neq 0. \tag{8.3}$$

The mixture cure model (8.1) can be written as

$$S_j^*(t) = 1 - e^{(-1)^j \gamma}(1 - \pi_0)\{1 - S(t)\}, \tag{8.4}$$

and the corresponding hazard function is given by

$$\lambda_j^*(t) = \frac{e^{(-1)^j \gamma}(1 - \pi_0)S(t)}{1 - e^{(-1)^j \gamma}(1 - \pi_0) + e^{(-1)^j \gamma}(1 - \pi_0)S(t)}\lambda(t). \tag{8.5}$$

This alternative implies that the unconditional failure distributions for two groups are proportional: $1 - S_2^*(t) = e^{2\gamma}(1 - S_1^*(t))$; this is called a proportional distributions alternative by Gray and Tsiatis (1989).

8.2.2 Asymptotic Distribution

To test hypothesis (8.3), the weighted log-rank score test can be used. This can be written in counting process notation as follows (see equation (5.2) in section 5.3):

$$U_w = \int_0^\infty W(t)\left\{\frac{Y_2(t)}{Y(t)}dN_1(t) - \frac{Y_1(t)}{Y(t)}dN_2(t)\right\},$$

where $W(t)$ is a weight function that converges in probability to $w(t)$, $N_j(t) = \sum_{i=1}^{n_j} \Delta_{ij}I(X_{ij} > t)$ is the number of observed failures by time t, $Y_j(t) = \sum_{i=1}^{n_j} I(X_{ij} > t)$ is the number of subjects at risk just before t in the jth group, where $j = 1, 2$, and $Y(t) = Y_1(t) + Y_2(t)$. If we define martingale processes such that $M_j(t) = N_j(t) - \int_0^t \lambda_j^*(t)Y_j(t)dt, j = 1, 2$, where $\lambda_j^*(t)$ is given in equation (8.5), then the weighted score test can be written as

$$\begin{aligned}U_w &= \int_0^\infty W(t)\left\{\frac{Y_2(t)}{Y(t)}dM_1(t) - \frac{Y_1(t)}{Y(t)}dM_2(t)\right\} \\ &+ \int_0^\infty W(t)\frac{Y_1(t)Y_2(t)}{Y(t)}\{\lambda_1^*(t) - \lambda_2^*(t)\}dt.\end{aligned}$$

Under the null hypothesis $H_0 : \gamma = 0$, we have $\lambda_1^*(t) = \lambda_2^*(t) = \lambda_0^*(t)$, where

$$\lambda_0^*(t) = \frac{(1 - \pi_0)S(t)}{\pi_0 + (1 - \pi_0)S(t)}\lambda(t);$$

thus, the weighted score test reduces to

$$U_w = \int_0^\infty W(t)\left\{\frac{Y_2(t)}{Y(t)}dM_1(t) - \frac{Y_1(t)}{Y(t)}dM_2(t)\right\}.$$

Hence, by the martingale property, the mean of U_w is 0 and the variance of U_w is given by

$$\mathrm{Var}(U_w) = E\int_0^\infty W^2(t)\frac{Y_1(t)Y_2(t)}{Y(t)}d\Lambda_0^*(t),$$

where $\Lambda_0^*(t) = \int_0^t \lambda_0^*(u)du$. We can show that

$$\frac{Y_1(t)Y_2(t)}{nY(t)} = \frac{n_1 n_2}{n^2} \frac{\{Y_1(t)/n_1\}\{Y_2(t)/n_2\}}{Y(t)/n} \rightarrow \omega_1 \omega_2 \frac{\pi_1(t)\pi_2(t)}{\pi(t)},$$

where $\omega_1 = \lim_{n\to\infty} n_1/n$, $\omega_2 = 1 - \omega_1$, $\pi_j(t) = P(X_{ij} > t)$, and $\pi(t) = \omega_1 \pi_1(t) + \omega_2 \pi_2(t)$. Note that $\pi_j(t) = P(T_{ij}^* > t)P(C_{ij} > t) = S_j^*(t)G(t)$, where $G(t)$ is the common survival distribution of the censoring time of the two groups and $S_1^*(t) = S_2^*(t) = S_0^*(t)$ under the null hypothesis, where $S_0^*(t) = \pi_0 + (1 - \pi_0)S(t)$; thus, by the martingale central limit theorem, $n^{-1/2}U_w \xrightarrow{D} N(0, \sigma_w^2)$, where

$$\sigma_w^2 = \omega_1 \omega_2 \int_0^\infty w^2(t)G(t)S_0^*(t)\lambda_0^*(t)dt.$$

As $S_0^*(t)\lambda_0^*(t) = (1 - \pi_0)S(t)\lambda(t)$, we then have

$$\sigma_w^2 = \omega_1 \omega_2 (1 - \pi_0) \int_0^\infty w^2(t)G(t)S(t)\lambda(t)dt. \qquad (8.6)$$

The variance σ_w^2 can be estimated by

$$\hat{\sigma}_w^2 = n^{-1} \int_0^\infty W^2(t)\frac{Y_1(t)Y_2(t)}{Y(t)}d\hat{\Lambda}_0^*(t),$$

where $d\hat{\Lambda}_0^*(t) = dN(t)/Y(t)$ and $N(t) = N_1(t) + N_2(t)$. Therefore, under the null hypothesis, the weighted log-rank test $L_w = n^{-1/2}U_w/\hat{\sigma}_w$ is asymptotically standard normal distributed. Thus, given a significance level α, we reject the null hypothesis if $|L_w| > z_{1-\alpha/2}$, where $z_{1-\alpha/2}$ is the $100(1 - \alpha/2)^{th}$ percentile of the standard normal distribution.

To derive the asymptotic distribution of the weighted log-rank test under the alternative, consider a sequence of local alternatives $H_1^{(n)} : S_j^{*(n)}(t) = 1 - e^{(-1)^j \gamma_n}(1 - \pi_0)\{1 - S(t)\}$, or

$$\lambda_j^{*(n)}(t) = \frac{e^{(-1)^j \gamma_n}(1 - \pi_0)S(t)}{1 - e^{(-1)^j \gamma_n}(1 - \pi_0) + e^{(-1)^j \gamma_n}(1 - \pi_0)S(t)}\lambda(t),$$

where $n^{1/2}\gamma_n = \gamma_a < \infty$, and define martingale processes as $M_j^{(n)}(t) = N_j(t) - \int_0^t Y_j(u)\lambda_j^{*(n)}(u)du$. Then, we have $U_w = U_{1w} + U_{2w}$, where

$$U_{1w} = \int_0^\infty W(t)\left\{\frac{Y_2(t)}{Y(t)}dM_1^{(n)}(t) - \frac{Y_1(t)}{Y(t)}dM_2^{(n)}(t)\right\}$$

and

$$U_{2w} = \int_0^\infty W(t)\frac{Y_1(t)Y_2(t)}{Y(t)}\{\lambda_1^{*(n)}(t) - \lambda_2^{*(n)}(t)\}dt.$$

As $\gamma_n \to 0$, $H_1^{(n)} \to H_0$, and $\lambda_j^{*(n)}(t) \to \lambda_0^*(t)$, by the martingale central limit theorem, $n^{-1/2}U_{1w}$ converges to a normal variable with mean 0 and variance

$$n^{-1}EU_{1w}^2 = E \int_0^\infty W^2(t) \left\{ \frac{Y_2^2(t)}{Y^2(t)} Y_1(t)\lambda_1^{*(n)}(t) + \frac{Y_1^2(t)}{Y^2(t)} Y_2(t)\lambda_2^{*(n)}(t) \right\} du/n$$

$$\to \omega_1\omega_2 \int_0^\infty w^2(t) \left\{ \omega_2 \frac{\pi_2^2(t)\pi_1(t)}{\pi^2(t)} \lambda_0^*(t) + \omega_1 \frac{\pi_1^2(t)\pi_2(t)}{\pi^2(t)} \lambda_0^*(t) \right\} dt$$

$$= \omega_1\omega_2 \int_0^\infty w^2(t) \frac{\pi_1(t)\pi_2(t)}{\pi(t)} \lambda_0^*(t) du$$

$$= \omega_1\omega_2 \int_0^\infty w^2(t)G(t)S_0^*(t)\lambda_0^*(t) dt = \sigma_w^2.$$

By Taylor's expansion of $\lambda_j^{*(n)}(t)$ at $\gamma_n = 0$, we have

$$\lambda_j^{*(n)}(t) \simeq \frac{(1-\pi_0)S(t)}{\pi_0 + (1-\pi_0)S(t)} \lambda(t) + \frac{(1-\pi_0)S(t)}{\{\pi_0 + (1-\pi_0)S(t)\}^2} \lambda(t)(-1)^j \gamma_n.$$

It then follows that

$$\lim_{n\to\infty} n^{1/2}\{\lambda_1^{*(n)}(t) - \lambda_2^{*(n)}(t)\} = \frac{2\gamma_a(\pi_0 - 1)S(t)\lambda(t)}{\{\pi_0 + (1-\pi_0)S(t)\}^2}.$$

By substituting this into U_{2w}, we show that $n^{-1/2}U_{2w}$ converges in probability to $\mu(w, \gamma_a)$, where

$$\mu(w, \gamma_a) = 2\omega_1\omega_2(\pi_0 - 1)\gamma_a \int_0^\infty w(t)\{S_0^*(t)\}^{-1}G(t)S(t)\lambda(t) dt. \tag{8.7}$$

Thus, under the local alternatives $H_1^{(n)}$, the weighted log-rank test is asymptotically normal distributed with mean $\mu(w, \gamma_a)/\sigma_w$ and unit variance, that is,

$$L_w = n^{-1/2}U_w/\hat{\sigma}_w \to N(\mu(w, \gamma_a)/\sigma_w, 1).$$

8.2.3   Sample Size Formula

Under local alternatives, as shown in the previous subsection, the weighted log-rank test $L_w = n^{-1/2}U_w/\hat{\sigma}_w$ converges in distribution to a normal variable with unit variance and mean $\mu(w, \gamma_a)/\sigma_w$, where $\mu(w, \gamma_a)$ and σ_w^2 are given by (8.7) and (8.6), respectively.

Therefore, on the basis of the limiting distribution of L_w, given a type I error of α, the study power of $1 - \beta$ must approximately satisfy the following equation:

$$1 - \beta \simeq \Phi\{\mu(w, \gamma_a)/\sigma_w - z_{1-\alpha/2}\}.$$

For a local alternative γ, we replace γ_a by $n^{1/2}\gamma$, and the sample size required to detect a local alternative γ can then be determined by

$$n = \frac{(z_{1-\alpha/2} + z_{1-\beta})^2 \sigma_w^2}{\mu(w, \gamma)^2}. \tag{8.8}$$

Substituting equations (8.6) and (8.7) into (8.8), the total sample size for the weighted log-rank test can be calculated by

$$n = \frac{(z_{1-\alpha/2} + z_{1-\beta})^2 \int_0^\infty w^2(t)G(t)S(t)d\Lambda(t)}{4\omega_1\omega_2(1 - \pi_0)\gamma^2[\int_0^\infty w(t)\{S_0^*(t)\}^{-1}G(t)S(t)d\Lambda(t)]^2}. \quad (8.9)$$

8.2.4 Optimal Log-Rank Test

We have shown in Chapter 5 that the log-rank test is optimal for the proportional hazards model. However, the cure model (8.1) does not satisfy the proportional hazards assumption; thus, the log-rank test is not an optimal test for this model, and a study design based on the log-rank test is not fully efficient. Therefore, it is desirable to find an optimal test for the cure model (8.1) under the local proportional distributions alternative. As the mean of the weighted log-rank test is proportional to

$$\int_0^\infty w(t)\{S_0^*(t)\}^{-1}h(t)dt,$$

where $h(t) = G(t)S(t)\lambda(t)$, by using the Cauchy-Schwartz inequality, we obtain the following inequality:

$$\int_0^\infty w(t)\{S_0^*(t)\}^{-1}h(t)dt \leq \left\{\int_0^\infty w^2(t)h(t)dt \int_0^\infty \{S_0^*(t)\}^{-2}h(t)dt\right\}^{1/2},$$

with equality iff $w(t) \propto \{S_0^*(t)\}^{-1}$. That is, the optimal weight function $w(t)$ is proportional to $\{S_0^*(t)\}^{-1}$, which minimizes the sample size given by formula (8.9). Thus, using the weight function $W(t) = \{K(t^-)\}^{-1}$, where $K(t^-)$ is the left-continuous version of the Kaplan-Meier estimate computed from the pooled sample of two groups, gives the asymptotically optimal test for the proportional distributions alternative. This weight function assigns more weight to late survival differences (the differences in cure rates). Hence, substituting $w(t) = \{S_0^*(t)\}^{-1}$ into formula (8.9), the sample size for the optimal log-rank test L_K is given by

$$n_K = \frac{(z_{1-\alpha/2} + z_{1-\beta})^2}{4\omega_1\omega_2(1 - \pi_0)\gamma^2 \int_0^\infty \{S_0^*(t)\}^{-2}G(t)S(t)d\Lambda(t)}, \quad (8.10)$$

and substituting $w(t) = 1$ into formula (8.9), the sample size for the standard log-rank test L is given by

$$n = \frac{(z_{1-\alpha/2} + z_{1-\beta})^2 \int_0^\infty G(t)S(t)d\Lambda(t)}{4\omega_1\omega_2(1 - \pi_0)\gamma^2[\int_0^\infty \{S_0^*(t)\}^{-1}G(t)S(t)d\Lambda(t)]^2}. \quad (8.11)$$

The asymptotic relative efficiency $\varrho = n/n_K$ (Randales and Wolfe, 1979) of the optimal test when compared to the standard log-rank test is given by

$$\varrho = \frac{\int_0^\infty \{S_0^*(t)\}^{-2}G(t)S(t)d\Lambda(t) \int_0^\infty G(t)S(t)d\Lambda(t)}{[\int_0^\infty \{S_0^*(t)\}^{-1}G(t)S(t)d\Lambda(t)]^2}. \quad (8.12)$$

In the special case when there is no censoring, that is when $G(t) = 1$, the asymptotic relative efficiency ϱ in (8.12) is reduced to

$$\varrho = \frac{(1 - \pi_0)^2}{\pi_0 [\log(\pi_0)]^2}.$$

8.2.5 Comparison

We investigated two important issues. First, we studied the relative efficiency of the optimal log-rank test versus the standard log-rank test. Second, we investigated the performance of the two sample size formulae under various design scenarios.

The relative efficiency ϱ given in equation (8.12) was calculated for selected cure rates under the exponential mixture cure model with a hazard parameter of $\lambda = 1$ for the latency distribution. We assumed a uniform accrual over $[0, \tau]$ and no follow-up period, with τ being determined by the percentage of censoring ranging from 0% to 50%. The results showed that when the cure rate π_0 was at most 10% and there was no censoring, the gain in efficiency of the optimal log-rank test relative to the standard log-rank test was more than 50%, whereas if the cure rate π_0 was at least 50%, the gain in efficiency was less than 5%. If the percentage of censoring was more than 50%, then the gain in efficiency was less than 10%, regardless of the cure rate (Table 8.1). We also investigated the relative efficiency through sample size calculations. Under the same assumptions, sample sizes were calculated for various combinations of the cure rates of two groups. The largest gain in efficiency was achieved when both the cure rate and the percentage of censoring were small (Table 8.2).

TABLE 8.1: The relative efficiency ϱ of the optimal log-rank test when compared to the standard log-rank test under the exponential mixture cure model $S(t) = \pi + (1 - \pi)e^{-\lambda t}$, with a hazard parameter of $\lambda = 1$ and a uniform accrual over the interval $[0, \tau]$, where τ is determined by the percentage of censoring

	Cure rate π_0								
Cens	0.1	0.2	0.3	0.4	0.5	0.6	0.7	0.8	0.9
None	1.528	1.235	1.127	1.072	1.041	1.022	1.011	1.004	1.001
10%	1.490	1.221	1.120	1.068	1.039	1.021	1.010	1.004	1.001
20%	1.399	1.190	1.105	1.061	1.035	1.019	1.009	1.004	1.001
30%	1.272	1.144	1.084	1.050	1.029	1.016	1.008	1.003	1.001
40%	1.166	1.099	1.061	1.037	1.022	1.012	1.006	1.002	1.001
50%	1.095	1.061	1.040	1.026	1.016	1.009	1.005	1.002	1.000

Note: Censoring time was uniformly distributed over $[0, \tau]$, with the value of τ being chosen so that the probability of the failure time being censored for a subject who was not cured was the specified censoring percentage. Abbreviations: Cens: censoring.

TABLE 8.2: Sample sizes for the optimal and standard log-rank tests for various cure rates in two groups with a nominal type I error of 5% and power of 90%

				Cure rate (π_1, π_2)			
	(.05, .15)	(.05, .2)	(.1, .2)	(.1, .3)	(.2, .4)	(.3, .5)	(.4, .6)
Cens				Sample size using test L			
0%	598	301	738	217	257	279	281
10%	766	379	916	263	304	323	321
20%	1067	513	1218	338	375	388	379
30%	1566	730	1697	453	481	483	460
40%	2323	1058	2415	623	632	616	573
50%	3479	1577	3509	881	860	813	740
Cens				Sample size using test L_K			
0%	394	215	554	177	230	261	270
10%	517	275	698	217	272	303	310
20%	766	391	964	286	341	367	367
30%	1233	597	1423	398	445	461	448
40%	1993	926	2144	569	597	594	562
50%	3180	1437	3262	831	828	794	729

Notes: Censoring time was uniformly distributed over $[0, \tau]$, with the value of τ being chosen so that the probability of the failure time being censored for a subject who was not cured was the specified censoring percentage. Abbreviation: Cens: censoring; L: standard log-rank test; L_K: optimal log-rank test. Here, sample sizes were calculated under the exponential mixture cure model $S(t) = \pi + (1 - \pi)e^{-\lambda t}$, with a hazard parameter of $\lambda = 1$ and a uniform accrual over the interval $[0, \tau]$, where τ is determined by the percentage of censoring.

To investigate the performance of the sample size formulae for the optimal and standard log-rank tests, we calculated sample sizes under the cure model (8.1), where the cure rates were set as shown in Table 8.3, and the conditional survival distribution was Weibull, $S(t) = e^{-\lambda t^\kappa}$, or log-logistic, $S(t) = \frac{1}{1+\lambda t^\kappa}$. The scale parameter λ was set to 0.4, and the shape parameter κ was set to 0.5, 1, or 2, reflecting a decreasing, constant, and increasing hazard function, respectively, for the Weibull distribution and a decreasing and single-mode hazard function for the log-logistic distribution. We assumed that subjects were recruited with a uniform distribution over the accrual period $t_a = 1$, with a follow-up period $t_f = 2$. We further assumed that no subject was lost to follow-up during the study. Then, the censoring time was uniformly distributed over the interval $[t_f, t_a + t_f]$. Therefore, given a two-sided nominal significance level of 0.05 and power of 90%, the required sample sizes were calculated for each design scenario under each distribution. The empirical type I errors and powers of the corresponding designs were simulated based on 100,000 runs. The simulation results presented in Table 8.3 can be summarized as follows. First, the empirical powers of both the optimal and standard log-rank tests were close to the nominal level of 90%; thus, the sample sizes were adequately estimated. Second, the empirical type I errors of both tests were close to the nominal level of 5%; thus, both tests preserved type I error well. Third, the sample sizes calculated from the optimal test were smaller than those calculated for the standard log-rank test.

Overall, the results showed that the derived sample size formulae provide adequate sample size estimation for trial design if the main interest is to detect the differences between the cure rates of two groups and that the optimal test is more efficient than the standard log-rank test, particularly when both cure rates and percentage censoring are small.

8.2.6   Example and R code

Example 8.1 *Trial design to test the difference in cure rates*

We will illustrate study design under a parametric cure model by using the data from the Eastern Cooperative Oncology Group (ECOG) trial e1684. This trial was a two-arm phase III clinical trial to compare the relapse-free survival (RFS) of patients with melanoma who were treated with high-dose interferon alpha-2b or placebo (observation arm) as postoperative adjuvant therapy. The trial accrued patients between 1984 and 1990 and remained blinded under analysis until 1993 (Kirkwood, et al., 1996). Researchers have studied this dataset extensively using mixture cure models (Corbière and Joly, 2007). There were 92 deaths among the 146 patients in the treatment group. The SAS macro 'PSPMCM' was applied to fit the treatment arm data under the Weibull cure model (Figure 8.2), with an estimated shape parameter κ of 1.018, a scale parameter λ of 0.836, and a cure rate of 35%. Suppose we wish to design a two-arm randomized phase III trial to detect a 20% difference between the cure rate in the arm that receives the new treatment and that in the control arm that receives the same therapy as the treatment arm of the ECOG trial, as illustrated by Figure 8.2, with a two-sided type I error of 0.05, power of 90% at the alternative, a uniform accrual with a 5-year accrual period and 5 years of follow-up, no loss to follow-up, and equal allocation between the two groups. Then, the required sample sizes calculated using formulae (8.10) and (8.11) under the Weibull mixture cure model are 266 and 280 patients, respectively. The corresponding simulated empirical type I error and power are 0.05 and 91.4% for the optimal log-rank test and 0.05 and 90.7% for the standard log-rank test. As the cure rate is relatively high, the gain in efficiency using the weighted log-rank test is only approximately 5% in this example. The R function 'SizeMC' is given below for the sample size calculation under the Weibull mixture cure model using formulae (8.10) and (8.11).

```
############################# Input parameters #############################
###   kappa is the shape parameter of the Weibull distribution;          ###
###   lambda is the hazard parameter of the Weibull distribution for the ###
```

TABLE 8.3: Sample sizes (n) and corresponding simulated empirical type I errors ($\hat{\alpha}$) and powers (EP) for the optimal and standard log-rank tests under the Weibull and log-logistic mixture cure models, with a scale parameter of $\lambda = 0.4$, a cure rate of $\pi_1 = 0.1$, nominal type I error of 0.05, power of 90%, and uniform accrual with accrual time $t_a = 1$ and follow-up time $t_f = 2$

Dist	Test	γ	$\kappa = 0.5$			$\kappa = 1$			$\kappa = 2$		
			n	$\hat{\alpha}$	EP	n	$\hat{\alpha}$	EP	n	$\hat{\alpha}$	EP
WB	L	1.5	841	.048	.905	510	.053	.905	222	.052	.914
		1.6	695	.049	.900	424	.050	.899	188	.052	.914
		1.7	580	.051	.901	355	.045	.906	161	.050	.922
		1.8	488	.050	.903	301	.050	.906	139	.051	.924
		1.9	415	.049	.905	258	.048	.907	121	.052	.921
		2.0	356	.051	.907	222	.053	.906	106	.050	.925
	L_K	1.5	827	.049	.901	490	.053	.904	195	.051	.919
		1.6	683	.045	.901	408	.048	.910	166	.055	.919
		1.7	571	.051	.902	343	.051	.902	143	.048	.925
		1.8	481	.049	.905	291	.050	.906	125	.052	.928
		1.9	410	.053	.904	250	.052	.909	110	.052	.926
		2.0	351	.052	.906	216	.047	.910	97	.052	.932
LG	L	1.5	1112	.048	.900	762	.052	.908	404	.048	.906
		1.6	916	.050	.907	630	.049	.903	337	.049	.908
		1.7	763	.047	.908	526	.053	.904	284	.051	.908
		1.8	641	.047	.905	443	.050	.907	241	.050	.916
		1.9	544	.049	.903	377	.050	.907	207	.049	.915
		2.0	465	.048	.900	324	.054	.907	180	.050	.912
	L_K	1.5	1100	.048	.902	746	.051	.903	382	.053	.907
		1.6	907	.049	.906	617	.045	.897	319	.053	.909
		1.7	755	.050	.908	516	.052	.898	270	.051	.914
		1.8	635	.048	.903	436	.051	.906	230	.050	.911
		1.9	539	.049	.908	371	.056	.903	198	.051	.910
		2.0	461	.053	.904	319	.049	.910	172	.050	.916

Note: Abbreviations: Cens: censoring; Dist: distribution; WB: Weibull; LG: log-logistic; L: standard log-rank test; L_K: optimal log-rank test. $\gamma = 0.5 \log\{(1 - \pi_2)/(1 - \pi_1)\}$ or $\pi_2 = 1 - (1 - \pi_1)e^{2\gamma}$.

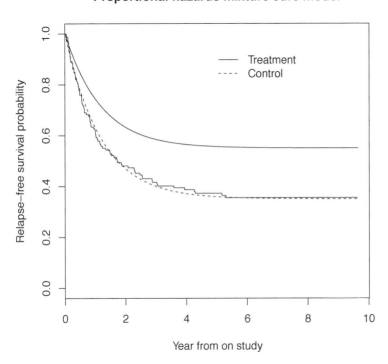

FIGURE 8.2: The step function is the Kaplan-Meier curve for relapse-free survival for ECOG trial e1684. The dash and solid lines are the hypothetical survival curves for the control and treatment groups.

```
###   control group; pi1 and pi2 are the cure rates for the control and      ###
###   treatment groups, respectively; p is the allocation ratio for the      ###
###   control group; ta and tf are the accrual and follow-up times;          ###
###   rho is parameter of weight function; alpha is the type I error.        ###
################################################################################
SizeMC=function(kappa, lambda, pi1, pi2, p, ta, tf, rho, alpha, power)
{ z0=qnorm(1-alpha/2); z1=qnorm(power); tau=ta+tf
  pi0=1-((1-pi1)*(1-pi2))^(1/2)
  eta=log((1-pi2)/(1-pi1))/2
  w=function(t){(pi0+(1-pi0)*S0(t))^rho}
  m=function(t){2*eta/(pi0+(1-pi0)*S0(t))}
  S0=function(t){exp(-lambda*t^kappa)}
  h0=function(t){kappa*lambda*t^(kappa-1)}
  G=function(t){1-punif(t, tf, tau)}
  f0=function(t){w(t)^2*G(t)*S0(t)*h0(t)}
  f1=function(t){w(t)*m(t)*G(t)*S0(t)*h0(t)}
  A=integrate(f0, 0, tau)$value
  B=integrate(f1, 0, tau)$value
  n=(z0+z1)^2*A/(p*(1-p)*(1-pi0)*B^2)
  ans=ceiling(n);return(ans)
}
SizeMC(kappa=1.018,lambda=0.836,pi1=0.35,pi2=0.55,p=0.5,ta=5,tf=5,
    rho=-1,alpha=0.05,power=0.9)# optimal log-rank test #
266
SizeMC(kappa=1.018,lambda=0.836,pi1=0.35,pi2=0.55,p=0.5,ta=5,tf=5,
    rho=0,alpha=0.05,power=0.9) # standard log-rank test #
280
```

8.2.7 Conclusion

For cancer clinical trials in which a portion of patients are cured, the main interest may be in demonstrating the differences between the cure rates in the two treatment groups. Sample size formulae have been derived for both the optimal and standard log-rank tests. Because the proposed cure model is not a proportional hazards model, the standard log-rank test is not fully efficient. Thus, a sample size calculation derived under the optimal test can ensure the efficacy of the study design. The optimal log-rank test is implemented in the standard statistical software R by using the 'survdiff' function with the option **rho** $= -1$. The simulation results demonstrated that the sample size formula for the optimal test provides adequate sample size estimation and is more efficient than the formula for the standard log-rank test.

8.3 Testing Differences in Short- and Long-Term Survival

8.3.1 Hypothesis Testing

Ewell and Ibrahim (1997) extended the work of Gray and Tsiatis (1989) to testing both short-term and long-term survival. Let $S_j^*(t)$ denote the overall survival function, and let $\lambda_j^*(t)$ denote its corresponding hazard function for group $j = 1, 2$. Similarly, let $S_j(t)$ denote the survival function of susceptible patients, and let $\lambda_j(t)$ and $\Lambda_j(t)$ denote its hazard and cumulative functions. The cure rate in group j is defined by π_j, where $0 \leq \pi_j < 1$. The mixture cure model is given by

$$S_j^*(t) = \pi_j + (1 - \pi_j)S_j(t) \tag{8.13}$$

and

$$\lambda_j^*(t) = \frac{(1 - \pi_j)S_j(t)}{\pi_j + (1 - \pi_j)S_j(t)}\lambda_j(t),$$

for $j = 1, 2$. Ewell and Ibrahim defined the following quantities:

$$\bar{\Lambda}(t) = [\Lambda_1(t)\Lambda_2(t)]^{1/2},$$
$$\eta = \frac{1}{2}\log\frac{\Lambda_2(t)}{\Lambda_1(t)},$$
$$\gamma = \frac{1}{2}\log\frac{1 - \pi_2}{1 - \pi_1}.$$

If we assume a proportional hazards (PH) model for the susceptible patients, that is, $\lambda_2(t) = \delta\lambda_1(t)$, we then have

$$\bar{\Lambda}(t) = \delta^{1/2}\Lambda_1(t), \quad \eta = \frac{1}{2}\log\delta.$$

Thus, the mixture cure model (8.13) can be written as

$$S_j^*(t) = 1 - e^{(-1)^j\gamma}(1 - \pi_0)\{1 - \bar{S}(t)^{e^{(-1)^j\eta}}\}, \tag{8.14}$$

where $\pi_0 = 1 - [(1 - \pi_1)(1 - \pi_2)]^{1/2}$ and $\bar{S}(t) = e^{-\bar{\Lambda}(t)}$, respectively, representing the cure rate and survival distribution under the null hypothesis.

For a survival trial in which a proportion of patients are cured, we are interested in testing

$$H_0 : \pi_2 = \pi_1 \quad \text{and} \quad S_2(t) = S_1(t), \tag{8.15}$$

which is equivalent to $H_0 : \eta = \gamma = 0$. Various alternative hypotheses are of interest: for $H_{1a} : \eta \neq 0, \gamma \neq 0$, there are differences in both the short-term survival and the cure fraction; for $H_{1b} : \eta \neq 0, \gamma = 0$, there is a difference in the short-term survival but not in the cure fraction; and for $H_{1c} : \eta = 0, \gamma \neq 0$, there is a difference in the cure fraction but not in the short-term survival.

8.3.2 Ewell and Ibrahim Formula

To test hypothesis (8.15), the weighted log-rank score test can be used. This can be written as

$$U_w = \int_0^\infty W(t)\left\{\frac{Y_2(t)}{Y(t)}dN_1(t) - \frac{Y_1(t)}{Y(t)}dN_2(t)\right\},$$

where $W(t)$ is a weight function that converges to $w(t)$, $N_j(t)$ is the number of observed failures by time t, $Y_j(t)$ is the number of subjects at risk before t in the jth group, where $j = 1, 2$, and $Y(t) = Y_1(t) + Y_2(t)$. As shown in Appendix E, by the martingale central limit theorem, under the null hypothesis H_0, $n^{-1/2}U_w \to N(0, \sigma_w^2)$, where

$$\sigma_w^2 = \omega_1\omega_2(1 - \pi_0) \int_0^\infty w^2(t)G(t)\bar{S}(t)\bar{\lambda}(t)dt, \qquad (8.16)$$

in which $\omega_1 = \lim_{n\to\infty} n_1/n$, $\omega_2 = 1 - \omega_1$, $\bar{\lambda}(t) = \delta^{1/2}\lambda_1(t)$, $\bar{S}(t) = e^{-\bar{\Lambda}(t)}$, and $G(t)$ is the common survival distribution of the censoring time.

The asymptotic distribution of the weighted log-rank test under the alternative can be derived under a sequence of local alternatives:

$$S_j^{*(n)}(t) = 1 - e^{(-1)^j\gamma_n}(1 - \pi_0)\{1 - \bar{S}(t)^{e^{(-1)^j\eta_n}}\},$$

where $n^{1/2}\eta_n = \eta_a$ and $n^{1/2}\gamma_n = \gamma_a$. By the martingale central limit theorem, the weighted log-rank score $n^{-1/2}U_w$ converges in distribution to a normal variable with variance σ_w^2 given by equation (8.16), and mean $\mu_w = \mu(w, \gamma_a, \eta_a)$, given as follow

$$\mu_w = 2\omega_1\omega_2(\pi_0 - 1)$$
$$\times \int_0^\infty w(t)\left\{\eta_a + \frac{\gamma_a + \eta_a\pi_0\log\bar{S}(t)}{\pi_0 + (1 - \pi_0)\bar{S}(t)}\right\}G(t)\bar{S}(t)\bar{\lambda}(t)dt. \qquad (8.17)$$

A consistent estimate of the variance σ_w^2 is given by

$$\hat{\sigma}_w^2 = n^{-1}\int_0^\infty W^2(t)\frac{Y_1(t)Y_2(t)}{Y(t)}d\hat{\Lambda}_0^*(t),$$

where $d\hat{\Lambda}_0^*(t) = dN(t)/Y(t)$ and $N(t) = N_1(t) + N_2(t)$. Thus, the weighted log-rank test $L_w = n^{-1/2}U_w/\hat{\sigma}_w$ converges in distribution to a normal variable with unit variance and mean $\mu(w, \gamma_a, \eta_a)/\sigma_w$ (see Appendix E for details of the derivation).

Therefore, on the basis of the limiting distribution of L_w, given a two-sided type I error of α, the study power of $1 - \beta$ must approximately satisfy the following equation:

$$1 - \beta = \Phi\{\mu(w, \gamma_a, \eta_a)/\sigma_w - z_{1-\alpha/2}\}. \qquad (8.18)$$

For local alternatives of γ and η, if we replace γ_a and η_a in equation (8.18) by $n^{1/2}\gamma$ and $n^{1/2}\eta$, respectively, the total sample size of two groups is then determined by

$$n = \frac{(z_{1-\alpha/2} + z_{1-\beta})^2\sigma_w^2}{\{\mu(w, \gamma, \eta)\}^2}. \qquad (8.19)$$

Substituting equations (8.16) and (8.17) into (8.19), the total sample size for the weighted log-rank test can be calculated by

$$n = \frac{(z_{1-\alpha/2} + z_{1-\beta})^2 \int_0^\infty w^2(t) G(t) \bar{S}(t) \bar{\lambda}(t) dt}{\omega_1 \omega_2 (1 - \pi_0) \{\int_0^\infty w(t) m(t) G(t) \bar{S}(t) \bar{\lambda}(t) dt\}^2}, \quad (8.20)$$

where $\bar{S}(t) = e^{-\bar{\Lambda}(t)}$, $\bar{\lambda}(t) = \delta^{1/2} \lambda_1(t)$, and $m(t)$ is given by

$$m(t) = 2 \left\{ \eta + \frac{\gamma + \eta \pi_0 \log \bar{S}(t)}{\pi_0 + (1 - \pi_0) \bar{S}(t)} \right\}. \quad (8.21)$$

The sample size formula for the standard log-rank test $(w(t) = 1)$ reduces to

$$n = \frac{(z_{1-\alpha/2} + z_{1-\beta})^2 \int_0^\infty G(t) \bar{S}(t) \bar{\lambda}(t) dt}{\omega_1 \omega_2 (1 - \pi_0) \{\int_0^\infty m(t) G(t) \bar{S}(t) \bar{\lambda}(t) dt\}^2}. \quad (8.22)$$

Remark 1: When $\pi_1 = \pi_2 = 0$, the mixture cure model (8.14) reduces to the standard PH model, with $\gamma = \pi_0 = 0$ and $m(t) = 2\eta = \log(\delta)$. Therefore, the sample size formula (8.22) for the standard log-rank test further reduces to

$$n = \frac{(z_{1-\alpha/2} + z_{1-\beta})^2}{\omega_1 \omega_2 [\log(\delta)]^2 \int_0^\infty G(t) \bar{S}(t) \bar{\lambda}(t) dt}.$$

This sample size formula is not the same as the Schoenfeld formula (Schoenfeld, 1981). However, numerical calculations showed that two formulae give almost identical sample size estimations under a balanced design (with equal treatment allocation).

Remark 2: A similar sample size formula for the weighted log-rank test was derived by Wang et al. (2012) under the proportional hazards mixture cure model. Using our notation, their formula for the standard log-rank test can be expressed as

$$n = \frac{(z_{1-\alpha/2} + z_{1-\beta})^2 \int_0^\infty G(t) S_1(t) \lambda_1(t) dt}{\omega_1 \omega_2 (1 - \pi_1) \{\int_0^\infty m_0(t) G(t) S_1(t) \lambda_1(t) dt\}^2}, \quad (8.23)$$

where $m_0(t)$ is given by

$$m_0(t) = \frac{\pi_1 \{\zeta + \log(\delta) \Lambda_1(t)\}}{\pi_1 + (1 - \pi_1) S_1(t)} - \log(\delta),$$

in which $\zeta = \log(\frac{\pi_2}{1-\pi_2}) - \log(\frac{\pi_1}{1-\pi_1})$. However, Wang's formula does not provide a correct sample size estimation when the alternative departs from the null (Wu, 2015). This is because the cure rate, survival distribution, and hazard function presented in Wang's formula are all given under the null hypothesis, whereas they are adjusted for the alternative hypothesis in the Ewell and Ibrahim formula.

Remark 3: A new sample size formula for the weighted log-rank test was derived by Xiong and Wu (2017) under the proportional hazards mixture cure model. The formula for the weighted log-rank test can be expressed as

$$n = \frac{(z_{1-\alpha/2} + z_{1-\beta})^2 \int_0^\infty w^2(t) q_1(t) G(t) S_1(t) d\Lambda_1(t)}{\omega_1 \omega_2 (1 - \pi_1)(1 - \pi_1 + \pi_1 e^\varsigma) \{\int_0^\infty w(t) q_2(t) G(t) S_1(t) d\Lambda_1(t)\}^2}, \quad (8.24)$$

where

$$q_1(t) = \frac{q(t)\{\omega_1(1 - \pi_1 + \pi_1 e^\varsigma) + \omega_2 \delta [S_1(t)]^{\delta-1}\}}{[\omega_1 + \omega_2 q(t)]^2},$$

$$q_2(t) = \frac{q(t)\{1 - \delta [S_1(t)]^{\delta-1} [q(t)(1 - \pi_1 + \pi_1 e^\varsigma)]^{-1}\}}{\omega_1 + \omega_2 q(t)},$$

and

$$q(t) = \frac{\pi_1 e^\varsigma + (1 - \pi_1)[S_1(t)]^\delta}{(1 - \pi_1 + \pi_1 e^\varsigma)[\pi_1 + (1 - \pi_1) S_1(t)]},$$

in which $\varsigma = \log(\frac{\pi_2}{1-\pi_2}) - \log(\frac{\pi_1}{1-\pi_1})$. This formula provides more accurate sample size estimation, particularly when the alternatives are far away from the null. The R code for the sample size calculation using formula (8.24) is given in Appendix D.

8.3.3 Simulation

To study the performance of the proposed sample size formula (8.22), we calculated sample sizes under the exponential mixture cure model, where the cure rate of the control group was set to $\pi_1 = 0.4$ and the latency distribution was exponential, that is $S(t) = e^{-\lambda t}$. The hazard parameter λ_1 of the control group was set to 0.1. We assumed that subjects were recruited with a uniform distribution over the accrual period of $t_a = 1$ (year), and that there was a relatively longer follow-up period of $t_f = 5$ or 10 (years). We further assumed that no subject was lost to follow-up during the study. Then, the censoring time was uniformly distributed over the interval $[t_f, t_a + t_f]$, that is, the censoring survival distribution $G(t) = 1$ if $t \le t_f$; $= (t_a + t_f - t)/t_a$ if $t_f \le t \le t_a + t_f$; $= 0$ otherwise. Therefore, given a two-sided nominal significance level of 0.05 and power of 90%, sample sizes were calculated under three hypothesis scenarios for different hazard ratios and cure rates at the alternative (see Table 8.4 for details). The empirical type I error and power of the corresponding designs were simulated based on 10,000 runs. The simulation results (Table 8.4) showed that empirical type I errors and powers of the standard log-rank test were close to the nominal levels of 0.05 and 90%, respectively, for all three scenarios.

To investigate the relative efficiency of the weighted log-rank test versus the standard log-rank test, we considered a class of Harrington-Fleming $\mathcal{G}^{\rho,\nu}$ weight functions (Harrington and Fleming, 1982). Sample sizes were calculated for both the weighted log-rank test and the standard log-rank test under the same scenarios as above, except that the cure rate of the control group was set to $\pi_1 = 0.1$. The results (Table 8.5) showed that a) the weighted log-rank test was not as efficient as the standard log-rank test for scenarios 1 and 2 and b) the weighted log-rank test with the weight function $\mathcal{G}^{-1,0}$ was more efficient than the standard log-rank test for scenario 3. In fact, the weight function $\mathcal{G}^{-1,0}$ is the optimal weight function for scenario 3, as shown in section 8.2.4.

8.3.4 Example and R code

Example 8.2 *Trial design to test the differences in short- and long-term survival*

We illustrated the application of the proposed sample size formula by using data from the Eastern Cooperative Oncology Group (ECOG) trial e1684 (see Example 8.1). Let us now design a randomized two-arm phase III trial to compare the relapse-free survival by using the treatment arm of the ECOG trial as the preliminary data for the control arm of the new trial design. The SAS macro 'PSPMCM' was applied to fit the treatment arm data under the Weibull cure model, with an estimated shape parameter of $\kappa = 1.018$, a scale parameter $\lambda_1 = 0.836$, and a cure rate of 35%. We then have the Weibull mixture cure model $S_1^*(t) = \pi_1 + (1 - \pi_1)S_1(t)$ for the control group, which matches well with the Kaplan-Meier curve, where $\pi_1 = 0.35$ and $S_1(t) = \exp(-0.836t^{1.018})$. For trial design under the PH mixture cure model, assume the alternatives for the three scenarios are as follows: 1) $\pi_2 > \pi_1$ and $\delta < 1$, to detect a hazard ratio of $\delta = 1/1.5$ and a 10% increase in the cure rate (i.e., $\pi_2 = 0.45$), as illustrated in Figure 8.3; 2) $\pi_2 = \pi_1$ and $\delta < 1$, to detect a hazard ratio of $\delta = 0.5$ and identical 35% cure rates for the two groups, as illustrated in Figure 8.4; and 3) $\pi_2 > \pi_1$ and $\delta = 1$, to detect a 15% increase in the cure rate (i.e., $\pi_2 = 0.50$) and to keep the hazard rates the same for the two groups (i.e., $\delta = 1$), as illustrated in Figure 8.5. With an equal allocation, an accrual period of $t_a = 4$ and follow-up time of $t_f = 3$, we can calculate the sample sizes by using formula (8.22) for the standard log-rank test. To achieve a power of 90% with a two-sided type I error of 0.05 under the Weibull mixture cure model, sample sizes of 470, 740, and 512 are required when using the standard log-rank test for scenarios 1, 2, and 3, respectively, and the corresponding empirical powers based on 10,000 simulation runs are 0.896, 0.890, and 0.913, respectively. The R function 'SizeEI' is given below for the sample size calculation under the Weibull mixture cure model using formula (8.22).

Scenario 1 for example 8.2

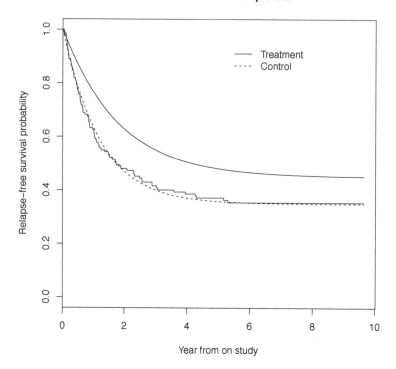

FIGURE 8.3: Hypothetical proportional hazards mixture cure model: The dash and solid lines are the hypothetical survival curves for the control and treatment groups, respectively. The step function is the Kaplan-Meier curve for relapse-free survival for ECOG trial e1684.

```
############################# Input parameters ##############################
### kappa is the shape parameter of the Weibull distribution;        ###
### lambda1 is the hazard parameter of the Weibull distribution for the ###
### control group; pi1 and pi2 are the cure rates for the control and  ###
### treatment groups, respectively; p is the allocation ratio for the  ###
### control group; ta and tf are the accrual and follow-up times;     ###
### HR is the hazard ratio of control vs treatment; alpha and beta are ###
### the type I and type II errors; rho and nu are parameters of the    ###
### Harrington-Fleming weight function.                               ###
#############################################################################
SizeEI=function(kappa,lambda1,pi1,pi2,p,ta,tf,HR,alpha,beta,rho,nu)
{ z0=qnorm(1-alpha/2); z1=qnorm(1-beta)
  tau=ta+tf; lambda2=lambda1/HR
  pi0=1-((1-pi1)*(1-pi2))^(1/2)
  lambda=sqrt(lambda1*lambda2)
  eta=-log(HR)/2
  psi=log((1-pi2)/(1-pi1))/2
```

TABLE 8.4: Sample sizes are calculated by formula (8.22) under the exponential mixture cure model with a nominal type I error of 0.05 and power of 90% (two-sided test and equal allocation)

Design	δ^{-1}/γ	n	$\hat{\alpha}$	EP	Design	n	$\hat{\alpha}$	EP
Scenario 1: $\eta \neq 0$ $\gamma \neq 0$								
$\pi_1 = 0.4$	1.2/0.4	1479	0.051	0.898	$\pi_1 = 0.4$	972	0.049	0.901
$\lambda_1 = 0.1$	1.3/0.5	860	0.052	0.899	$\lambda_1 = 0.1$	570	0.048	0.898
$t_a = 1$	1.4/0.6	580	0.052	0.905	$t_a = 1$	385	0.052	0.902
$t_f = 5$	1.5/0.7	427	0.052	0.906	$t_f = 10$	283	0.049	0.901
	1.6/0.8	334	0.050	0.906		220	0.054	0.905
	1.7/0.9	272	0.049	0.905		179	0.053	0.904
	1.8/1.0	229	0.051	0.905		150	0.050	0.910
Scenario 2: $\eta \neq 0$ $\gamma = 0$								
$\pi_1 = 0.4$	1.4/0.0	2064	0.051	0.906	$\pi_1 = 0.4$	1655	0.050	0.898
$\lambda_1 = 0.1$	1.5/0.0	1449	0.050	0.908	$\lambda_1 = 0.1$	1144	0.051	0.899
$t_a = 1$	1.6/0.0	1098	0.052	0.897	$t_a = 1$	855	0.047	0.901
$t_f = 5$	1.7/0.0	877	0.053	0.901	$t_f = 10$	674	0.045	0.893
	1.8/0.0	727	0.050	0.897		553	0.049	0.897
	1.9/0.0	620	0.048	0.893		466	0.049	0.891
	2.0/0.0	540	0.050	0.902		402	0.050	0.897
Scenario 3: $\eta = 0$ $\gamma \neq 0$								
$\pi_1 = 0.4$	1.0/1.0	636	0.053	0.903	$\pi_1 = 0.4$	362	0.053	0.907
$\lambda_1 = 0.1$	1.0/1.1	523	0.049	0.906	$\lambda_1 = 0.1$	300	0.051	0.910
$t_a = 1$	1.0/1.2	438	0.050	0.906	$t_a = 1$	252	0.050	0.910
$t_f = 5$	1.0/1.3	373	0.050	0.902	$t_f = 10$	216	0.050	0.905
	1.0/1.4	323	0.050	0.908		188	0.047	0.915
	1.0/1.5	283	0.050	0.912		165	0.049	0.910
	1.0/1.6	250	0.054	0.912		147	0.048	0.913

Note: $\gamma = 0.5 \log\{(1 - \pi_2)/(1 - \pi_1)\}$ or $\pi_2 = 1 - (1 - \pi_1)e^{2\gamma}$; $\eta = \frac{1}{2}\log(\delta)$. In the calculations, we assumed a uniform accrual with accrual time $t_a = 1$ and follow-up period $t_f = 5, 10$. The corresponding empirical type I errors and powers are estimated based on 10,000 simulation runs.

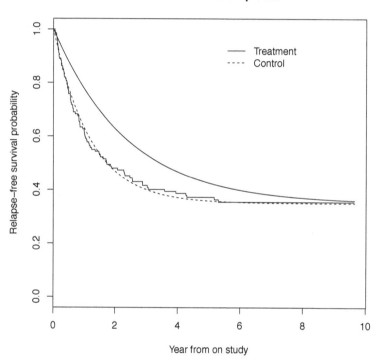

FIGURE 8.4: Hypothetical proportional hazards mixture cure model: The dash and solid lines are the hypothetical survival curves for the control and treatment groups, respectively. The step function is the Kaplan-Meier curve for relapse-free survival for ECOG trial e1684.

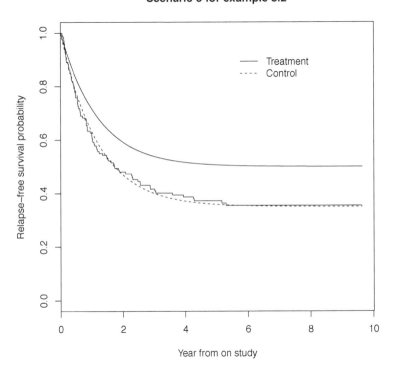

FIGURE 8.5: Hypothetical proportional hazards mixture cure model: The dash and solid lines are the hypothetical survival curves for the control and treatment groups, respectively. The step function is the Kaplan-Meier curve for relapse-free survival for ECOG trial e1684.

```
S1=function(t){exp(-lambda1*t^kappa)} #survival dist. of control#
S2=function(t){exp(-lambda2*t^kappa)} #survival dist. of treatment#
S0=function(t){1-(1-pi0)*(1-exp(-lambda*t^kappa))}
G=function(t){1-punif(t, tf, tau)}  #uniform censoring dist.#
fb=function(t){kappa*lambda*t^(kappa-1)*exp(-lambda*t^kappa)}
Fb=function(t){1-exp(-lambda*t^kappa)}
h0=function(t){(1-pi0)*fb(t)}
m=function(t){2*(eta*(1+pi0*log(1-Fb(t))/S0(t))+psi/S0(t))}
w=function(t){S=p*(pi1+(1-pi1)*S1(t))+(1-p)*(pi2+(1-pi2)*S2(t))
    ans=S^rho*(1-S)^nu; return(ans)} #G^(rho, nu) weight function#
g0=function(t){w(t)*m(t)*G(t)*fb(t)}
g1=function(t){w(t)^2*G(t)*fb(t)}
A=integrate(g0, 0, tau)$value
B=integrate(g1, 0, tau)$value
n=(z0+z1)^2*B/(p*(1-p)*(1-pi0)*A^2)
ans=ceiling(n); return(ans)
}
SizeEI(kappa=1.018,lambda1=0.836,pi1=0.35,pi2=0.45,p=0.5,ta=4,tf=3,
    HR=1.5,alpha=0.05,beta=0.1,rho=0,nu=0)
470
SizeEI(kappa=1.018,lambda1=0.836,pi1=0.35,pi2=0.35,p=0.5,ta=4,tf=3,
    HR=2.0,alpha=0.05,beta=0.1,rho=0,nu=0)
740
SizeEI(kappa=1.018,lambda1=0.836,pi1=0.35,pi2=0.50,p=0.5,ta=4,tf=3,
    HR=1.0,alpha=0.05,beta=0.1,rho=0,nu=0)
512
```

8.3.5 Conclusion

A sample size formula was derived for the weighted log-rank test under the proportional hazards mixture cure model. The simulation results showed that the derived formula provides accurate sample size estimation. The efficiency of a Harrington-Fleming $\mathcal{G}^{\rho,\nu}$-weighted log-rank test was explored. For both scenarios 1 and 2, the $\mathcal{G}^{\rho,\nu}$-weighted log-rank test may not be as efficient as the standard log-rank test. However, the $\mathcal{G}^{-1,0}$ weighted log-rank test is more efficient than the standard log-rank test for scenario 3. In fact, $\mathcal{G}^{-1,0}$ is the optimal weight function for scenario 3, as shown by Gray and Tsiatis (1989) and Wu (2016). It would be interesting to investigate the optimal weight function for scenarios 1 and 2. Wu and Gilbert (2002) proposed a new class of weighted log-rank test statistics that emphasizes early and/or late survival differences. However, further research is necessary to determine whether the weighted log-rank test proposed by Wu and Gilbert is optimal for scenarios 1 and 2.

TABLE 8.5: Sample sizes are given to compare the efficiency of the weighted log-rank test to that of the standard log-rank test, with the sample sizes being calculated under the exponential mixture cure model using formula (8.22) with a nominal type I error of 0.05 and power of 90% (two-sided test and equal allocation)

Design	δ^{-1}/γ	Weight function					
		$\mathcal{G}^{0,0}$	$\mathcal{G}^{0,1}$	$\mathcal{G}^{1,0}$	$\mathcal{G}^{1,1}$	$\mathcal{G}^{-1,0}$	$\mathcal{G}^{-1,1}$
Scenario 1: $\eta \neq 0 \; \gamma \neq 0$							
$\pi_1 = 0.1$	1.2/0.4	1366	1780	1441	1594	1425	2065
$\lambda_1 = 0.1$	1.3/0.5	722	948	756	850	752	1094
$t_a = 1$	1.4/0.6	459	605	479	544	478	694
$t_f = 10$	1.5/0.7	325	428	338	386	337	488
	1.6/0.8	246	324	256	293	255	367
	1.7/0.9	195	256	202	233	202	289
	1.8/1.0	160	210	166	191	165	236
Scenario 2: $\eta \neq 0 \; \gamma = 0$							
$\pi_1 = 0.1$	1.4/0.0	807	1151	822	1004	870	1366
$\lambda_1 = 0.1$	1.5/0.0	566	804	576	705	607	948
$t_a = 1$	1.6/0.0	428	607	436	534	458	711
$t_f = 10$	1.7/0.0	342	483	347	426	364	562
	1.8/0.0	283	399	287	353	300	462
	1.9/0.0	241	338	245	301	255	390
	2.0/0.0	210	294	213	262	221	337
Scenario 3: $\eta = 0 \; \gamma \neq 0$							
$\pi_1 = 0.1$	1.0/1.0	1495	1565	1725	1504	1422	1701
$\lambda_1 = 0.1$	1.0/1.1	1154	1214	1326	1164	1100	1318
$t_a = 1$	1.0/1.2	908	959	1038	919	867	1041
$t_f = 10$	1.0/1.3	726	770	826	737	694	835
	1.0/1.4	589	627	666	600	564	680
	1.0/1.5	484	518	545	494	464	561
	1.0/1.6	402	432	450	412	386	468

Notes: $\gamma = 0.5 \log\{(1 - \pi_2)/(1 - \pi_1)\}$ or $\pi_2 = 1 - (1 - \pi_1)e^{2\gamma}$; $\eta = \frac{1}{2}\log(\delta)$. In the calculations, we assumed a uniform accrual with accrual time $t_a = 1$, follow-up period $t_f = 10$, and no loss to follow-up.

9

A General Group Sequential Procedure

A survival trial usually takes a long time to finish, and data are accumulated gradually over the course of the study. For ethical reasons, such trials are usually monitored for early stopping. The stopping rule is devised based on the planned interim analysis, which is a statistical analysis conducted during a clinical trial. A primary goal of the interim analysis is to determine whether the trial should stop if the efficacy and/or futility of the treatment being evaluated is established. Because of the nature of a human clinical trial, it is usually not feasible to monitor the trial for each patient. Thus, interim analysis is usually planned for a group of patients. The statistical methodology developed to monitor a group of patients at each interim look time point is called a group sequential procedure. Group sequential monitoring methods have been developed in the last few decades by Haybittle (1971), Pocock (1977), O'Brien and Fleming (1979), Lan and DeMets (1983), Whitehead and Stratton (1983), Xiong (1995), Jennison and Turnbull (1997), and many others. Several comprehensive reviews of these methods are available (Jennison and Turnbull 2000, references therein).

In the monitoring process of a sequential trial, the statistically appropriate measure of how far a trial has progressed is the amount of statistical information accumulated, which is usually measured by information time. The information time and the Brownian motion process play important roles in trial monitoring. Although the information time is key to determining the rejection and acceptance regions at each interim analysis, the Brownian motion property makes computation of the rejection and acceptance regions much simpler.

9.1 Brownian Motion

A sequential test is a stochastic process over the course of the study period, say $[0, \tau]$. Let U_t be such a test statistic evaluated at calendar time t for the interim look, where $t \in [0, \tau]$. Suppose that the process $\{U_t, t \in [0, \tau]\}$ satisfies the conditions

- $E(U_t) = \mu I(t),$

- $\mathrm{Var}(U_t) = I(t)$,

- $\mathrm{Cov}(U_t, U_s) = I(t)$, $t \leq s$,

where $I(t), t \in [0, \tau]$ is usually called the information of the test statistic U_t at calendar time t. Let $t^* = I(t)/I(\tau) \in [0, 1]$ denote the information fraction or information time at calendar time t; thus, $B_{t^*} = U_t/\sqrt{I(\tau)}$ is a process of information time t^* over interval $[0, 1]$ that satisfies the following:

- $E(B_{t^*}) = \theta t^*$,

- $\mathrm{Var}(B_{t^*}) = t^*$,

- $\mathrm{Cov}(B_{t^*}, B_{s^*}) = t^*$, $t^* \leq s^*$,

where $\theta = \mu I^{1/2}(\tau)$ is called the drift parameter. Suppose a group sequential study with up to K interim looks at information times $0 < t_1^* < \cdots < t_K^* = 1$ and the process $B_{t^*}, t^* \in [0, 1]$ satisfies the following:

- $B_{t_1^*}, B_{t_2^*}, \ldots, B_{t_K^*}$ have a multivariate normal distribution,

- $E(B_{t^*}) = \theta t^*$,

- $\mathrm{Cov}(B_{t_{k_1}^*}, B_{t_{k_2}^*}) = t_{k_1}^*$, if $t_{k_1}^* \leq t_{k_2}^*$.

Such a process, $\{B_{t^*}, t^* \in [0, 1]\}$, is called a Brownian motion process (Figure 9.1). Brownian motion properties imply that for $t_{k_1}^* < t_{k_2}^*$, $B_{t_{k_1}^*}$ and $B_{t_{k_2}^*} - B_{t_{k_1}^*}$ are uncorrelated (also independent under the multivariate normal distribution). This is usually called an independent increment structure. As we will show, many sequential test statistics can be normalized as Brownian motion processes that have an independent increment structure, and this will be important in simplifying the calculations for the group sequential boundaries.

9.2   Sequential Conditional Probability Ratio Test

A general sequential procedure based on a Brownian motion process has been developed by Xiong et al. (2003). In this section, we will introduce this sequential procedure for survival trial monitoring. Let $\{B_{t^*} : 0 < t^* \leq 1\}$ be the Brownian motion $B_{t^*} \sim N(\theta t^*, t^*)$, and let B_1 be the B_{t^*} at the final stage with full information $t^* = 1$. The hypothesis of interest is

$$H_0 : \theta \leq 0 \quad vs. \quad H_1 : \theta > 0.$$

The joint distribution of (B_{t^*}, B_1) has a bivariate distribution with mean $\mu = (\theta t^*, \theta)'$ and a variance-covariance matrix $\Sigma = (\sigma_{ij})_{2 \times 2}$ with $\sigma_{11} = \sigma_{12} = $

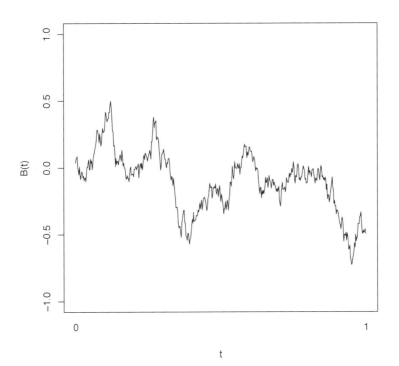

FIGURE 9.1: Graphic representation of a Brownian motion process.

$\sigma_{21} = t^*$ and $\sigma_{22} = 1$. Therefore, according to multivariate conditional distribution theory (e.g., Anderson, 1958), the conditional density $f(B_{t^*}|B_1)$ is the normal density of $N(B_1 t^*, (1 - t^*)t^*)$, that is,

$$f(B_{t^*}|B_1 = s) = \frac{1}{\sqrt{2\pi t^*(1 - t^*)}} e^{-\frac{(B_{t^*} - st^*)^2}{2t^*(1 - t^*)}}.$$

Let $z_{1-\alpha}$ be the critical value of B_1 for rejecting the null hypothesis for the fixed sample test, then, the conditional maximum likelihood ratio for the stochastic process on information time t^* is defined as follow:

$$L(t^*, B_{t^*}|z_{1-\alpha}) = \frac{\max_{\{s > z_{1-\alpha}\}} f(B_{t^*}|B_1 = s)}{\max_{\{s \le z_{1-\alpha}\}} f(B_{t^*}|B_1 = s)}$$

(Xiong, 1995) and we can show that

$$L(t^*, B_{t^*}|z_{1-\alpha}) = \begin{cases} e^{\frac{(B_{t^*} - z_{1-\alpha}t^*)^2}{2t^*(1 - t^*)}}, & B_{t^*} > z_{1-\alpha}t^* \\ e^{-\frac{(B_{t^*} - z_{1-\alpha}t^*)^2}{2t^*(1 - t^*)}}, & B_{t^*} \le z_{1-\alpha}t^* \end{cases}$$

Taking the logarithm, the log-likelihood ratio can be simplified as

$$\log(L(t^*, B_{t^*}|z_{1-\alpha})) = \pm\frac{(B_{t^*} - z_{1-\alpha}t^*)^2}{2(1 - t^*)t^*}, \tag{9.1}$$

which has a positive sign if $B_{t^*} > z_{1-\alpha}t^*$ and a negative sign if $B_{t^*} < z_{1-\alpha}t^*$. Suppose the kth interim look is planned at information time t_k^*, where $0 < t_1^* < \cdots < t_K^* = 1$, and the sequential test should stop when the likelihood is too great or too small. For a given $a, b > 0$, with a positive sign in (9.1), the inequality $\log\{L(t_k^*, B_{t_k^*}|z_{1-\alpha})\} \ge b$ is equivalent to $B_{t_k^*} - z_{1-\alpha}t_k^* \ge \{2bt_k^*(1 - t_k^*)\}^{1/2}$, or $B_{t_k^*} \ge b_k$; with a negative sign in (9.1), the inequality $\log\{L(t_k^*, B_{t_k^*}|z_{1-\alpha})\} \le -a$ is equivalent to $z_{1-\alpha}t_k^* - B_{t_k^*} \ge \{2at_k^*(1 - t_k^*)\}^{1/2}$, or $B_{t_k^*} \le a_k$, where

$$a_k = z_{1-\alpha}t_k^* - \{2at_k^*(1 - t_k^*)\}^{1/2}; \quad b_k = z_{1-\alpha}t_k^* + \{2bt_k^*(1 - t_k^*)\}^{1/2}, \tag{9.2}$$

for $k = 1, ..., K$, and t_k^* is the information time at the kth look at calendar time t_k. In these equations, a and b are boundary coefficients. The symmetric sequential boundaries are generated if we let $a = b$. The appropriate a and b can be determined by choosing an appropriate discordance probability (Xiong, 1995; Xiong et al., 2003). The nominal critical p-values for testing H_0 are

$$P_{\bar{a}_k} = 1 - \Phi(\bar{a}_k); \quad P_{\bar{b}_k} = 1 - \Phi(\bar{b}_k),$$

where $\bar{a}_k = a_k/\sqrt{t_k^*}$ and $\bar{b}_k = b_k/\sqrt{t_k^*}$. The observed p-value at the kth look is

$$P_{B_{t_k^*}} = 1 - \Phi(B_{t_k^*}/\sqrt{t_k^*}).$$

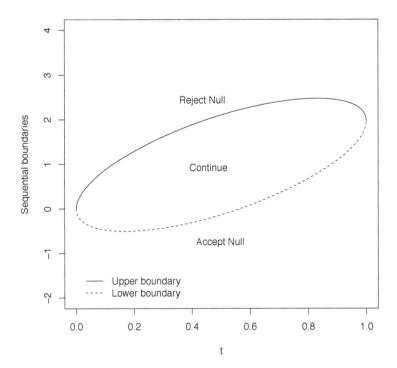

FIGURE 9.2: Graphic representation of the sequential boundaries given in equation (9.2) based on a one-sided SCPRT.

The stopping rule for the trial can be executed by stopping the trial when, for the first time, $P_{B_{t_k^*}} \geq P_{\bar{a}_k}$ (accept H_0 and stop for futility) or $P_{B_{t_k^*}} \leq P_{\bar{b}_k}$ (reject H_0 and stop for efficacy) (Figure 9.2).

This general sequential procedure is called the sequential conditional probability ratio test (SCPRT). Xiong (1995) has shown that the power function of the SCPRT is virtually the same as that of the fixed sample test. The SCPRT has two unique features: (1) the maximum sample size of the sequential test is the same as the sample size of the fixed sample test; (2) the probability of discordance, or the probability that the conclusion of the sequential test would be reversed if the experiment were not stopped according to the stopping rule but continued to the planned end, can be controlled to an arbitrarily low level. All these features make the SCPRT more practical and attractive for use in designing a sequential trial.

For a two-sided hypothesis with a significance level of α:

$$H_0 : \theta = 0 \quad \text{vs.} \quad H_1 : \theta \neq 0.$$

which is equivalent to the following two one-sided hypotheses with a one-sided significance level $\alpha/2$ for each test,

$$H_0^+ : \theta \leq 0 \quad \text{vs.} \quad H_1^+ : \theta > 0.$$

and

$$H_0^- : \theta \geq 0 \quad \text{vs.} \quad H_1^- : \theta < 0.$$

As we discussed before, the SCPRT's lower and upper boundaries for $B_{t_k^*}$ for the hypothesis H^+ are

$$a_k^+ = z_{1-\alpha/2} t_k^* - \{2at_k^*(1 - t_k^*)\}^{1/2}; \quad b_k^+ = z_{1-\alpha/2} t_k^* + \{2at_k^*(1 - t_k^*)\}^{1/2}, (9.3)$$

for $k = 1, ..., K$, where K is the total number of looks, and $0 < t_1^* < \cdots < t_K^* = 1$ are the information times of the interim looks and the final look. The nominal critical p-values for testing H_0 are

$$P_{a_k^+} = 1 - \Phi(a_k^+/\sqrt{t_k^*}); \quad P_{b_k^+} = 1 - \Phi(b_k^+/\sqrt{t_k^*}). \tag{9.4}$$

The observed p-values at the kth look for the one-sided test H^+ are

$$P_{B_{t_k^*}}^+ = 1 - \Phi(B_{t_k^*}/\sqrt{t_k^*}). \tag{9.5}$$

Thus, the stopping rule for monitoring the trial based on the one-sided hypothesis H^+ can be executed by stopping the trial when, for the first time, $P_{B_{t_k^*}}^+ \geq P_{a_k^+}$ (accept H_0^+ and stop for futility) or $P_{B_{t_k^*}}^+ \leq P_{b_k^+}$ (reject H_0^+ and stop for efficacy).

For the hypothesis H^-, similarly, we can derive the lower and upper boundaries for $B_{t_k^*}$ as follows:

$$a_k^- = -z_{1-\alpha/2} t_k^* - \{2at_k^*(1 - t_k^*)\}^{1/2}; \quad b_k^- = -z_{1-\alpha/2} t_k^* + \{2at_k^*(1 - t_k^*)\}^{1/2},$$

for $k = 1, ..., K$. The nominal critical p-values are

$$P_{a_k^-} = \Phi(a_k^-/\sqrt{t_k^*}); \quad P_{b_k^-} = \Phi(b_k^-/\sqrt{t_k^*}). \tag{9.6}$$

The observed p-values at the kth look for one-sided test H^- are

$$P_{B_{t_k^*}}^- = \Phi(B_{t_k^*}/\sqrt{t_k^*}); \tag{9.7}$$

The stopping rule for the trial can be executed by stopping the trial when, for the first time, $P_{B_{t_k^*}}^- \geq P_{b_k^-}$ (accept H_0^- and stop for futility) or $P_{B_{t_k^*}}^- \leq P_{a_k^-}$ (reject H_0^- and stop for efficacy). Finally, the stopping rule for the two-sided test H can be executed by stopping the trial when, for the first time, both one-sided tests accept H_0 and stop for futility or both one-sided tests reject H_0 and stop for efficacy (Figure 9.3).

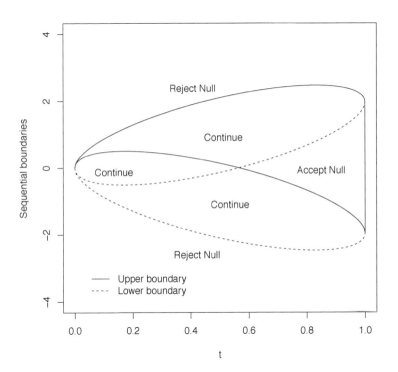

FIGURE 9.3: Graphic representation of the sequential boundaries based on a two-sided SCPRT.

9.3   Operating Characteristics

Let $B_{t^*} \sim N(\theta t^*, t^*)$ be a Brownian motion process with the time variable t^* over interval $[0, 1]$ and drift parameter θ. Let $0 < t_1^* < \cdots < t_K^* = 1$ be the information times of the looks for a sequential test, with a total of K looks (including the final look with $t_K^* = 1$). Let $a_k < b_k$ be the lower and upper boundaries for B_{t^*} at time t_k^* for $k = 1, \cdots, K-1$, and $a_K = b_K$. It is important to know the operating characteristics of a sequential test. The lower and upper boundary crossing probability at the kth look can be calculated as follows:

$$PL_k(\theta) \quad = \quad P(\cap_{i=1}^{k-1}(\bar{a}_i < S_{t_i^*} < \bar{b}_i) \cup (S_{t_k^*} < \bar{a}_k)|\theta)$$

and

$$PU_k(\theta) \quad = \quad P(\cap_{i=1}^{k-1}(\bar{a}_i < S_{t_i^*} < \bar{b}_i) \cup (S_{t_k^*} > \bar{b}_k)|\theta),$$

where $\bar{a}_k = a_k/\sqrt{t_k^*}$, $\bar{b}_k = b_k/\sqrt{t_k^*}$ and $S_{t_k^*} = B_{t_k^*}/\sqrt{t_k^*}$ for $k = 1, \ldots K$. Then, the boundary crossing probability at the kth look is given by $CP_k(\theta) = PL_k(\theta) + PU_k(\theta)$. The power function of a sequential test is given by

$$P(\theta) = \sum_{k=1}^{K} CP_k(\theta). \tag{9.8}$$

The expected stopping time is given by

$$E_\theta(T) = \sum_{k=1}^{K} t_k^* CP_k(\theta), \tag{9.9}$$

where T is the stopping time of the trial. For censored survival data with staggered entry, the number of patients enrolled by calendar time t during the accrual period over interval $[0, t_a]$ is a function of t denoted by $N_a(t)$. For a uniform accrual over interval $[0, t_a]$, let N be the maximum sample size for a sequential trial, the function $N_a(t)$ is given as follows:

$$N_a(t) = \begin{cases} N(\frac{t}{t_a}) & \text{if } 0 < t < t_a \\ N & \text{if } t \geq t_a \end{cases}$$

The expected sample size of the sequential trial can then be calculated by

$$E_\theta[N_a(T)] = \sum_{k=1}^{K} N_a(t_k) CP_k(\theta), \tag{9.10}$$

where t_k is the calendar time at which the corresponding information time t_k^* is calculated. These operating characteristics can be calculated by using R function 'pmvnorm' because $(S_{t_1^*}, \ldots, S_{t_K^*})$ have a multivariate normal distribution with mean $E(S_{t_k^*}) = \theta\sqrt{t_k^*}$ and covariance $\mathrm{Cov}(S_{t_k^*}, S_{t_{k'}^*}) = t_k^* \wedge t_{k'}^*/(\sqrt{t_k^*}\sqrt{t_{k'}^*})$.

9.4   Probability of Discordance

Appropriate boundaries should be chosen such that the probability of the conclusion obtained by the sequential test being reversed by the test at the planned end is small, but not unnecessarily so. Let D be the event in which the conclusion at an interim time t is reversed at the final time $t^* = 1$. Let $\rho(\theta) = P_\theta(D)$, which is the discordance probability, given a true θ, and let $\rho_{max} = max_\theta \rho(\theta)$, which is the maximum discordance probability. Let $\rho_s = P_\theta(D|B_1 = s)$, which is the conditional probability of discordance, given the final-stage observation $B_1 = s$, and it does not depend on θ because B_1 is a sufficient statistic for θ, and let $\rho = max_s \rho_s$, which is the maximum conditional probability of discordance. The boundary coefficients a and b are determined by choosing appropriate value of ρ or ρ_{max}, which provide intuitive benchmarks for designing a sequential trial. The values of the symmetric boundary coefficient a for the balanced information time given the maximum conditional probability of discordance, are given by Xiong et al. (2003, Table 1).

9.5   SCPRT Design

An SCPRT procedure to test $H_0 : \theta \le 0$ vs. $H_1 : \theta > 0$ based on Brownian motion statistics $\{B_{t^*}, t^* \in [0,1]\}$ can be summarized as follows. We first calculate the sample size for a reference fixed sample test, according to the significance level of α and power of $1 - \beta$ at the alternative $\theta = \theta_1$. Given the number of looks K (including the final look), and the maximum conditional discordance probability, ρ (or the maximum discordance probability ρ_{max}), we can determine the boundary coefficients a and b by using the methods discussed in the previous section and calculate the SCPRT boundaries by using equation (9.2). The information time can be calculated based on the test statistics discussed in the next several chapters. It is necessary only to compare sequentially the p-values of the tests (as fixed sample tests) with the upper and lower critical significance levels at t_k^*. We recommend using $\rho = 0.02$, which leads to a reasonable maximum discordance probability ($\rho_{max} = 0.0054$) and results in an SCPRT boundary that is efficient and preserves the accordance of the conclusions from the test at the early stopping time and the test at the planned end. To calculate the operating characteristics of the sequential tests, it should first be noted that the cutoff value at the final stage $t_K^* = 1$ is $a_K = b_K = z_{1-\alpha}$, the drift at the null hypothesis is $\theta_0 = 0$, and the drift at the alternative hypothesis is $\theta_1 = z_{1-\alpha} + z_{1-\beta}$, all of which are the same as the corresponding values for the fixed test at the final stage with information time $t_K^* = 1$. Substituting θ_0 and θ_1 into equations (9.8), (9.9), and (9.10), we can compute the sequential type I error $P(\theta_0)$, the power $P(\theta_1)$, and the expected stopping time and expected sample size by $E_\theta(T)$ and $E_\theta[N_a(T)]$, respectively, under the null and alternative hypotheses for the SCPRT design. The SCPRT procedure has been implemented in a user-friendly software SCPRTinfWin (Xiong, 2007) which can be downloaded from http://www.stjuderesearch.org/site/depts/biostats/scprt.

10

Sequential Survival Trial Design

10.1 Introduction

In cancer clinical trials, the primary interest is in comparing the survival distributions of the treatment groups. The nonparametric log-rank test is the most popular test statistic used for trial design and monitoring. The Brownian motion property of the log-rank test makes it easy to monitor such trials by using a group sequential procedure (Tsiatis, 1982; Sellke and Siegmund, 1983; Slud, 1984; Kim and Tsiatis, 1990). However, Tsiatis et al. (1995) also derived the Brownian motion property of the score and Wald tests for general parametric survival models. Thus, sequential trials can also be designed under parametric models.

The exponential and Weibull distributions are the two most frequently used parametric models. In general, a survival trial designed under the exponential or Weibull model can also be designed under the proportional hazards model using the log-rank test. However, a parametric test derived under the exponential or Weibull model has better small-sample properties than the nonparametric log-rank test because the latter has to be general and, thus, information from continuous quantities derived from a specific parametric model cannot be included for inference (Wu and Xiong, 2015). The maximum sample size is usually large for a phase III group sequential trial. However, the available data could be small in the early stages of interim monitoring; therefore, a study with a group sequential design under the Weibull model may perform better than a general proportional hazards model in the early stages.

In the next section, we will develop a sequential parametric MLE test for trial design and monitoring under the Weibull model.

10.2 Sequential Procedure for the Parametric Model

Assume that the failure time T_j of a subject from the jth group follows the Weibull distribution with a common shape parameter κ and a scale parameter λ_j, where $j = 1$ and 2 represent the control and treatment groups, respectively, that is, T_j has a survival distribution function

$$S_j(t) = e^{-\lambda_j t^\kappa},$$

and we are interested in the following one-sided hypothesis:

$$H_0 : \delta \geq 1 \ \ vs. \ \ H_1 : \delta < 1,$$

where $\delta = \lambda_2/\lambda_1$ is the hazard ratio.

Now, suppose that during the accrual phase of the trial, n_j subjects of the jth group are enrolled in the study, and let $\{T_{ij}, i = 1, \ldots, n_j\}$ denote a random sample of T_j for $j = 1$ and 2, and let C_{ij} denote the censoring time of the ith subject of the jth group, with both failure times and censoring times being measured from the time of study entry, Y_{ij}. We assume that the failure times T_{ij} are independent of the censoring times C_{ij} and entry times Y_{ij}, and that $\{(Y_{ij}, T_{ij}, C_{ij}); i = 1, \cdots, n_j\}$ are independent and identically distributed for $j = 1$ and 2. When the data are examined at calendar time $t \leq \tau$, where τ is the study duration, we observe the failure times $X_{ij}(t) = T_{ij} \wedge C_{ij} \wedge (t - Y_{ij})^+$ and failure indicators $\Delta_{ij}(t) = I(T_{ij} \leq C_{ij} \wedge (t - Y_{ij})^+), i = 1, \cdots, n_j, j = 1, 2,$ where x^+ is the positive part of x.

The right censored survival times in a sequential trial for five patients are illustrated in Figure 10.1, in which the time of entry to the trial is represented by a $\bullet$, subjects 1, 2, and 4 die ($\times$) during the course of the study, and subject 3 is lost to follow-up ($\circ$) and subject 5 is still alive ($\diamond$) at the end of the study. Suppose two interim looks are planned at calendar times t_1 and t_2, respectively, before the end of the study. Then, the first three subjects are included in the first interim analysis. The observed survival time for the third subject at the first interim analysis is $t_1 - Y_3$. All five subjects are included in the second interim analysis, and the survival time for the fifth subject is $t_2 - Y_5$.

10.2.1   Sequential Wald Test

Based on the observed data $\{X_{ij}(t), \Delta_{ij}(t), i = 1, \cdots, n_j, j = 1, 2\}$, the observed likelihood function at time t is proportional to

$$L(\lambda_1, \lambda_2; t) = \lambda_1^{d_1(t)} \lambda_2^{d_2(t)} e^{-\lambda_1 U_1(t) - \lambda_2 U_2(t)}$$

(see, e.g., Cox and Oakes, 1984, Chapter 3 or Appendix A), where $d_j(t) = \sum_{i=1}^{n_j} \Delta_{ij}(t)$ is the total number of events observed in the jth group by time t, and $U_j(t) = \sum_{i=1}^{n_j} X_{ij}^\kappa(t)$ is the cumulative follow-up time by time t penalized by the Weibull shape parameter κ.

To drive the test statistics, we convert (λ_1, λ_2) to (ψ, χ), where $\psi = \log(\lambda_1/\lambda_2)$ and $\chi = \lambda_2$. Then, the log-likelihood at time t for (ψ, χ) is given by

$$\ell(\psi, \chi; t) = d_1(t) \log(\chi) + \psi d_1(t) + d_2(t) \log(\chi) - \chi e^\psi U_1(t) - \chi U_2(t).$$

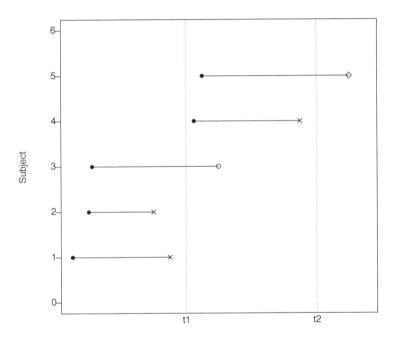

FIGURE 10.1: Graphic representation of survival data in a sequential trial.

By solving the following score equations:

$$\ell_\psi(\psi, \chi; t) = d_1(t) - \chi e^\psi U_1(t),$$

$$\ell_\chi(\psi, \chi; t) = \frac{d_1(t)}{\chi} + \frac{d_2(t)}{\chi} - e^\psi U_1(t) - U_2(t),$$

the maximum likelihood estimates of ψ and χ at time t are

$$\hat\psi(t) = \log\left\{ \frac{U_2(t) d_1(t)}{U_1(t) d_2(t)} \right\} \quad \text{and} \quad \hat\chi(t) = \frac{d_2(t)}{U_2(t)}.$$

The observed Fisher information matrix, a negative second derivatives matrix of $\ell(\psi, \chi)$ with respect to ψ and χ, evaluated at $(\psi, \chi) = (\hat\psi(t), \hat\chi(t))$, is given by

$$J(\hat\psi, \hat\chi; t) = \frac{1}{n} \begin{pmatrix} d_1(t) & U_2(t) d_1(t) d_2^{-1}(t) \\ U_2(t) d_1(t) d_2^{-1}(t) & U_2^2(t) d_2^{-2}(t)(d_1(t) + d_2(t)) \end{pmatrix},$$

and the variance of $\hat\psi(t)$ can then be estimated by $J^{\psi\psi}(t) = n(d_1^{-1}(t) + d_2^{-1}(t))$, which is the $(1,1)$ entry in the inverse of the Fisher information matrix $J^{-1}(\hat\psi, \hat\chi; t)$. Therefore, the sequential Wald test statistic $\hat\psi(t)$ is given by

$$Z(t) = n^{1/2}(\hat\psi(t) - \psi)\{J^{\psi\psi}(t)\}^{-1/2}.$$

Under the null hypothesis $H_0 : \delta = 1$, or $\psi = -\log(\delta) = 0$, the sequential test statistic $Z(t)$ reduces to

$$Z(t) = \log\{U_2(t) d_1(t)/U_1(t) d_2(t)\}(d_1^{-1}(t) + d_2^{-1}(t))^{-1/2},$$

which is approximately standard normal distributed. To derive the group sequential design, let

$$U(t) = \log\{U_2(t) d_1(t)/U_1(t) d_2(t)\}(d_1^{-1}(t) + d_2^{-1}(t))^{-1}. \tag{10.1}$$

Then, under the local alternative, the statistic $U(t)$ is approximately normal with mean $-\log(\delta) V(t)$ and variance $V(t)$, and it has an independent increment structure, where $V(t) = (d_1^{-1}(t) + d_2^{-1}(t))^{-1}$. The above results can be derived from the work of Tsiatis et al. (1995), who proved the results for general parametric survival models. Thus, $B_{t^*} = U(t)/V^{1/2}(\tau) \sim N(\theta t^*, t^*)$ is approximately a Brownian motion with drift parameter $\theta = -\log(\delta) V^{1/2}(\tau)$ and information time $t^* = V(t)/V(\tau)$, where $V(\tau)$ is the value of $V(t)$ at $t = \tau$. Furthermore, it is easy to verify that $Z(t) = B_{t^*}/\sqrt{t^*}$.

10.2.2 SCPRT for the Parametric Model

To develop a group sequential method for the test statistic $Z(t)$ under the Weibull model, we will apply the SCPRT procedure. Because the required maximum sample size for the sequential test using the SCPRT is the same as for the reference fixed sample test, the maximum sample size for the sequential test $Z(t)$ can be calculated by formula (4.2). Note that $Z(t) = U(t)/V^{1/2}(t) = B_{t^*}/\sqrt{t^*}$; thus, we need only apply the SCPRT procedure to the test statistic $B_{t^*} = U(t)/V^{1/2}(\tau) \sim N(\theta t^*, t^*)$, which is a Brownian motion in information time $t^* = V(t)/V(\tau)$ over $[0, 1]$, and the drift parameter $\theta = -\log(\delta)V^{1/2}(\tau)$. The information time $t^* = V(t)/V(\tau)$ is a random variable and is unknown until the end of the study; thus, it cannot be used for the interim analysis. As

$$V(t) \sim D(t) = \left(\frac{1}{n_1 p_1(t)} + \frac{1}{n_2 p_2(t)} \right)^{-1}, \tag{10.2}$$

where $p_j(t) = P(\Delta_{ij}(t) = 1)$, $j = 1, 2$, the information time $t^* = V(t)/V(\tau)$ can be estimated by

$$t_D^* = D(t)/D(\tau),$$

where

$$D(t) = n \left(\frac{1}{\omega_1 p_1(t)} + \frac{1}{\omega_2 p_2(t)} \right)^{-1},$$

and $D(\tau) = D(t)|_{t=\tau}$.

To calculate the information time, assume that subjects are accrued over an accrual period of length t_a, with a follow-up time t_f, giving a study duration of $\tau = t_a + t_f$, and that the entry time Y is uniformly distributed over $[0, t_a]$, with no patient lost to follow-up. Then, the administrative censoring distribution $G(t)$ is a uniform distribution over interval $[t_f, t_a + t_f]$. It follows that

$$\begin{aligned}
p_j(t) &= P(T + Y < t) \\
&= \int_0^\infty P(T + Y < t | Y = u) dG(u) \\
&= \frac{1}{t_a} \int_0^{t \wedge t_a} P(T < t - u) du \\
&= \frac{1}{t_a} \int_0^{t \wedge t_a} \{1 - S_j(t - u)\} du,
\end{aligned}$$

where $S_j(t) = e^{-\lambda_j t^\kappa}$. Thus, the information time t_D^* can be calculated at any interim look planned at calendar time t within the study duration $[0, \tau]$.

Suppose a total of K interim looks are planned at calendar time $t_1, \ldots, t_K$. As $B_{t_k^*} = U(t_k)/V^{1/2}(\tau) \sim N(\theta t_k^*, t_k^*)$ and has a Brownian motion property, then, based on the SCPRT procedure, the symmetric lower and upper boundaries for $B_{t_k^*}$ at the kth look are given by

$$a_k = z_{1-\alpha} t_k^* - \{2at_k^*(1 - t_k^*)\}^{1/2}; \quad b_k = z_{1-\alpha} t_k^* + \{2at_k^*(1 - t_k^*)\}^{1/2}, \tag{10.3}$$

for $k = 1, \ldots, K$, where $t_k^* = D(t_k)/D(\tau)$ is the information time at the kth look at calendar time t_k. The nominal critical p-values for testing H_0 are

$$P_{\bar{a}_k} = 1 - \Phi(\bar{a}_k); \quad P_{\bar{b}_k} = 1 - \Phi(\bar{b}_k),$$

where $\bar{a}_k = a_k/\sqrt{t_k^*}$ and $\bar{b}_k = b_k/\sqrt{t_k^*}$. The observed p-value at the kth look for the test statistic $Z(t)$ is given by

$$P_{Z_{t_k}} = 1 - \Phi(B_{t_k^*}/\sqrt{t_k^*}) = 1 - \Phi(Z_{t_k}), \qquad (10.4)$$

where $Z_{t_k} = Z(t_k)$. The stopping rule for the trial can be executed by stopping the trial when, for the first time, $P_{Z_{t_k}} \geq P_{\bar{a}_k}$ (accept H_0 and stop for futility) or $P_{Z_{t_k}} \leq P_{\bar{b}_k}$ (reject H_0 and stop for efficacy) (Wu and Xiong, 2015).

Example 10.1 *A study for rhabdoid tumor*

Rhabdoid tumors are aggressive pediatric malignant neoplasms with a poor prognosis. Over a 5-year period, St. Jude Children's Research Hospital accrued 14 pediatric patients with recurrent or refractory non-CNS rhabdoid tumors that were treated with conventional chemotherapy. The median event-free survival was only approximately 1 year, with an event being defined as disease relapse or death. All 14 patients had events within approximately 3 years. The Weibull model was fitted to the data, resulting in an estimate (standard error) of the shape parameter of $\kappa = 1.37(0.28)$ and a median event-free survival time of $m_1 = 0.936$ years, which provides a model that is more satisfactory than the exponential model (Figure 10.2).

Now, suppose that we would like to design a multicenter randomized two-arm trial to assess the effectiveness of the small molecule inhibitor alisertib (the experimental treatment) relative to that of conventional chemotherapy (the control) for this group of patients. Patients will be randomized with equal allocation to each treatment group. The hypothesis of the planned study is $H_0 : m_2 \leq m_1$ vs. $H_1 : m_2 > m_1$. The investigators would like to detect a half-year increase in the median event-free survival of the alisertib treatment group when compared to that of the conventional chemotherapy group, that is $m_2 = m_1 + 0.5 = 1.436$ and $\delta = \lambda_2/\lambda_1 = (m_1/m_2)^\kappa = 0.5565$. Assuming this multicenter trial has the capacity to enroll and treat 20 patients per year (assuming uniform accrual), then, given a type I error of 5%, power of 90%, and 2 years of follow-up ($t_f = 2$), the required total accrual time is $t_a = 5.3$ years, calculated by equation (4.6). Therefore, the study duration is $\tau = t_a + t_f = 7.3$ years, and the total sample size is 106 patients (53 per group). Now, assuming the interim and final looks are planned at calendar times $t_1 = 4$, $t_2 = 5$, and $t_3 = \tau = 7.3$ years, the corresponding information time at each planned interim look t_k can be calculated by $t_k^* = D(t_k)/D(\tau)$, where $D(t) = n(\omega_1^{-1}p_1^{-1}(t) + \omega_2^{-1}p_2^{-1}(t))^{-1}$ with

$$p_j(t) = \frac{1}{t_a}\int_0^{t \wedge t_a} \{1 - S_j(t - u)\}du,$$

$S_j(t) = e^{-\log(2)(\frac{t}{m_j})^\kappa}$, and $\omega_1 = \omega_2 = 0.5$. By calculation, the corresponding information times are $t_1^* = 0.511, t_2^* = 0.706$, and $t_3^* = 1$. Assuming

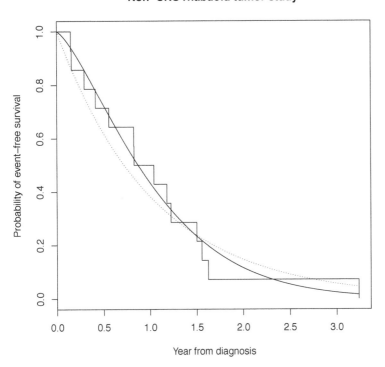

FIGURE 10.2: The step function is a Kaplan-Meier curve. The solid and dotted curves are the fitted Weibull and exponential survival distributions, respectively.

TABLE 10.1: The empirical operating characteristics of the three-stage SCPRT design for the example were estimated based on 100,000 simulation runs under the Weibull distribution

At the kth interim look	$k = 1$	$k = 2$	$k = 3$	Total
Type I error				
Nominal	0.0028	0.0031	0.0446	0.0500
Empirical	0.0031	0.0029	0.0453	0.0514
Power				
Nominal	0.2494	0.2066	0.4435	0.8995
Empirical	0.2499	0.2106	0.4429	0.9034
Probability of stopping under the null				
Nominal	0.3412	0.2405	0.4184	1.0000
Empirical	0.3446	0.2456	0.4098	1.0000
Probability of stopping under the alternative				
Nominal	0.2554	0.2136	0.5311	1.0000
Empirical	0.2557	0.2182	0.5261	1.0000

the maximum conditional probability of discordance $\rho = 0.02$, the boundary coefficient is $a = 2.593$ for $K = 3$ (Xiong et al., 2003), and the maximum probability of discordance is $\rho_{max} = 0.0043$. The lower and upper boundaries calculated from (10.3) are $(a_1, a_2, a_3) = (-0.298, 0.124, 1.645)$ and $(b_1, b_2, b_3) = (1.979, 2.199, 1.645)$, respectively. The acceptance and rejection nominal critical significance levels are (0.6615, 0.4415, 0.050) and (0.0028, 0.0044, 0.050).

We performed 100,000 simulation runs to evaluate the operating characteristics of the proposed group sequential design. The empirical (nominal) type I error and power of the sequential test are 0.0514 (0.0505) and 0.9034 (0.8995), respectively. The empirical (nominal) probabilities of stopping under the null and alternative hypotheses are 0.3446 (0.3412) and 0.2557(0.2554) at the first look, and 0.2456(0.2405) and 0.2182(0.2136) at the second look, and 0.4098(0.4184) and 0.5261(0.5311) at the third look, respectively. The details of the operating characteristics for the proposed group sequential design are shown in Table 10.1.

10.3 Sequential Procedure for the Proportional Hazard Model

The parametric sequential procedure discussed in the previous section is restricted under the Weibull distribution. The proportional hazards model is the most popular model for survival trial design and monitoring. To consider sequential trial design, we will formulate the sequential log-rank test statistics by using counting process notation as follows. For notational convenience, we use the binary covariate $Z = 1/0$ as the group indicator, 1 for the control group (group 1), and 0 for the treatment group (group 2). (Note: here Z is defined to make the notation consistent with the previous definition of the log-rank test, so that the log-rank test has a positive expectation under the alternative). Let $\lambda_1(x)$ and $\lambda_2(x)$ be the hazard functions of the control and treatment groups, respectively, then the proportional hazards model $\lambda_2(x) = \delta\lambda_1(x)$ can be written in a Cox model as follows:

$$\lambda(x|Z) = \lambda_2(x)e^{\gamma Z},$$

where $\gamma = -\log\{\lambda(x|Z = 0)/\lambda(x|Z = 1)\} = -\log(\delta)$ is the negative log-hazard ratio of the treatment group versus the control group.

10.3.1 Sequential Log-Rank Test

Suppose that during the accrual phase of the trial, a total of n subjects in two groups are enrolled in the study, and let T_i and C_i denote, respectively, the failure time and censoring time of the ith subject, being measured from the time of study entry Y_i. Let Z_i be the control group indicator for the ith patient. We assume that the failure time T_i is independent of the censoring time C_i and entry time Y_i, that $\{(Y_i, T_i, C_i); i = 1, \cdots, n\}$ are independent and identically distributed within each group, and that the censoring distributions of the two treatment groups are the same. When the data are examined at calendar time $t \leq \tau$, we observe the time to failure $X_i(t) = T_i \wedge C_i \wedge (t - Y_i)^+$ and the failure indicator $\Delta_i(t) = I(T_i \leq C_i \wedge (t - Y_i)^+), i = 1, \cdots, n$. Based on of the observed data $\{X_i(t), \Delta_i(t), Z_i, i = 1, \cdots, n\}$, let $N_i(t, x) = \Delta_i(t)I\{X_i(t) \leq x\}$ and $Y_i(t, x) = I(X_i(t) \geq x)$. Then, the weighted sequential log-rank score statistic at calendar time t is given by

$$U_w(t) = \sum_{i=1}^n W_n(t, X_i(t))\Delta_i(t)\{Z_i - \bar{Z}(t, X_i(t))\}$$

$$= \sum_{i=1}^n \int_0^t W_n(t, x)\{Z_i - \bar{Z}(t, x)\}N_i(t, dx),$$

where

$$\bar{Z}(t, x) = \frac{\sum_{i=1}^n Z_i Y_i(t, x)}{\sum_{i=1}^n Y_i(t, x)},$$

and $W_n(t, x)$ is a weight function that converges to $w(t, x)$ in probability. By the martingale central limit theorem, we can obtain the following results.

Theorem 10.1 *Under the contiguous alternatives* H_{1n} : $\lambda_n(x|Z) = e^{\gamma_{1n}Z}\lambda_2(x)$, *where* γ_{1n} *is a sequence of constants satisfying* $n^{1/2}\gamma_{1n} = b < \infty$, *the process* $U_w(t)$ *converges weakly to a Gaussian process with mean* $b\mu_w(t)$ *and covariance* $\sigma_w^2(t, s)$ *at* (t, s), *where*

$$\mu_w(t) = \int_0^t w(t, x)\bar{z}(t, x)\{1 - \bar{z}(t, x)\}\pi(t, x)d\Lambda_2(x)$$

and

$$\sigma_w^2(t, s) = \int_0^{t \wedge s} w(t, x)w(s, x)\bar{z}(t \wedge s, x)\{1 - \bar{z}(t \wedge s, x)\}\pi(t \wedge s, x)d\Lambda_2(x).$$

Proof 10.1 *Consider a sequence of contiguous alternatives* $H_{1n} : \lambda_n(x|Z) = e^{\gamma_{1n}Z}\lambda_2(x)$, *where* γ_{1n} *is a sequence of constants satisfying* $n^{1/2}\gamma_{1n} = b < \infty$. *If we further define an* $\mathcal{F}_{t,x}$-*martingale sequence for each* t *by*

$$M_i^{(n)}(t, x) = N_i(t, x) - \int_0^x Y_i(t, u)e^{\gamma_{1n}Z_i}d\Lambda_2(u),$$

where $\mathcal{F}_{t,x} = \sigma\{N_i(t, u), Y_i(t, u), Z_i; u \leq x, i = 1, \ldots, n\}$, *then the weighted sequential log-rank score statistic is given by*

$$U_w(t) = U_M(t) + U_D(t),$$

where

$$U_M(t) = \sum_{i=1}^n \int_0^t W_n(t, x)\{Z_i - \bar{Z}(t, x)\}M_i^{(n)}(t, dx)$$

and

$$U_D(t) = \sum_{i=1}^n \int_0^t W_n(t, x)\{Z_i - \bar{Z}(t, x)\}\left\{e^{\gamma_{1n}Z_i} - 1\right\}Y_i(t, x)d\Lambda_2(x).$$

By a Taylor series expansion,

$$e^{\gamma_{1n}Z_i} = 1 + \gamma_{1n}Z_i + O(\gamma_{1n}^2)$$

and $W_n(t, x) \xrightarrow{P} w(t, x)$, *we obtain*

$$n^{-1/2}U_M(t) = n^{-1/2}\sum_{i=1}^n \int_0^t w(t, x)\{Z_i - \bar{Z}(t, x)\}M_i^{(n)}(t, dx) + o_p(1)$$

and

$$n^{-1/2}U_D(t) = n^{1/2}\gamma_{1n}\int_0^t w(t, x)\bar{Z}(t, x)\{1 - \bar{Z}(t, x)\}\{n^{-1}\sum_{i=1}^n Y_i(t, x)\}d\Lambda_2(x) + o_p(1).$$

Furthermore, as

$$n^{1/2}\gamma_{1n} = b, \quad n^{-1}\sum_{i=1}^{n} Y_i(t,x) \xrightarrow{P} \pi(t,x), \text{ and } \bar{Z}(t,x) \xrightarrow{P} \bar{z}(t,x),$$

where $\pi(t,x) = P_{H_0}(X(t) \geq x)$ and $\bar{z}(t,x) = E_{H_0}(Z|X(t) \geq x)$, we have

$$n^{-1/2}U_D(t) \to b\mu_w(t),$$

where

$$\mu_w(t) = \int_0^t w(t,x)\bar{z}(t,x)\{1 - \bar{z}(t,x)\}\pi(t,x)d\Lambda_2(x).$$

Therefore,

$$n^{-1/2}U_w(t) = n^{-1/2}\sum_1^n \int_0^t \{Z_i - \bar{z}(t,x)\}w(t,x)M_i^{(n)}(t,dx) + b\mu_w(t) + o_p(1).$$

By the martingale central limit theorem, $n^{-1/2}U_w(t)$ converges weakly to a Gaussian process with mean $b\mu_w(t)$ and covariance $\sigma_w^2(t,s)$, which is given by

$$\sigma_w^2(t,s) = \int_0^{t\wedge s} w(t,x)w(s,x)\bar{z}(t\wedge s,x)\{1 - \bar{z}(t\wedge s,x)\}\pi(t\wedge s,x)d\Lambda_2(x).$$

Now let us consider the standard log-rank score test (when $W_n(t,x) = 1$):

$$U(t) = \sum_{i=1}^{n} \int_0^t \{Z_i - \bar{Z}(t,x)\}N_i(t,dx), \tag{10.5}$$

and its variance estimate is $n^{-1}V(t)$, where

$$V(t) = \sum_{i=1}^{n} \Delta_i(t)\bar{Z}(t,X_i(t))\{1 - \bar{Z}(t,X_i(t))\}. \tag{10.6}$$

Thus, the sequential log-rank test is given by

$$L(t) = \frac{U(t)}{\sqrt{V(t)}},$$

and the following corollary holds for the standard sequential log-rank test $L(t)$.

Corollary *Under the contiguous alternatives $H_{1n} : \lambda_n(x|Z) = e^{\gamma_{1n}Z}\lambda_2(x)$, where $n^{1/2}\gamma_{1n} = b < \infty$,*
(i) $B_{t^*} = U(t)/\sqrt{V(\tau)} \xrightarrow{D} N(\theta t^*, t^*)$, which is a Brownian motion with information time $t^* = V(t)/V(\tau)$, and the drift parameter $\theta = -\log(\delta)V^{1/2}(\tau)$.

(ii) The asymptotic distribution of the log-rank test for the fixed test at $t = \tau$ is approximately normal with mean of $b\sigma(\tau)$ and unit variance, that is,

$$L(\tau) = U(\tau)/\sqrt{V(\tau)} \xrightarrow{D} N(b\sigma(\tau), 1),$$

where $\sigma^2(\tau)$ is given by

$$\sigma^2(\tau) = \omega_1\omega_2 \int_0^\tau \pi(\tau, x)d\Lambda_2(x).$$

Proof 10.2 *The standard log-rank test has a weight function $W_n(t, x) = 1$. Then, $\mu_w(t)$ and $\sigma_w^2(t)$ reduce to*

$$\mu(t) = \sigma^2(t) = \int_0^t \bar{z}(t, x)\{1 - \bar{z}(t, x)\}\pi(t, x)d\Lambda_2(x),$$

which can be consistently estimated by

$$n^{-1}V(t) = n^{-1}\sum_1^n \Delta_i(t)\bar{Z}(t, X_i(t))\{1 - \bar{Z}(t, X_i(t))\}.$$

Because Z is independent of $X(t)$, then $\bar{z}(t, x) = E(Z) = \omega_1$. Thus, $\sigma^2(t)$ further reduces to

$$\sigma^2(t) = \omega_1\omega_2 \int_0^t \pi(t, x)d\Lambda_2(x),$$

where $\omega_2 = 1 - \omega_1$. Therefore,

$$n^{-1/2}U(t) \sim N(b\sigma^2(t), \sigma^2(t)),$$

and it has an independent increment structure. Because $n^{-1}V(t)$ is a consistent estimate of the $\sigma^2(t)$,

$$B_{t^*} = U(t)/\sqrt{V(\tau)} \sim N(\theta t^*, t^*)$$

is a Brownian motion with information time $t^* = V(t)/V(\tau)$, where the drift parameter $\theta = -\log(\delta)V^{1/2}(\tau)$. The asymptotic distribution of the log-rank test for the fixed test at $t = \tau$ is approximately normal with mean of $b\sigma(\tau)$ and unit variance, that is,

$$L(\tau) = U(\tau)/\sqrt{V(\tau)} \sim N(b\sigma(\tau), 1),$$

where $\sigma^2(\tau)$ is given by

$$\sigma^2(\tau) = \omega_1\omega_2 \int_0^\tau \pi(\tau, x)d\Lambda_2(x).$$

10.3.2 Information Time

Information time plays an important role in trial monitoring. It is key to determining the rejection and acceptance regions at each interim analysis.

For the log-rank test, several information times have been proposed in the literature (Lan and Lachin, 1990). For example, the exact information time for the log-rank test is defined as the ratio of the variance at calendar time t to that at the end of the trial, that is, $t^* = V(t)/V(\tau)$, where $V(t)$ is the variance estimate at calendar time t given by (10.6). However, t^* cannot be used in practice because $V(\tau)$ is unknown until the end of the study. We can replace the final variance $V(\tau)$ by its projected final variance $\tilde{V} = (z_{1-\alpha} + z_{1-\beta})^2/[\log(\delta)]^2$ (Collett, 2003) to define the information time $\hat{t}^* = V(t)/\tilde{V}$, which is usually used at earlier stages of the trial monitoring; if at a later stage $V(t) > \tilde{V}$, then this information time cannot be used either.

A convenient information time commonly used in practice is derived from an approximation of $V(t) \simeq \omega_1\omega_2 d^0(t)$, where $d^0(t)$ is the observed total number of events for two groups at calendar time t. Hence the following information time can be used as an approximation of t^*:

$$t_{d^0}^* = d^0(t)/d^0(\tau). \tag{10.7}$$

However, $d^0(\tau)$ is also unknown until the end of the study. We can replace $d^0(\tau)$ by the projected total number of events $\tilde{d} = (z_{1-\alpha} + z_{1-\beta})^2/\{\omega_1\omega_2[\log(\delta)]^2\}$. One way to overcome this difficulty is to design the trial as an event-driven trial. That is, the trial accrual is stopped when the projected number of events has been observed.

Lan and Zucker (1993) proposed an information for the log-rank test at calendar time t given by

$$I(t) = \left(\frac{1}{n_1(t)} + \frac{1}{n_2(t)}\right)^{-1} \frac{d(t)}{n(t)}, \tag{10.8}$$

where $d(t)$ is the expected total number of events in two groups at time t, $n_i(t)$ is the sample size at time t in the ith group, and $n(t) = n_1(t) + n_2(t)$. Only when a subject has had an event by time t, the information of their survival is complete. Thus, we can modify $I(t)$ in (10.8) by replacing $n_i(t)$ by $d_i(t)$ and $n(t)$ by $d(t) = d_1(t) + d_2(t)$; then,

$$I(t) \simeq \left(\frac{1}{d_1(t)} + \frac{1}{d_2(t)}\right)^{-1}, \tag{10.9}$$

where $d_i(t)$ is the expected number of events by time t in the ith group, $i = 1, 2$. Thus, the information time $t^* = V(t)/V(\tau) \simeq I(t)/I(\tau)$ at calendar time t can be approximated by

$$t_D^* = D(t)/D(\tau), \tag{10.10}$$

where $D(t) = (d_1^{-1}(t) + d_2^{-1}(t))^{-1}$ and $D(\tau) = (d_1^{-1}(\tau) + d_2^{-1}(\tau))^{-1}$.

To calculate the information time defined by (11.11) under a uniform accrual, the expected number of events in the ith group up to time t can be calculated by $d_i(t) = n\omega_i p_i(t)$, where

$$p_i(t) \quad = \quad \frac{1}{t_a} \int_0^{t \wedge t_a} \{1 - S_i(t-u)\} du \qquad (10.11)$$

and $D(\tau) = (z_{1-\alpha} + z_{1-\beta})^2/[\log(\delta)]^2$. Here, the survival distribution $S_1(t)$ for the control group can be estimated from historical data by a parametric survival distribution or a spline version of the survival distribution without a specific model assumption, and $S_2(t) = [S_1(t)]^\delta$ under the PH model assumption.

If the trial is planned as an event-driven trial with K interim analyses, that is the trial stops accrual when $d_K = d_{1K} + d_{2K}$ events have been observed, and assuming the kth interim look is planned for when $d_k = d_{1k} + d_{2k}$ events have occurred, where $k = 1, \ldots, K$, then the information time at the kth interim look can be calculated by

$$t_k^* = D_k/D_K, \qquad (10.12)$$

where $D_k = (d_{1k}^{-1} + d_{2k}^{-1})^{-1}$ and $D_K = (d_{1K}^{-1} + d_{2K}^{-1})^{-1}$. Note: It is easy to see that $D_K = (z_{1-\alpha} + z_{1-\beta})^2/[\log(\delta)]^2$.

Example 10.2 *A clinical trial for carcinoma of the oropharynx*

We will illustrate the information time calculation by using the data from a clinical trial conducted by the Radiation Therapy Oncology Group in the United States to investigate treatments of carcinoma of the oropharynx. We will use the data from six of the larger institutions that participated in this trial, as recorded by Kalbfleisch and Prentice (2002, Appendix II). Subjects were recruited to the study between 1968 and 1972 and randomized to a standard radiotherapy treatment (group C) or an experimental treatment in which the radiotherapy was supplemented by chemotherapy (group E). The major endpoint was patient survival, and patients were followed until around the end of 1973.

The conduct of the study did not follow a group sequential plan but, for purposes of illustration, Jennison and Turnbull (2000) have reconstructed the patient survival data for five interim analyses at times 720, 1080, 1440, 1800, and 2160 days from the beginning of 1968. This reconstructed data is presented in Table 10.2. We use formula (10.12) to calculate the information times at each interim analysis, and these are shown in the last column of Table 10.2. For example, the information time at the first interim look $k = 1$ can be calculated as

$$t_1^* = (1/13 + 1/14)^{-1}/(1/69 + 1/73)^{-1} = 0.190.$$

TABLE 10.2: Information times for carcinoma trial

	Analysis	Number of Patients		Number of Deaths		Information Time
k	Date	$n_{E,k}$	$n_{C,k}$	$d_{E,k}$	$d_{C,k}$	t_k^*
1	12/69	38	45	13	14	0.190
2	12/70	56	70	30	28	0.408
3	12/71	81	93	44	47	0.641
4	12/72	95	100	63	66	0.908
5	12/73	95	100	69	73	1.000

10.3.3 SCPRT for the PH Model

To develop a group sequential method for the sequential log-rank test statistic $L(t)$, we will apply the SCPRT procedure presented in Chapter 9. Because the required sample size for the sequential test using the SCPRT is the same as for the reference fixed sample test, the total sample size for a sequential trial design based on the log-rank test can be calculated by the Schoenfeld formula or by one of the other formulae discussed in previous chapters. Note that $L(t) = U(t)/V^{1/2}(t) = B_{t^*}/\sqrt{t^*}$; thus, we need only apply the SCPRT procedure to the test statistic $B_{t^*} = U(t)/V^{1/2}(\tau) \sim N(\theta t^*, t^*)$, which is a Brownian motion in information time $t^* = V(t)/V(\tau)$ over $[0, 1]$, and the drift parameter $\theta = -\log(\delta)V^{1/2}(\tau)$. The information time $t^* = V(t)/V(\tau)$ is a random variable and is unknown until the end of the study; however, it can be estimated by

$$t_D^* = D(t)/D(\tau), \tag{10.13}$$

where

$$D(t) = n\left(\frac{1}{\omega_1 p_1(t)} + \frac{1}{\omega_2 p_2(t)}\right)^{-1}$$

and $D(\tau) = (z_{1-\alpha} + z_{1-\beta})^2/[\log(\delta)]^2$. Suppose that a total of K interim looks are planned at calendar time $t_1, \ldots, t_K$. Then, based on the SCPRT procedure, the symmetric lower and upper boundaries for $B_{t_k^*}$ at the kth look are given by

$$a_k = z_{1-\alpha}t_k^* - \{2at_k^*(1 - t_k^*)\}^{1/2}; \quad b_k = z_{1-\alpha}t_k^* + \{2at_k^*(1 - t_k^*)\}^{1/2},$$

for $k = 1, \ldots, K$, where $t_k^* = D(t_k)/D(\tau)$ is the information time at the kth look at calendar time t_k. The nominal critical p-values for testing H_0 are

$$P_{\bar{a}_k} = 1 - \Phi(\bar{a}_k); \quad P_{\bar{b}_k} = 1 - \Phi(\bar{b}_k),$$

where $\bar{a}_k = a_k/\sqrt{t_k^*}$ and $\bar{b}_k = b_k/\sqrt{t_k^*}$ are the boundaries of $L(t_k)$. The observed p-value at the kth look for the test statistic $L(t)$ is given by

$$P_{L_{t_k}} = 1 - \Phi(B_{t_k^*}/\sqrt{t_k^*}) = 1 - \Phi(L_{t_k}).$$

where $L_{t_k} = L(t_k)$. The stopping rule for monitoring the trial can be executed by stopping the trial when, for the first time, $P_{L_{t_k}} \geq P_{\bar{a}_k}$ (accept H_0 and stop for futility) or $P_{L_{t_k}} \leq P_{\bar{b}_k}$ (reject H_0 and stop for efficacy) (Wu and Xiong, 2017).

Example 10.3 *Continuation of Example 10.2*

We will use Example 10.2 to illustrate the SCPRT boundary calculation. First, we input the information time $t^* = (0.190, 0.408, 0.641, 0.908, 1.000)$ into the user-friendly software SCPRTinfWin (Xiong, 2007), with a maximum conditional probability of discordance of $\rho = 0.02$, to calculate the boundary coefficient $a = 3.209$ for a 5-stage group sequential design with an unequally spaced information time and a one-sided type I error of $\alpha = 0.05$. SCPRT-infWin calculates the lower and upper boundaries and the nominal critical p-values, which are shown in Table 10.3.

Example 10.4 *Sequential Survival Trial Design*

To illustrate randomized phase III survival trial design with unbalanced treatment allocation and compare it to the commonly used method implemented in the commercially available software EAST 6, let us assume that the overall survival is exponentially distributed for both the control and treatment groups. Assume that the 3-year survival probability for the control group is 50%, and that investigators expect the treatment might improve the 3-year survival probability to 60%, and that there is a uniform accrual with accrual period $t_a = 5$ (years), follow-up time $t_f = 3$ (years), and study duration $\tau = 8$ (years). Also assume that no subjects are lost to follow-up and that 30% of patients are randomized to the control group and 70% of patients to the treatment group. Then, the trial can be designed to detect a hazard ratio of $\delta = \log(0.6)/\log(0.5) = 0.737$ for the one-sided hypothesis with type I error of 0.05 and power of 90%. Thus, the total number of deaths and the sample size calculated for a fixed sample test using the Schoenfeld formula (the same as calculated in EAST) are $d_S(\tau) = 438$ and $N_S = 697$, and by the Rubinstein formula they are $d_R = 413$ and $N_R = 656$. Now suppose that the trial will be monitored for both futility (reject H_1) and efficacy (reject H_0) based on a 7-stage group sequential design at calendar time $t = 2, 3, 4, 5, 6, 7$ and 8 years. Then, the traditional information times calculated by (10.7) are $t_{d^0}^* = (0.106, 0.225, 0.378, 0.559, 0.735, 0.880, 1.000)$. If we input this information time into EAST, the total number of deaths and the sample size required for this 7-stage group sequential design increase to 499 and 794, respectively, by using the O'Brien-Fleming boundaries and to 664 and 1057, respectively, by using the Pocock boundaries. The information times calculated by (10.10) are $t_D^* = (0.109, 0.231, 0.386, 0.568, 0.743, 0.885, 1.000)$, and the required number of deaths and the sample size for the SCPRT are the same as for the fixed sample test. The symmetric Pocock and O'Brien-Fleming boundaries and boundary crossing probabilities calculated in EAST by using Lan-DeMets error spend-

TABLE 10.3: Sequential boundaries and nominal significance levels for a carcinoma trial

k	Date	$d_{E,k}$	$d_{C,k}$	t_k^*	a_k	b_k	$\bar{a}_k$	$\bar{b}_k$	P_{a_k}	P_{b_k}
1	12/69	13	14	0.190	-0.681	1.306	-1.562	2.996	0.9410	0.0014
2	12/70	30	28	0.408	-0.574	1.916	-0.899	2.999	0.8156	0.0014
3	12/71	44	47	0.641	-0.161	2.270	-0.201	2.835	0.5797	0.0023
4	12/72	63	66	0.908	0.761	2.226	0.799	2.336	0.2122	0.0098
5	12/73	69	73	1.000	1.645	1.645	1.645	1.645	0.0500	0.0500

ing functions are given in Table 10.4. On using the SCPRT, implemented in the user-friendly software SCPRTinfWin (Xiong, 2007), a probability of discordance of $\rho = 0.02$ is given, with a maximum probability of discordance of $\rho_{max} = 0.0056$, to calculate the boundary coefficient $a = 3.496$ for a 7-stage group sequential design with an unequally spaced information time. Inputting the number of interim looks $K = 7$ and the information time t_D^* at each stage into SCPRTinfWin gives the symmetric group sequential futility and efficacy boundaries and boundary crossing probabilities shown in Table 10.4. The actual significance level and power for this 7-stage group sequential design based on the SCPRT are 0.051 and 0.899, respectively, and are very close to the nominal levels of type I error of 5% and power of 90%. The expected sample size, study duration, and number of events under the alternative H_1 calculated from EAST 6 and SCPRTinfWin are also shown in Table 10.4. The operating characteristics of the three designs can be summarized as follows. First, the SCPRT requires the smallest maximum sample size and smallest maximum number of deaths, which are the same as for the fixed sample test. Second, the SCPRT also requires the smallest expected sample size. However, Pocock's method requires the smallest expected study duration and expected number of deaths, and O'Brien-Fleming's method requires the expected study duration to be larger than that required for the Pocock's method but smaller than that for the SCPRT. This is because Pocock's method has the highest stopping probabilities in the early stages, O'Brien-Fleming's method has the highest stopping probabilities in the middle stages, and the SCPRT has the highest stopping probabilities in the later stages of the trial.

Overall, the group sequential design based on the SCPRT enabled a smaller number of patients to be enrolled in the study when compared to methods implemented in EAST. The SCPRT has two advantages over other sequential methods. First, the maximum sample size of the SCPRT is the same as that for the fixed sample test, whereas other methods require the sample size to be increased. Second, the probability of discordance can be controlled to an arbitrarily low level, whereas it cannot be prespecified at the design stage when using other sequential procedures. The R function 'SCPRTinf' is given below to calculate the SCPRT boundaries, crossing probabilities and stopping probabilities under the null and alternative, respectively.

```
############################ Input parameters ############################
### ts is the information time; a is boundary coefficient which can be    ###
### calculated by using SCPRTinfWin software;                             ###
### alpha and beta are the type I error and type II error.                ###
##########################################################################
library(mvtnorm)
SCPRTinf=function(ts, a, alpha, beta){
 k=length(ts)
 z0=qnorm(1-alpha)
 z1=qnorm(1-beta)
 lb=ub=NULL
 for (i in 1:k){
```

TABLE 10.4: Operating characteristics of a 7-stage group sequential design based on the Pocock and O'Brien-Fleming boundaries and using the Lan-DeMets error spending function implemented in EAST and the SCPRT procedure for Example 10.4

	Pocock				O'Brien-Fleming				SCPRT			
	Boundaries		Stopping Prob.		Boundaries		Stopping Prob.		Boundaries		Stopping Prob.	
	Reject		Under		Reject		Under		Reject		Under	
t	H_0	H_1	H_0	H_1	H_0	H_1	H_0	H_1	H_0	H_1	H_0	H_1
2	2.393	-0.953	0.179	0.128	5.907	-3.901	0.000	0.000	3.039	-1.953	0.027	0.021
3	2.316	-0.313	0.247	0.203	3.970	-1.795	0.036	0.007	3.109	-1.528	0.050	0.037
4	2.219	0.315	0.261	0.255	2.984	-0.522	0.267	0.144	3.094	-1.050	0.096	0.069
5	2.150	0.889	0.185	0.217	2.396	0.384	0.362	0.356	2.978	-0.498	0.169	0.128
6	2.124	1.351	0.087	0.122	2.064	0.997	0.208	0.287	2.759	0.077	0.218	0.189
7	2.125	1.716	0.032	0.053	1.887	1.400	0.090	0.143	2.444	0.651	0.204	0.215
8	2.129	2.129	0.010	0.021	1.777	1.777	0.037	0.062	1.645	1.645	0.236	0.341
	N_{max} 1057	D_{max} 8.0	d_{max} 664		N_{max} 794	D_{max} 8.0	d_{max} 499		N_{max} 656	D_{max} 8.0	d_{max} 413	
	$E[N_a(T)]$ 836	$E(T)$ 4.25	$E[d(T)]$ 289		$E[N_a(T)]$ 769	$E(T)$ 5.61	$E[d(T)]$ 326		$E[N_a(T)]$ 628	$E(T)$ 6.4	$E[d(T)]$ 323	

```
   lb[i]=(z0*ts[i]-(2*a*ts[i]*(1-ts[i]))^(1/2))/sqrt(ts[i])
   ub[i]=(z0*ts[i]+(2*a*ts[i]*(1-ts[i]))^(1/2))/sqrt(ts[i])}
covmatrix=matrix(rep(0,(k+1)*(k+1)),ncol=k+1,byrow=T)
tij=c(0, ts)
for (i in 1:(k+1)) {
 for (j in 1:(k+1)) {
  covmatrix[i,j]=(1/2)*(tij[i]+tij[j]-(abs(tij[i]-tij[j])))/sqrt(tij[i]*tij[j])}}
### calculate nominal incremental boundary crossing probabilities #####
### 1. under the null ### 1.1 efficacy
pce0=NULL
pce0[1]=1-pnorm(ub[1])
for (i in 2:k){
 covm=covmatrix[2:(i+1),2:(i+1)]
 pce0[i]=pmvnorm(lower=c(lb[1:(i-1)],ub[i]),upper=c(ub[1:(i-1)],Inf),
 sigma=covm)[1]}
### 1.2 futility
pcf0=NULL
pcf0[1]=pnorm(lb[1])
for (i in 2:k){
 covm=covmatrix[2:(i+1),2:(i+1)]
 pcf0[i]=pmvnorm(lower=c(lb[1:(i-1)],-Inf),upper=c(ub[1:(i-1)],lb[i]),
 sigma=covm)[1]}
### calculate nominal incremental boundary crossing probabilities #####
### 2. under the alternative ### 2.1 efficacy
etam=z0+z1
pce1=NULL
pce1[1]=1-pnorm(ub[1],mean=etam*sqrt(ts[1]))
for (i in 2:k){
 lmean=etam*sqrt(ts[1:i])
 covm=covmatrix[2:(i+1),2:(i+1)]
 pce1[i]=pmvnorm(lower=c(lb[1:(i-1)],ub[i]),upper=c(ub[1:(i-1)],Inf),
 mean=lmean,sigma=covm)[1]}
### 2.2 futility
pcf1=NULL
pcf1[1]=pnorm(lb[1],mean=etam*sqrt(ts[1]))
for (i in 2:k){
 lmean=etam*sqrt(ts[1:i])
 covm=covmatrix[2:(i+1),2:(i+1)]
 pcf1[i]=pmvnorm(lower=c(lb[1:(i-1)],-Inf),upper=c(ub[1:(i-1)],lb[i]),
 mean=lmean,sigma=covm)[1]}
SL=EP=SP0=SP1=NULL
for (i in 1:k){
  SL[i]=pce0[i]
  EP[i]=pce1[i]
  SP0[i]=pce0[i]+pcf0[i]
  SP1[i]=pce1[i]+pcf1[i]}
SL[k+1]=sum(SL); SL=round(SL,4)
EP[k+1]=sum(EP); EP=round(EP,4)
SP0[k+1]=sum(SP0); SP0=round(SP0,4)
SP1[k+1]=sum(SP1); SP1=round(SP1,4)
ans=list(lb=round(lb,4),ub=round(ub,4),SL=SL,EP=EP,SP0=SP0,SP1=SP1)
return(ans)}
SCPRTinf(ts=c(.109,.231,.386,.568,.743,.885,1),a=3.496,alpha=0.05,beta=0.1)
$lb  ## lower bound #
-1.9529 -1.5282 -1.0500 -0.4983  0.0773  0.6507  1.6449
$ub  ## upper bound #
3.0390 3.1094 3.0939 2.9776 2.7583 2.4441 1.6449
```

```
$SL  ## upper boundary crossing probabilty under the null ##
0.0012 0.0008 0.0007 0.0010 0.0019 0.0047 0.0409 0.0513
$EP  ## upper boundary crossing probabilty under the alternative ##
0.0191 0.0351 0.0675 0.1258 0.1845 0.2041 0.2625 0.8986
$SP0 ## stopping probability under the null ##
0.0266 0.0504 0.0964 0.1686 0.2178 0.2042 0.2360 1.0000
$SP1 ## stopping probability under the alternative ##
0.0208 0.0365 0.0690 0.1282 0.1892 0.2151 0.3411 1.0000
```

11

Sequential Survival Trial Design Using Historical Controls

11.1   Introduction

Randomized clinical trials (RCTs) are the gold standard for clinical trials comparing treatment groups. When randomization is not feasible because of ethical concerns, patient preference, or regulatory acceptability, historical control trials (HCTs) are an alternative. A strong argument for using HCTs is that all patients can receive the new treatment. The major benefits of HCTs include their contribution to medical knowledge and the potential cost savings with respect to sample size and length of study. However, HCTs may suffer from patient selection bias because patients with more favorable prognoses may be more likely to be selected to receive the new treatment. HCTs may also suffer from outcome evaluation bias due to changes in the experimental environment, as well as in technology, and have been criticized accordingly (Pocock, 1976; Gehan, 1982; Gehan and Freireich, 1981).

Despite these facts, HCTs have been widely applied in clinical research. In randomized trials, factors such as age, race, and gender that may be confounded with treatment effects are balanced with respect to their marginal or joint frequencies in the control and experimental groups through randomization. Obviously, an HCT lacks this mechanism and, hence, in the application of HCTs, it is important to make sure that the patient eligibility criteria for the experimental group are the same as or at least similar to those of the historical control study. If it is not possible to guarantee minimal selection bias in the design phase, or it is difficult to implement balance in the trial process, the potential confounding effects of factors with unbalanced frequencies should be investigated in later analyses.

Sample size calculations for designing HCTs have been discussed by Makuch and Simon (1980) for binary endpoints and by Dixon and Simon (1988) and Emrich (1989) for exponential survival endpoints. When assessing the power of these designs, these authors assumed the true control treatment effect to be equal to the observed effect in the historical control group. However, Korn and Freidlin (2006) reported that these popular methods do not preserve the power and type I error when considering the uncertainty in the historical control data. Several publications have discussed sample size calculations for HCTs by taking into account the uncertainty in the true historical control treatment effect (Chang et al., 1999; Xiong et al., 2007).

HCTs are often monitored by interim analysis in order to stop accrual if patients in the experimental group have poorer outcomes than those in the historical control group. Monitoring clinical trials with historical controls poses a statistical problem of comparing two outcomes in a situation wherein data from the experimental group are sequentially collected and compared with all data from historical controls at each interim analysis. Thus, the widely used variable information time, defined as the ratio of the number of events to be observed at an interim analysis to the total number of events in the entire trial (Lan and Lachin, 1990), is not appropriate for HCTs. A few studies have examined the monitoring of clinical trials that use historical controls. For example, Chang et al. (1999) proposed a two-stage design for binary outcomes and Xiong et al. (2007) developed a multistage group sequential procedure for monitoring HCTs with binary, continuous, and survival endpoints. However, the sample size and information time calculations developed by Xiong at al. (2007) for survival endpoints are not convenient for such an application. Recently, Wu and Xiong (2016) have developed a convenient group sequential procedure to design survival HCTs, wherein a sequential log-rank test using historical controls is defined. Based on this sequential log-rank test, we derived sample size calculations for sequential HCT designs. Furthermore, a transformed information time was derived to define the sequential boundary based on the SCPRT procedure.

11.2 Sequential Log-Rank Test with Historical Controls

Suppose there are two groups, a historical control group and an experimental group, designated as group 1 and group 2, respectively. Assuming the survival distributions of the two groups satisfy the proportional hazards model

$$S_2(t) = [S_1(t)]^\delta, \tag{11.1}$$

where δ is the unknown hazard ratio, the hypothesis of improvement in the survival distribution of the treatment group as compared to that of the historical control group, can be expressed as

$$H_0 : \delta \geq 1 \quad \text{vs.} \quad H_1 : \delta < 1. \tag{11.2}$$

A well-known test statistic for the above hypothesis is the log-rank test. We introduce a sequential log-rank test statistic for HCTs as follows. Suppose there are k distinct event (or failure) times, $t_1 < t_2 \cdots < t_k$, among the two groups. An event time is measured from the time of enrollment in the study to the time of an event for a patient. At an event time t_j, d_{1j} events occur for the historical control group and d_{2j} events occur for the experimental group, with n_{1j} and n_{2j} subjects being at risk in the two groups, respectively, just before t_j. Thus, there are $d_j = d_{1j} + d_{2j}$ events at t_j among a total of $n_j = n_{1j} + n_{2j}$ subjects. Let τ be the study duration for the experimental group and t $(< \tau)$ be the calendar time from the start of study enrollment to the interim look, and let $n_{2j}(t)$ and $d_{2j}(t)$ represent, respectively, the parts of n_{2j} and d_{2j} with calendar times of entry no later than t. Let $n_j(t) = n_{1j} + n_{2j}(t)$, $d_j(t) = d_{1j} + d_{2j}(t)$, and $e_{2j}(t) = n_{2j}(t)d_j(t)/n_j(t)$. Then, the log-rank score at an interim look at calendar time t is

$$U(t) = \sum_{j=1}^{r} \{e_{2j}(t) - d_{2j}(t)\}, \tag{11.3}$$

which is approximately normal, with a mean of $-\log(\delta)V(t)$ and variance of $V(t)$, where the variance $V(t)$ is given by

$$V(t) = \sum_{j=1}^{k} \frac{n_{1j}n_{2j}(t)d_j(t)(n_j(t) - d_j(t))}{n_j^2(t)(n_j(t) - 1)}.$$

The sequential log-rank test at calendar time t is given by

$$L(t) = U(t)/V^{1/2}(t). \tag{11.4}$$

Then, $B_{t^*} = U(t)/V^{1/2}(\tau) \sim N(\theta t^*, t^*)$ is approximately a Brownian motion with drift parameter $\theta = -\log(\delta)V^{1/2}(\tau)$ and information time $t^* = V(t)/V(\tau)$, where $V(\tau)$ is the value of $V(t)$ at $t = \tau$. The difference between the two-sample sequential log-rank test and the historical control sequential log-rank test is that at an interim analysis, the two-sample sequential log-rank test uses only the data up to the calendar time t from both groups, whereas the sequential log-rank test for the HCTs uses all the data from the historical control group but only the data up to time t from the experimental group.

Remark 1: Because the sequential log-rank test for HCTs uses all the data from the historical control group but only the data up to time t from the experimental group, the sequential log-rank test $L(t)$ has to be defined by using the observed and expected number of events from the treatment group. Thus, definition of the log-rank score (11.3) using expected minus observed number of events is to make its sign the same as the log-rank test defined in previous chapters.

11.2.1 Sample Size Calculation

For a randomized two-arm trial, we have shown that the expected number of events in each group satisfies

$$D_1(\tau)^{-1} + D_2(\tau)^{-1} = \frac{[\log(\delta)]^2}{(z_{1-\alpha} + z_{1-\beta})^2} \tag{11.5}$$

for the log-rank test statistic (the Rubinstein formula). Because the historical control data are obtained from previous trials, the total number of events $D_1 = D_1(\tau)$ for the historical control group is known. Therefore, to design a historical control trial, we need only calculate the number of events or sample size for the experimental group by assuming no further follow-up for the historical control group or that the historical control data were frozen at the design stage. Thus, for HCTs, the sample size formula (11.5) can be written as

$$D_1^{-1} + D_2^{-1}(\tau) = \frac{[\log(\delta)]^2}{(z_{1-\alpha} + z_{1-\beta})^2}, \tag{11.6}$$

where D_1 is the total number of events observed in the historical control data, which is known, and $D_2(\tau)$ is the expected total number of events for the experimental group. The expected total number of events for the experimental group, based on the log-rank test $L(\tau)$, can be solved by equation (11.6) as

$$D_2(\tau) = \left\{ \frac{[\log(\delta)]^2}{(z_{1-\alpha} + z_{1-\beta})^2} - D_1^{-1} \right\}^{-1}, \tag{11.7}$$

and the sample size for the experimental group is given by

$$n_2 = D_2(\tau)/p_2(\tau), \tag{11.8}$$

where $p_2(\tau)$ is the probability of a subject from the experimental group having an event during the study.

To calculate the sample size using formula (11.8), we have to calculate $p_2(\tau)$. We assume that subjects are recruited with a uniform distribution over the accrual period t_a and are followed for time t_f and that the study duration is $\tau = t_a + t_f$. We further assume that no subjects are lost to follow-up. Then the distribution of the censoring due to the distributed accrual is uniform over the interval $[t_f, t_a + t_f]$. Thus, $p_2(\tau)$ can be calculated by

$$p_2(\tau) = 1 - \frac{1}{t_a} \int_{t_f}^{t_a + t_f} S_2(t) dt, \tag{11.9}$$

where $S_2(t) = [S_1(t)]^\delta$ and $S_1(t)$ is the survival distribution of the historical control group, which can be estimated from the historical data by a parametric survival distribution, a Kaplan-Meier curve, or a spline version of the survival distribution without a specific model assumption.

11.2.2 Information Time

The information time $t^* = V(t)/V(\tau)$ derived from a randomized trial for the two-sample log-rank test cannot be used because $V(\tau)$ is unknown until the end of the study. The widely used information time defined as the ratio of the number of events to be observed at an interim analysis to the total number of events in the entire trial is not appropriate for HCTs because the total number of events in the historical controls is known and remains the same at each stage of the interim analysis. However, as we discussed in previous chapters, the information time $t^* = V(t)/V(\tau)$ can be approximated by

$$t_D^* = D(t)/D(\tau), \tag{11.10}$$

where $D(t) = (D_1^{-1}(t) + D_2^{-1}(t))^{-1}$ and $D_i(t)$ is the expected number of events by time t in the ith group.

For HCTs, at calendar time t of an interim analysis, the data cumulated up to time t from the experimental group are compared to all the data from the historical controls. Thus, D_1 is not dependent on the time of an interim analysis. Therefore, we can calculate the information time at the planned calendar time t for the interim analysis by the formula $t_D^* = D(t)/D(\tau)$, where $D(t) = (D_1^{-1} + D_2^{-1}(t))^{-1}$ and $D(\tau) = (D_1^{-1} + D_2^{-1}(\tau))^{-1}$, which can be rewritten as

$$t_D^* = \frac{(1+\xi)I}{1+\xi I}, \tag{11.11}$$

where $I = D_2(t)/D_2(\tau)$ is the information time for the experimental group and $\xi = D_2(\tau)/D_1$ is the ratio of the projected number of events for the experimental group to the observed number of events for the historical control group. The information time t_D^* combining the information from the experimental group and the historical control group is called the transformed information time. Because D_1 is known from the historical control data, the information time t_D^* can be estimated by letting $D_2(t) = n_2 p_2(t)$, which is the expected number of events in the experimental group up to time t, where $p_2(t)$ can be calculated by the following equation under the uniform accrual distribution:

$$p_2(t) = \frac{1}{t_a} \int_0^{t \wedge t_a} \{1 - S_2(t-u)\} du, \tag{11.12}$$

where $S_2(t) = [S_1(t)]^\delta$.

If the trial is designed as a maximum information trial, that is, the trial will continue until a pre-specified number of events $D_2(\tau)$ has been observed for the experimental group, then the information time at the kth look planned at the number of events D_{2k} for the experimental group can be calculated by

$$t_k^* = \frac{(1+\xi)I_k}{1+\xi I_k}, \tag{11.13}$$

where $I_k = D_{2k}/D_2(\tau)$ and $\xi = D_2(\tau)/D_1$. Given t_k^* and using equation (11.11) in reverse, we can obtain the calendar time t_k at the kth stage corresponding to the information time t_k^*. As shown in a later example, the calendar time t_k of the kth stage is indicative for calculating the sequential test statistic $L(t_k)$ by (11.4).

11.2.3   Group Sequential Procedure

In this section, we will apply an SCPRT procedure (Xiong, 1995) to the log-rank test $L(t)$ to derive the sequential boundaries for HCTs. The SCPRT sequential design based on information time has been implemented in a user-friendly software, SCPRTinfWin, developed by Xiong (2007).

We apply the SCPRT to the test statistic $B_{t^*} = U(t)/V^{1/2}(\tau) \sim N(\theta t^*, t^*)$, which is a Brownian motion in information time $t^* = V(t)/V(\tau)$ on $[0, 1]$, and the drift parameter $\theta = -\log(\delta)V^{1/2}(\tau)$. The sequential boundaries are given by

$$a_k = z_{1-\alpha}t_k^* - \{2at_k^*(1-t_k^*)\}^{1/2}; \quad b_k = z_{1-\alpha}t_k^* + \{2at_k^*(1-t_k^*)\}^{1/2} \tag{11.14}$$

for $k = 1, ..., K$, where $t_k^* = V(t_k)/V(\tau)$ is the information time which can be estimated by information time defined by equation (11.11) at the kth look at calendar time t_k. The nominal critical p-values for testing H_0 are

$$P_{\bar{a}_k} = 1 - \Phi(\bar{a}_k); \quad P_{\bar{b}_k} = 1 - \Phi(\bar{b}_k),$$

where $\bar{a}_k = a_k/\sqrt{t_k^*}$ and $\bar{b}_k = b_k/\sqrt{t_k^*}$ are the boundaries of $L(t_k)$. The observed p-value at the kth look can be calculated from the test statistic $L(t_k)$ by applying all observations up to stage k:

$$P_{L_{t_k}} = 1 - \Phi(L_{t_k}),$$

where $L_{t_k} = L(t_k)$. The stopping rule for the trial can be executed by stopping the trial when, for the first time, $P_{L_{t_k}} \geq P_{\bar{a}_k}$ (accept H_0 and stop for futility) or $P_{L_{t_k}} \leq P_{\bar{b}_k}$ (reject H_0 and stop for efficacy).

Remark 2: For HCTs, the trials are often stopped for futility; thus, a one-sided sequential boundary (lower boundary) should be used in this situation. The SCPRT procedure has the feature that part or all of its upper and lower sequential boundaries can be omitted with very little effect on its significance level and power of testing; only the expected sample size of the sequential design may be substantially changed. Therefore, one can simply omit the upper boundary to obtain a one-sided lower boundary for futility monitoring. However, in trials of a new drug, it is also important to know as early as possible if the trial is highly promising; thus, the upper boundary can serve as an efficacy report without the need to stop the trial.

Example 11.1 *Continuation of the PBC trial*

In this section, we illustrate a survival HCT design using the DPCA arm of the PBC trial (see Example 4.2) as our historical control group. The survival distribution of the DPCA arm was estimated by a Kaplan-Meier curve, and a logspline version of the survival distribution was fitted using the R function **oldlogspline** *(Figure 5.2). Assume that the survival distribution of the experimental group $S_2(t)$ satisfies the proportional hazards model*

$$S_2(t) = [S_1(t)]^\delta,$$

where δ is the hazard ratio of the historical control group vs. the experimental group. The study aim is to test the following hypothesis:

$$H_0 : \delta \geq 1 \quad vs. \quad H_1 : \delta < 1,$$

with significance level $\alpha = 0.05$ and power of $1 - \beta = 90\%$ to detect an alternative hazard ratio $\delta = 0.5714$. Thus, the required number of deaths is

$$D_2(\tau) = \left\{ \frac{[\log(0.5714)]^2}{(1.645 + 1.282)^2} - 65^{-1} \right\}^{-1} = 48.$$

To calculate the sample size, we assume that subjects are recruited with a uniform distribution over the accrual period $t_a = 5$ years and followed for a period of $t_f = 4$ years, with no subjects being lost to follow-up. Then, the censoring distribution incurred by delayed entries is a uniform distribution over the interval $[t_f, t_a + t_f]$. For a patient in group 2, the probability of death during the trial can be calculated by numerical integration using the spline version of the survival distribution $S_1(t)$ as follows:

$$p_2(\tau) = 1 - \frac{1}{t_a} \int_{t_f}^{t_a + t_f} [S_1(t)]^{0.5714} dt = 0.239.$$

Thus, the trial requires enrollment of $n_2 = D_2(\tau)/p_2(\tau) = 201$ patients. The empirical power and type I error are 89.6% and 0.049, respectively, based on $100,000$ simulated trials from the fitted spline distribution. Suppose three interim looks are planned at 20, 30, and 48 events. Then, we have $\xi = D_2(\tau)/D_1 = 48/65 = 0.738$, $I_1 = D_{21}/D_2(\tau) = 20/48 = 0.417$, $I_2 = D_{22}/D_2(\tau) = 30/48 = 0.625$, and $I_3 = D_{23}/D_2(\tau) = 1$. Thus, the transformed information times calculated by the formula

$$t_k^* = \frac{(1 + \xi)I_k}{1 + \xi I_k}$$

are given as $t^* = (t_1^*, t_2^*, t_3^*) = (0.554, 0.743, 1)$. If we input the type I error $\alpha = 0.05$, power of $1 - \beta = 90\%$, number of interim looks $K = 3$ (including the final look), and information time $t^* = (0.554, 0.743, 1)$ at each stage in the software SCPRTinfWin, and given a maximum conditional discordance probability $\rho = 0.02$, the software can calculate the boundary coefficient $a = 2.595$, the lower boundaries $(\bar{a}_1, \bar{a}_2, \bar{a}_3) = (-0.297, 0.264, 1.645)$ and the upper boundaries $(\bar{b}_1, \bar{b}_2, \bar{b}_3) = (2.746, 2.572, 1.645)$ by (11.14), the nominal critical p-values for the lower boundaries $(P_{\bar{a}_1}, P_{\bar{a}_2}, P_{\bar{a}_3}) = (0.6168, 0.3963, 0.05)$, and those for the upper boundaries $(P_{\bar{b}_1}, P_{\bar{b}_2}, P_{\bar{b}_3}) = (0.0030, 0.0050, 0.05)$. To monitor the trial at the kth interim look, the survival data collected up to the kth interim look from the experimental group is combined with all the data from the historical control group to calculate the sequential test statistic $L_{t_k} = L(t_k)$ by (11.4), where t_k is the calendar time at the kth stage that is either being observed when the cumulative number of events has just reached the predetermined number *or is being calculated as described at the end of section 11.2.2. The observed p-values are*

$$P_{L_{t_k}} = 1 - \Phi(L_{t_k}), \quad k = 1, 2, 3.$$

At the kth stage, we stop the trial for futility if $P_{L_{t_k}} \geq P_{\bar{a}_k}$, and we stop the trial for efficacy (or report efficacy) if $P_{L_{t_k}} \leq P_{\bar{b}_k}$. The operating characteristics for the proposed three-stage group sequential design are shown in Table 11.1. The R functions for sample size and sequential boundaries calculation are given below for the historical control trial design.

```
############################## Input parameters ##############################
###   Input data datPBC can be obtained from the appendix D.1;            ###
###   D1 is the total number of events for the historical control;        ###
###   delta is the hazard ratio; ta and tf are the accrual/follow-up time; ###
###   alpha and beta are the type I error and type II error.              ###
##############################################################################
library(polspline)
time=datPBC$time
status=datPBC$status
fit=oldlogspline(time[status == 1], time[status == 0], lbound = 0)
F=function(x) {poldlogspline(x, fit)}
f=function(x) {doldlogspline(x, fit)}

SizeHC=function(D1,delta,ta,tf,alpha,beta)
{S1=function(t){ans=1-F(t)} ## historical control dist
 S2=function(t){ans=S1(t)^delta}
 tau=tf+ta
 z0=qnorm(1-alpha) ## one-sided test
 z1=qnorm(1-beta)
 D2=ceiling((log(delta)^2/(z0+z1)^2-1/D1)^(-1))
 p2=1-integrate(S2, tf, ta+tf)$value/ta
 n2=ceiling(D2/p2)
 return(c(D2=D2, n2=n2))}
SizeHC(D1=65,delta=0.5714,ta=5,tf=4,alpha=0.05,beta=0.1)
 D2  n2
 48 201


############################## Input parameters ##############################
###   Ds is the vector of number of events for planned interim analyses;  ###
###   D1 and D2 are the total number of events for the historical control ###
###   and treatment, respectively; ts is the transformed information time; ###
###   a is boundary coefficient which can be calculated by using SCPRTinfWin ###
###   software; alpha and beta are the type I error and type II error.    ###
##############################################################################
library(mvtnorm)
SCPRTinfTHC=function(Ds, D1, D2, a, alpha, beta){
 k=length(Ds)
 z0=qnorm(1-alpha)
 z1=qnorm(1-beta)
 xi=D2/D1
 I=ts=lb=ub=NULL
 for (i in 1:k){
   I[i]=Ds[i]/D2
   ts[i]=(1+xi)*I[i]/(1+xi*I[i])
   lb[i]=(z0*ts[i]-(2*a*ts[i]*(1-ts[i]))^(1/2))/sqrt(ts[i])
```

```
  ub[i]=(z0*ts[i]+(2*a*ts[i]*(1-ts[i]))^(1/2))/sqrt(ts[i])}
 covmatrix=matrix(rep(0,(k+1)*(k+1)),ncol=k+1,byrow=T)
 tij=c(0, ts)
 for (i in 1:(k+1)) {
  for (j in 1:(k+1)) {
  covmatrix[i,j]=0.5*(tij[i]+tij[j]-(abs(tij[i]-tij[j])))/sqrt(tij[i]*tij[j])}}
 ### calculate nominal incremental boundary crossing probabilities #####
 ### 1. under the null ### 1.1 efficacy
 pce0=NULL
 pce0[1]=1-pnorm(ub[1])
 for (i in 2:k){
  covm=covmatrix[2:(i+1),2:(i+1)]
  pce0[i]=pmvnorm(lower=c(lb[1:(i-1)],ub[i]),upper=c(ub[1:(i-1)],Inf),
  sigma=covm)[1]}
 ### 1.2 futility
 pcf0=NULL
 pcf0[1]=pnorm(lb[1])
 for (i in 2:k){
  covm=covmatrix[2:(i+1),2:(i+1)]
  pcf0[i]=pmvnorm(lower=c(lb[1:(i-1)],-Inf),upper=c(ub[1:(i-1)],lb[i]),
  sigma=covm)[1]}
 ### calculate nominal incremental boundary crossing probabilities #####
 ### 2. under the alternative ### 2.1 efficacy
 etam=z0+z1
 pce1=NULL
 pce1[1]=1-pnorm(ub[1],mean=etam*sqrt(ts[1]))
 for (i in 2:k){
  lmean=etam*sqrt(ts[1:i])
  covm=covmatrix[2:(i+1),2:(i+1)]
  pce1[i]=pmvnorm(lower=c(lb[1:(i-1)],ub[i]),upper=c(ub[1:(i-1)],Inf),
  mean=lmean,sigma=covm)[1]}
 ### 2.2 futility
 pcf1=NULL
 pcf1[1]=pnorm(lb[1],mean=etam*sqrt(ts[1]))
 for (i in 2:k){
  lmean=etam*sqrt(ts[1:i])
  covm=covmatrix[2:(i+1),2:(i+1)]
  pcf1[i]=pmvnorm(lower=c(lb[1:(i-1)],-Inf),upper=c(ub[1:(i-1)],lb[i]),
  mean=lmean,sigma=covm)[1]}
 SL=EP=SP0=SP1=NULL
 for (i in 1:k){
   SL[i]=pce0[i]
   EP[i]=pce1[i]
   SP0[i]=pce0[i]+pcf0[i]
   SP1[i]=pce1[i]+pcf1[i]}
 SL[k+1]=sum(SL); SL=round(SL,4)
 EP[k+1]=sum(EP); EP=round(EP,4)
 SP0[k+1]=sum(SP0); SP0=round(SP0,4)
 SP1[k+1]=sum(SP1); SP1=round(SP1,4)
 ans=list(ts=round(ts,4),lb=round(lb,4),ub=round(ub,4),SL=SL,EP=EP,
          SP0=SP0,SP1=SP1)
 return(ans)}
SCPRTinfTHC(Ds=c(20,30,48),D1=65,D2=48,a=2.595,alpha=0.05,beta=0.1)
$ts ## transformed information time #
0.5539 0.7434 1.0000
$lb ## lower bound #
-0.2974  0.2643  1.6449
```

```
$ub ## upper bound #
2.7458 2.5722 1.6449
$SL ## upper boundary crossing probabilty under the null ##
0.0030 0.0034 0.0440 0.0504
$EP ## upper boundary crossing probabilty under the alternative ##
0.2851 0.2125 0.4018 0.8995
$SP0 ## stopping probability under the null ##
0.3861 0.2400 0.3739 1.0000
$SP1 ## stopping probability under the alternative ##
0.2918 0.2205 0.4878 1.0000
```

11.3   Conclusion

In this chapter, we have derived the sample size calculation for survival HCTs. A transformed information time that is not only based on the information time of the experimental group but also uses the information from the historical control group has also been derived for trial monitoring. It is simple and convenient to use the transformed information time to derive the sequential boundaries for the HCTs based on the SCPRT procedure. With this monitoring procedure, data from the experimental group are sequentially collected and compared with all data from the historical control group. This allows investigators to monitor the trial at any calendar time during enrollment and follow-up or at the time a prespecified number of events is reached, which was predetermined as an interim look. A user-friendly software, SCPRTinfWin, is available for HCT design. For the purpose of study design, we need only the number of events from the historical control data in order to calculate the sample size. However, for trial monitoring and final data analysis, we need the full data from the historical control group to calculate the sequential test statistic. In practice, the historical control data are usually available from previous trials conducted by the same institution or sponsor. If no such historical control data is available, we need to extract the relevant data from the published literature. Guyot et al. (2012) have proposed a method to reconstruct the survival data from published Kaplan-Meier survival curves. Thus, designing survival trials with historical controls is feasible by using control data from the published literature.

   In an HCT trial, the distributions of covariates of patients may differ between the historical control group and the experimental group, and this difference may lead to bias in the results. One possible practical solution to prevent this bias is to first identify influential covariates of treatment effect through analysis of historical data and then enroll the experimental group according to the stratifications of the covariates identified from the historical control group. If the matched enrollment approach mentioned above is difficult or impossible to implement in the trial, then one may use the Cox regression model to adjust for confounding factors and the score test based on the partial likelihood can be used for testing.

TABLE 11.1: Operating characteristics of the three-stage historical control design for the sequential log-rank test $L(t)$ based on 10,000 simulation runs under the logspline distribution with uniform censoring distribution over $[t_f, t_a + t_f]$, nominal type I error of 0.05, and power of 90% for Example 11.1, where $t_a = 5$ and $t_f = 4$

At the kth interim look	$k = 1$	$k = 2$	$k = 3$	Total
Type I error				
Empirical of $L(t)$	0.0029	0.0034	0.0441	0.0504
Nominal	0.0030	0.0034	0.0440	0.0504
Power				
Empirical of $L(t)$	0.2385	0.2293	0.4257	0.8935
Nominal	0.2851	0.2125	0.4018	0.8995
Probability of stopping under the null				
Empirical of $L(t)$	0.3939	0.2352	0.3709	1.0000
Nominal	0.3861	0.2400	0.3739	1.0000
Probability of stopping under the alternative				
Empirical of $L(t)$	0.2460	0.2377	0.5163	1.0000
Nominal	0.2918	0.2205	0.4878	1.0000

12

Some Practical Issues in Survival Trial Design

Sample size calculations for survival trials are based on the test statistics, assumption of the underlying survival model, accrual distribution, design parameters, and treatment effect size. The aim of this chapter is to make the reader aware of the non-robustness of the test statistics, parametric survival distribution and proportional hazards model assumptions, and the sensitivity to the design parameters and accrual distribution of the sample size calculation. The most popular assumption for survival trial design is the exponential distribution or proportional hazards model with uniform accrual and no loss to follow-up and cross-over. Usually, these simplified assumptions reflect the reality closely enough that the methods produce reasonably accurate sample sizes. Many times, however, the complexity of cancer survival trials leads to violations of the assumptions that result in unacceptably inaccurate sample size calculations and severe power loss for the trials (Wittes, 2002). In the literature, some simple adjustments for loss to follow-up and cross-over treatments have been proposed. However, such simple adjustments are usually conservative and inaccurate. Formal sample size calculations for complex trial are available, e.g., the Lakatos Markov chain approach, and should be used for such survival trial design.

12.1 Parametric vs. Nonparametric Model

Sample size calculation under a parametric model, such as the exponential or Weibull model, is simple, and the parametric test statistic derived under the exponential or Weibull has better small sample properties and more power than the nonparametric log-rank test. However, it is restricted under the parametric model. Both the test statistics and sample size calculation are sensitive to the underlying model assumption. If the exponential or Weibull model is assumed, the validity of this assumption is quite critical for the power and sample size calculation. Given that even a slight deviation may cause a severe power loss (Abel et al. 2015), it is usually very difficult to justify the underlying distribution assumption. Thus, sample size formulae derived from the nonparametric log-rank test are frequently used for survival trial design, and sample size calculation under the nonparametric model, such as using a Kaplan-Meier curve or spline survival distribution, is preferred. The log-rank test is not sensitive to the underlying survival distribution assumption and the Kaplan-Meier curve or spline distribution makes no assumption of the parametric form.

12.2 Nonproportional Hazards Model

Sample size is usually calculated under the proportional hazards model assumption. However, the proportional hazards assumption can be violated because patients may not comply with the assigned treatment, resulting in noncompliance and drop-in which can cause the hazard rate to vary during the trial or due to delayed treatment effect. The Schoenfeld, Rubinstein, and Freedman formulae do not provide valid sample size calculations under the nonproportional hazards model. However, the Lakatos Markov chain approach is valid for the nonproportional hazards model and can adjust for noncompliance and drop-in, as well as for complex trial designs.

12.3 Accrual Patterns

The most commonly assumed accrual distribution used for trial design is the uniform accrual distribution. However, in practice, the accrual rate is hardly constant or piecewise constant throughout the accrual period. For example, in a phase III trial comparing adjuvant treatments for colon cancer, the accrual rate was not constant and showed an increasing pattern during the early period (Van Cutsem et al., 2009). Barthel et al. (2006) also gave examples of trials in which the actual accrual rates were higher in the later period of accrual. In contrast, for trials dealing with small populations or rare diseases, the limited number of cases can be exhausted quickly and further enrollment may slow down (Maki, 2006). Misspecification of the accrual pattern will result in an under- or overpowered study. Thus, during the design stage, one should identify the accrual pattern based on historical data, and then use the specified accrual distribution to calculate the sample size by either the Schoenfeld formula or the Lakatos Markov chain approach.

12.4 Mixed Populations

Failure to account for a true positive cure rate in a subgroup of patients when planning a trial may result in a very serious error. In particular, the conventional Schoenfeld approach is inadequate when planning a trial in which there is a positive cure rate, as in the adjuvant treatment of cancer. Instead, a sample size calculation developed under the proportional hazards mixture cure model should be employed for the trial design by using the weighted log-rank test.

12.5 Loss to Follow-Up

In survival trials, it is expected that some patients will be lost to follow-up due to their moving out of the country or ceasing to return for follow-up visits, etc. Under the random censorship model, it is assumed that these loss to follow-up times are random and independent of the failure times and treatment. Then, to achieve the desired power, the required sample size N^* is usually adjusted by a factor of $1/(1-r)$ from the calculated sample size N, without accounting for loss to follow-up (Donner, 1984), that is,

$$N^* = \frac{N}{1 - r},$$

where r is the rate (percentage) of loss to follow-up. However, such simple adjustment is conservative and inaccurate. For example, Table 12.1 presents the probabilities of loss to follow-up for the exponential model for the control $(\lambda_1 = 0.3)$ and treatment $(\lambda_2 = 0.2)$ for various loss to follow-up hazard rates of η in a study with equal allocation, accrual period $t_a = 3$, follow-up time $t_f = 2$, type I error of 5%, and power of 90%. Sample sizes unadjusted $(\eta = 0)$ and adjusted $(\eta \neq 0)$ for the loss to follow-up by using the Schoenfeld formula (N_S), Lakatos method (N_L), and simple adjustment $N_S^* = 368/(1 - r)$ are given in the last column of Table 12.1, where 368 is the sample size calculated by the Schoenfeld formula without adjustment for the loss to follow-up. This shows that the sample sizes calculated using simple adjustment are overestimated, particular when the rate of loss to follow-up is high. Thus, simple adjustment is conservative and not recommended for adjusting for loss to follow-up. Therefore, a formal sample size calculation, such as the Lakatos Markov chain method, which can adjust for the loss to follow-up, should be used.

TABLE 12.1: Probability of death and loss to follow-up with death hazard rate $\lambda_1 = 0.3$, $\lambda_2 = 0.2$ and various loss to follow-up hazard rates $\eta_1 = \eta_2 = \eta$; $t_a = 3$, $t_f = 2$, type I error of 5%, and power of 90% (equal allocation and one-sided test)

η	$E(\xi\|\lambda_1, \eta)$	$E(\xi\|\lambda_2, \eta)$	average (r)	N_S(EP)	N_L(EP)	N_S^*
0	0	0	0	368 (.896)	370 (.897)	368
0.025	0.051	0.060	0.056	382 (.899)	384 (.896)	390
0.05	0.099	0.115	0.107	397 (.903)	399 (.901)	413
0.075	0.143	0.166	0.155	411 (.901)	413 (.900)	436
0.10	0.185	0.213	0.199	426 (.902)	428 (.904)	460
0.125	0.223	0.256	0.240	441 (.897)	444 (.901)	484
0.15	0.259	0.297	0.278	457 (.899)	459 (.903)	510
0.175	0.292	0.334	0.313	472 (.899)	475 (.900)	536
0.20	0.324	0.369	0.347	488 (.897)	491 (.898)	564

Note: $E(\xi|\lambda_1, \eta)$ and $E(\xi|\lambda_2, \eta)$ are the probabilities of loss to follow-up for control and treatment, respectively; $r = \{E(\xi|\lambda_1, \eta) + E(\xi|\lambda_2, \eta)\}/2$; N_S, sample size calculated using the Schoenfeld formula; N_L, sample size calculated using the Lakatos formula; N_S^*, sample size calculated using simple adjustment; EP, empirical power based on 10,000 simulation runs.

12.6 Noncompliance and Drop-In

For both theoretical and practical reasons, one of the problems in randomized trials is noncompliance and/or drop-in. Patients who participate in trials do not always adhere to their assigned treatment. They may forget to take their assigned medicine; they may overdose; or they may stop taking their medication, either because they experience side effects or because they feel better. Noncompliance can dilute the treatment effect, resulting in a loss of power to detect differences between treatment groups. For example, if some patients cross over to the other treatment group, then the overall difference between the treatment groups could be altered. Therefore, the expected degree of noncompliance should be taken into account at the design stage. A typical approach to adjusting for noncompliance is based principally on the dilution of the expected value of the treatment effect, that is, inflating the sample size (N) by a factor of $1/(1 - \zeta_1 - \zeta_2)^2$, where ζ_1 and ζ_2 are the proportions of drop-in and noncompliant patients, respectively (Lachin and Foulkes, 1986), and

$$N^* = \frac{N}{(1 - \zeta_1 - \zeta_2)^2}.$$

However, this method will provide a conservative adjustment because a noncompliant patient in one group is assumed to be subject to the hazard rate

TABLE 12.2: Sample sizes under the exponential model after adjusting for drop-in and noncompliance

Case	HR	Π_1^C(%)	Π_2^C(%)	N_L	N^*
1	0.6	0	0	206	206
2	0.6	0	5	212	214
3	0.6	0	10	218	223
4	0.6	0	20	232	242
5	0.6	0	30	248	266
6	0.6	10	10	232	241
7	0.6	20	10	247	263
8	0.6	30	10	266	290
9	0.6	20	20	262	289
10	0.6	30	30	300	355

Note: HR, hazard ratio; Π_1^C, proportion of drop-in by end of trial; Π_2^C, proportion of noncompliance by end of trial; N_L, sample size calculated using the Lakatos formula; N^*, sample size calculated using simple adjustment.

for the other group over the entire study. Hence, this approach is also not recommended. The Lakatos Markov chain approach can be used for dealing with noncompliance by adjusting the expected overall event rate in each treatment group to take account of the noncompliance anticipated in the trial.

Example 12.1 *Adjusting drop-in and noncompliance*

Assume a randomized trial has two years of uniform accrual, two years of follow-up, exponential survival, and one-year median survival in the control group ($m_1 = 1$). Sample sizes are calculated for 90% power with a two-sided type I error of 5% and equal allocation. Other design parameters are given in Table 12.2, where HR is the hazard ratio in favor of the experimental group; and Π_1^C and Π_2^C are the proportions of drop-in and noncompliance by the end of the trial. We calculate the sample sizes by using the Lakatos Markov chain method (N_L) and by using simple adjustment (N^*), and the results are recorded in Table 12.2. It can be seen that the simple adjustment is conservative and overestimates the sample size.

12.7 Competing Risk

In survival data analysis, a patient may have several distinct causes of failure. For example, in cancer clinical trials, the endpoint of interest is time to death. Although death due to cancer is the primary interest, a patient may die from other causes not related to cancer, for example, car accident or cardiovascular disease. Death due to other causes is the competing event because it prevents the observation of any subsequent cancer-related death. The probability of failure of an event of interest can be altered when competing events exist. Thus, the sample size calculation in the absence of any competing event cannot be used directly when a competing event exists.

We will briefly introduce sample size calculation in the presence of competing risk. Let T be the time to failure, J be the cause of failure, and $J = 1$ denote the failure cause of interest; then, the cumulative incidence function or subdistribution for failure due to the cause of interest is defined by

$$F_1(t) = P(T \leq t, J = 1),$$

and the subdistribution hazard function $\lambda_1(t)$ is given by

$$\lambda_1(t) = -\frac{d\log\{1 - F_1(t)\}}{dt}.$$

Let $\lambda_{1E}(t)$ and $\lambda_{1C}(t)$ be the subdistribution hazard functions for the treatment and control groups, respectively. Assuming proportional subdistribution hazards leads to

$$\lambda_{1E}(t) = \delta_s \lambda_{1C}(t)$$

where δ_s is called the subdistribution hazard ratio. Then, the testing hypothesis for equal cumulative incidence functions between the treatment and control groups is the same as the following:

$$H_0 : \delta_s = 1 \quad vs. \quad H_1 : \delta_s \neq 1.$$

Gray's test (Gray, 1988) can be used to test the above hypothesis. Then, given two-sided type I error α and power of $1 - \beta$, the required number of events of interest can be calculated by

$$d = \frac{(z_{1-\alpha/2} + z_{1-\beta})^2}{\omega_1 \omega_2 [\log(\delta_s)]^2},$$

where ω_1 and $\omega_2 = 1 - \omega_1$ are the proportions of subjects assigned to the treatment and control groups, respectively. The total number of subjects n can be calculated by $n = d/P$, where P is the probability of observing the event of interest during the trial. To calculate P, let $F_{1C}(t)$ be the cumulative incidence function estimated from historical data and assume uniform accrual over interval $[0, t_a]$, and follow-up time t_f, with no loss of follow-up. Then, using Simpson's rule, the probability of observing the event of interest in the control during the trial is given by

$$P_C = \frac{1}{6}\{F_{1C}(t_f) + 4F_{1C}(0.5t_a + t_f) + F_{1C}(t_a + t_f)\}.$$

Under the proportional subdistribution hazards assumption, the cumulative incidence function of treatment is given by $F_{1E}(t) = 1 - [1 - F_{1C}(t)]^{\delta_s}$. Thus, similarly, the probability of observing the event of interest in the treatment group during the trial is given by

$$P_E = \frac{1}{6}\{F_{1E}(t_f) + 4F_{1E}(0.5t_a + t_f) + F_{1E}(t_a + t_f)\}.$$

Then, $P = w_1 P_E + w_2 P_C$ and the sample size $n = d/P$. For further details, please see Pintilie (2003) or the book by Pintilie (2006).

A

Likelihood Function for the Censored Data

Suppose that during the accrual phase of the trial n subjects are enrolled in the study, and let T_i and C_i denote, respectively, the event time and censoring time of the ith subject, both were measured from the entry time. Let us further assume that the event time T_i is independent of the censoring time C_i, and that $\{(Y_i, T_i); i = 1, \cdots, n\}$ are independent and identically distributed. we observe the time to event $X_i = T_i \wedge C_i$ and the event indicator $\Delta_i = I(T_i \leq C_i), i = 1, \cdots, n$. In general, we use the notations $f(t)$ and $S(t)$ to define the density and survival distribution functions of the event time T_i and we use $g(t)$ and $G(t)$ to define the density and survival distribution functions of the censoring time C_i. We then consider the probability distribution of the pair (X_i, Δ_i):

$$
\begin{aligned}
P(X_i = t_i, \Delta_i = 0) &= P(C_i = t_i, T_i > t_i) \\
&= P(C_i = t_i)P(T_i > t_i) \\
&= g(t_i)S(t_i)
\end{aligned}
$$

and

$$
\begin{aligned}
P(X_i = t_i, \Delta_i = 1) &= P(T_i = t_i, C_i > t_i) \\
&= P(T_i = t_i)P(C_i > t_i) \\
&= f(t_i)G(t_i)
\end{aligned}
$$

Thus, the likelihood of the observed data $\{X_i = t_i, \Delta_i; i = 1, \ldots, n\}$ is given by

$$
\prod_{i=1}^{n} \{g(t_i)S(t_i)\}^{1-\Delta_i}\{f(t_i)G(t_i)\}^{\Delta_i} = \prod_{i=1}^{n} g(t_i)^{1-\Delta_i}G(t_i)^{\Delta_i} \prod_{i=1}^{n} f(t_i)^{\Delta_i}S(t_i)^{1-\Delta_i}.
$$

Assuming non-informative censoring, the first product in this expression will not involve any parameters that are relevant to the distribution of the survival times, and so the product can be regarded as a constant. Hence, the likelihood is proportional to

$$
\prod_{i=1}^{n} f(X_i)^{\Delta_i} S(X_i)^{1-\Delta_i}.
$$

B

Probability of Failure under Uniform Accrual

Assume that subjects are accrued over an accrual period of length t_a, with an additional follow-up time t_f, the study duration $\tau = t_a + t_f$, and the entry time is uniformly distributed over $[0, t_a]$, with no patient loss to follow-up or drop out, Then, the censoring distribution $G(t)$ is a uniform distribution over the interval $[t_f, t_a + t_f]$, that is, $G(t) = 1$ if $t \le t_f$; $= (t_a + t_f - t)/t_a$ if $t_f \le t \le t_a + t_f$; $= 0$ otherwise. Note that $S(t) = \exp\{-\Lambda(t)\}$; and by performing integration calculations, we obtain

$$
\begin{aligned}
p &= \int_0^\infty G(t)S(t)d\Lambda(t) \\
&= \int_0^{t_f} S(t)d\Lambda(t) + \frac{1}{t_a}\int_{t_f}^\tau (\tau - t)S(t)d\Lambda(t) \\
&= -\int_0^{t_f} dS(t) - \frac{1}{t_a}\int_{t_f}^\tau (\tau - t)dS(t) \\
&= 1 - S(t_f) - \frac{\tau}{t_a}[S(\tau) - S(t_f)] + \frac{1}{t_a}\int_{t_f}^\tau t\, dS(t).
\end{aligned}
$$

By integration by parts,

$$
\int_{t_f}^\tau t\, dS(t) = \tau S(\tau) - t_f S(t_f) - \int_{t_f}^\tau S(t)dt.
$$

Substituting this into the previous equation, we obtain

$$
p = 1 - \frac{1}{t_a}\int_{t_f}^{t_a + t_f} S(t)dt.
$$

C

Verification of the Minimum Sample Size Conditions

Minimizing the sample size: It can be shown that

$$
\frac{1}{\omega_1 p_1} + \frac{1}{\omega_2 p_2} - (\frac{1}{\sqrt{p_1}} + \frac{1}{\sqrt{p_2}})^2
$$
$$
= \zeta^{-1}[(1+\zeta)p_1^{-1} + \zeta(1+\zeta)p_2^{-1} - \zeta(p_1^{-1/2} + p_2^{-1/2})^2]
$$
$$
= \zeta^{-1}[\zeta^2 p_2^{-1} - 2\zeta p_1^{-1/2} p_2^{-1/2} + p_1^{-1}]
$$
$$
= \zeta^{-1} p_2^{-1}[\zeta^2 - 2\zeta\sqrt{p_2/p_1} + p_2/p_1]
$$
$$
= \zeta^{-1} p_2^{-1}[\zeta - \sqrt{p_2/p_1}]^2 \geq 0,
$$

with equality if and only if $\zeta = \sqrt{p_2/p_1}$. Thus, the optimal sample size ratio of the sample size formula (5.15) is $\hat{\zeta} = \sqrt{p_2/p_1}$.

Minimizing the expected number of events: It can be shown that

$$
\frac{[\omega_1 p_1 + \omega_2 p_2]^2}{\omega_1 \omega_2 p_1 p_2} - 4
$$
$$
= \frac{\zeta^2 p_1^2 - 2\zeta p_1 p_2 - p_2^2}{\zeta p_1 p_2}
$$
$$
= \frac{(\zeta p_1 - p_2)^2}{\zeta p_1 p_2} \geq 0,
$$

with equality if and only if $\zeta = p_2/p_1$. Thus, the minimum expected number of events based on the sample size formula (5.15) is achieved at $\hat{\zeta} = p_2/p_1$.

D

R Codes for the Sample Size Calculations

D.1 R code for the sample size calculation under the Weibull model, Kaplan-Meier curve or spline distribution using the Schoenfeld formula

```
library(survival)
library(logspline)
time=c(1.10, 12.33,  2.77,  5.27,  6.58,  9.82,  0.36, 11.59,  1.84, 11.18,
      10.78,  0.61,  6.29, 12.24,  3.70, 12.48,  6.18,  7.12,  6.54,  2.74,
       3.93,  3.73,  8.99, 12.22,  6.09, 11.96, 10.94, 11.48, 11.07,  3.21,
       9.47,  5.01,  3.26,  0.19,  4.63, 10.16,  6.96,  9.79, 11.10,  4.54,
       0.54,  4.77,  7.37,  1.06, 10.72,  2.05, 10.55, 10.47,  8.49,  8.45,
       8.83,  7.08,  5.77,  6.44,  2.68,  9.14,  2.97,  6.27,  1.41,  5.57,
       9.03,  2.66,  8.41,  2.26,  2.84,  8.87,  8.07,  8.63,  8.49,  8.19,
       3.55,  8.38,  8.36,  8.21,  2.09,  7.86,  3.16,  7.84,  0.38,  6.78,
       5.63,  2.95,  4.61,  7.38,  7.05,  7.28,  7.24,  4.09,  7.07,  7.00,
       7.00,  6.92,  4.32,  6.39,  6.86,  6.69,  6.71,  6.38,  6.47,  6.48,
       4.36,  6.22,  5.70,  6.18,  5.95,  2.48,  5.97,  5.94,  5.95,  3.38,
       0.92,  5.33,  5.54,  2.74,  0.95,  5.35,  5.29,  5.23,  5.16,  1.90,
       5.02,  4.96,  4.63,  3.93,  2.01,  4.88,  3.99,  4.85,  4.84,  2.02,
       4.66,  4.42,  4.66,  4.42,  0.49,  3.26,  4.30,  4.18,  3.96,  3.70,
       4.06,  3.87,  0.11,  3.84,  3.86,  3.38,  2.19,  3.73,  2.47,  3.57,
       2.40,  1.46,  3.54,  3.48,  3.37,  3.16,  2.57,  2.30)
status=c(1, 0, 1, 1, 1, 1, 1, 0, 1, 1, 0, 1, 1, 0, 1, 0, 1, 1, 1, 1, 1, 1,
         1, 0, 1, 0, 0, 1, 0, 1, 0, 1, 1, 1, 1, 0, 1, 1, 0, 1, 1, 1, 1, 1,
         0, 1, 0, 0, 0, 1, 1, 1, 1, 0, 1, 0, 1, 1, 1, 0, 0, 1, 0, 1, 1, 0,
         0, 0, 0, 0, 1, 0, 0, 0, 1, 0, 1, 0, 1, 0, 1, 1, 1, 1, 0, 0, 0, 0, 1,
         0, 0, 0, 0, 1, 0, 0, 0, 0, 0, 0, 0, 1, 0, 0, 1, 0, 0, 0, 1,
         1, 0, 0, 1, 1, 0, 0, 0, 0, 1, 0, 0, 1, 0, 0, 0, 0, 0, 0, 0,
         0, 0, 1, 1, 0, 0, 0, 0, 0, 0, 1, 0, 0, 0, 1, 0, 0, 0, 0, 0, 0, 0,
         0, 0, 0, 0)
datPBC=data.frame(time=time, status=status)
########################## Input parameters ############################
###   m0 and m1 are the median survival times for the control and treatment  ###
###   groups; eta is the hazard rate of exponential loss to follow-up;       ###
###   ta and tf are the accrual time and follow-up time; alpha and beta are  ###
###   the type I and II error and power=1-beta; omega1 is the sample size     ###
###   allocation ratio of control; data are a data.frame form.               ###
########################################################################
SizeSch=function(m0, m1, eta, ta, tf, alpha, beta, omega1, data)
{tau=tf+ta
 z0=qnorm(1-alpha/2)
 z1=qnorm(1-beta)
 ########## fit KM curve ##############
 surv=Surv(time, status)
 fitKM<- survfit(surv ~ 1, data = dat)
```

```
p0<-c(1, summary(fitKM)$surv)    # KM survival probability ###
t0<-c(0, summary(fitKM)$time)    # ordered failure times ###
outKM<-data.frame(t0=t0,p0=p0)
KM<-function(t){
  t0=outKM$t0; p0=outKM$p0; k=length(t0)
  if (t>=t0[k] || t<0) {ans<-0}
  for (i in 1:(k-1)){
    if (t>=t0[i] & t<t0[i+1]) {S0=p0[i]}}
  return(S0)}
######## fit Weibull ###############
fitWB=survreg(formula=surv~1, dist="weibull")
scale=as.numeric(exp(fitWB$coeff))
shape=1/fitWB$scale; kappa=shape
lambda0=log(2)/m0^kappa
WB=function(t){exp(-lambda0*t^kappa)}
####### fit spline curve ##########
fitSP=oldlogspline(time[status==1],time[status==0],lbound=0)
SP=function(t) {1-poldlogspline(t, fitSP)}
fp=function(t) {doldlogspline(t, fitSP)}
####### sample size calculation #####
delta=(m0/m1)^kappa
G=function(t){1-punif(t, tf, tau)}
S0=function(t){WB(t)}
S1=function(t){WB(t)^delta}
h0=function(t){kappa*lambda0*t^(kappa-1)}
h1=function(t){delta*kappa*lambda0*t^(kappa-1)}
f0=function(t){exp(-eta*t)*G(t)*S0(t)*h0(t)}
f1=function(t){exp(-eta*t)*G(t)*S1(t)*h1(t)}
p0=integrate(f0, 0, tau)$value
p1=integrate(f1, 0, tau)$value
PWB=omega1*p0+(1-omega1)*p1
S0=function(t){SP(t)}
S1=function(t){SP(t)^delta}
h0=function(t){fp(t)/SP(t)}
h1=function(t){delta*fp(t)/SP(t)}
p0=integrate(f0, 0, tau)$value
p1=integrate(f1, 0, tau)$value
PSP=omega1*p0+(1-omega1)*p1
S0=function(t){ans=exp(-eta*t)*KM(t); return(ans)}
S1=function(t){ans=exp(-eta*t)*KM(t)^delta; return(ans)}
a0=(tf/6)*(S0(0)+4*S0(0.5*tf)+S0(tf))
a1=(ta/6)*(S0(tf)+4*S0(0.5*ta+tf)+S0(ta+tf))
a2=(ta/6)*(tf*S0(tf)+4*(0.5*ta+tf)*S0(0.5*ta+tf)+(ta+tf)*S0(ta+tf))
b0=(tf/6)*(S1(0)+4*S1(0.5*tf)+S1(tf))
b1=(ta/6)*(S1(tf)+4*S1(0.5*ta+tf)+S1(ta+tf))
b2=(ta/6)*(tf*S1(tf)+4*(0.5*ta+tf)*S1(0.5*ta+tf)+(ta+tf)*S1(ta+tf))
p0=1-eta*a0-((1+eta*(ta+tf))*a1-eta*a2)/ta
p1=1-eta*b0-((1+eta*(ta+tf))*b1-eta*b2)/ta
PKM=omega1*p0+(1-omega1)*p1
d0=(z0+z1)^2/(omega1*(1-omega1)*log(delta)^2)
nWB=ceiling(d0/PWB)      # sample size formula under Weibull model#
nSP=ceiling(d0/PSP)      # sample size formula under spine curve#
nKM=ceiling(d0/PKM)      # sample size formula under KM curve#
d=ceiling(d0)
ans=list(c(nWB=nWB, nKM=nKM, nSP=nSP))
return(ans)}
SizeSch(m0=9,m1=14,eta=0,ta=6,tf=3,alpha=0.05,beta=0.1,omega1=0.5,
```

```
        data=datPBC)
nWB nKM nSP
519 517 508
SizeSch(m0=9,m1=14,eta=0.025,ta=6,tf=3,alpha=0.05,beta=0.1,omega1=0.5,
        data=datPBC)
nWB nKM nSP
563 561 552
```

D.2 R code for the information time and sample size calculation under the exponential model

```
############################# Input parameters #############################
### s1 and s2 are the survival probabilities at time point x for group 1   ###
### and group 2, respectively; x is the landmark time point;               ###
### pi is the proportion of patients assign to group 1: ta and tf are the  ###
### accrual and follow-up times; alpha and beta are type I and II errors;  ###
### t is the calendar time at which to calculate the information time.     ###
### Note: one can calculate the sample size and information time for any    ###
### distribution by changing the survival distribution function S1.        ###
#############################################################################
SIZEinfTime=function(s1, s2, x, pi, ta, tf, alpha, beta, t)
{z0=qnorm(1-alpha);  z1=qnorm(1-beta)
 lambda1=-log(s1)/x;  HR=log(s1)/log(s2)
 S1=function(t){ans=exp(-lambda1*t); return(ans)}
 S2=function(t){ans=S1(t)^(1/HR);return(ans)}
 dsc=ceiling((z0+z1)^2/(pi*(1-pi)*(log(HR))^2))#expected number of events#
 p1=1-integrate(S1, tf, ta+tf)$value/ta
 p2=1-integrate(S2, tf, ta+tf)$value/ta
 P0=pi*p1+(1-pi)*p2
 Nsc=ceiling((z0+z1)^2/(pi*(1-pi)*(log(HR))^2*P0))## Schoenfeld  formua#
 Nxw=ceiling((z0+z1)^2*P0/(pi*(1-pi)*(log(HR))^2*p1*p2))##Rubinstein formula##
 a=t-min(t,ta); b=min(t,ta)
 pt1=b/ta-integrate(S1, a, t)$value/ta
 pt2=b/ta-integrate(S2, a, t)$value/ta
 dt=Nsc*(pi*pt1+(1-pi)*pt2)
 dtau=(z0+z1)^2/(pi*(1-pi)*log(HR)^2)
 Dt=Nxw*(1/(pi*pt1)+1/((1-pi)*pt2))^(-1)
 Dtau=(z0+z1)^2/log(HR)^2
 td=round(dt/dtau,3) ### information time td based on traditional method #
 tD=round(Dt/Dtau,3) ### information time tD based on new method  #
 ans=data.frame(dsc=dsc, Nsc=Nsc, Nxw=Nxw, td=td, tD=tD)
 return(ans)
}
SIZEinfTime(s1=0.5, s2=0.6, x=3, pi=0.3, ta=5, tf=3, alpha=0.05, beta=0.1, t=1)
dsc Nsc Nxw    td    tD
438 697 656 0.028 0.029
# dsc and Nsc are the number of events and sample size calculated using ###
# the Schoenfeld formula; Nxw is the sample size calculated using the #####
# Rubinstein formula; td and tD are the inforamtion times calculated using#
# formulae (10.7) and (10.10). #
```

D.3 R code for the sample size calculation based on the Lakatos Markov chain model

```
############################# Input parameters #############################
```

```
### ploss is a vector of probability of loss to follow-up for both groups; ###
### pc is a vector of probability of having an event in control group;     ###
### k is a vector of hazard ratio;                                          ###
### pnoncmpl is a vector of probability of noncompliance;                   ###
### pdropin is a vector of probability of drop-in;                          ###
### rectime is a vector of accrual times (in unit time);                    ###
### recratio is a vector of accrual rates over the accrual times;           ###
### logr is a vector of weight of the log-rank test;                        ###
### ratio is a vector of sample size allocation ratio;                      ###
### simul =0/1: staggered entry (0) or simultaneously entry (1);            ###
### sbdv is the number of intervals to be divided for each unit time;       ###
### alpha is type I error for a two-sided test and beta is type II error.   ###
##############################################################################
SizeLak=function(ploss, pc, k, pnoncmpl, pdropin, rectime,
          recratio, logr, ratio, simul, sbdv, alpha, beta)
{options(digits=10)
 years=length(ploss)
 n_intrvl=sbdv
 nn=years*n_intrvl;
 trans=trans_a=diag(4)
 distr_e=as.matrix(c(0,0,1,0))
 distr_c=as.matrix(c(0,0,0,1))
 dstr_e=dstr_c=NULL
 logr0=NULL
 pe=NULL
 for (i in 1:years){
   pe[i]=1-(1-pc[i])^k[i]}
 if (simul==1) {
  for (i in 1:years){
   ls=1-(1-ploss[i])^(1/n_intrvl)
   dro=1-(1-pnoncmpl[i])^(1/n_intrvl)
   dri=1-(1-pdropin[i])^(1/n_intrvl)
   pc1=1-(1-pc[i])^(1/n_intrvl)
   pe1=1-(1-pe[i])^(1/n_intrvl)
   for (j in 1:n_intrvl){
    trans[,3]=c(ls,pe1, 1-(ls+pe1+dro), dro)
    trans[,4]=c(ls,pc1, dri, 1-(ls+pc1+dri))
    distr_e=trans%*%distr_e
    distr_c=trans%*%distr_c
    dstr_e=cbind(dstr_e, distr_e)
    dstr_c=cbind(dstr_c, distr_c)
    logr0=cbind(logr0,logr[i])}}}
 else {
   ad_cens=rep(0, nn)
   rcrt_sum=0
   wk=c(0, round(rectime*n_intrvl))
   rcrt=rep(0, nn)
   for (i in 1:length(rectime)){
    rcrt[(wk[i]+1):wk[i+1]]=rep(recratio[i], wk[i+1]-wk[i])}
   for (j in 1:nn){
    rcrt_sum=rcrt_sum + rcrt[j]
    ad_cens[nn+1-j]=rcrt[j]/rcrt_sum}
   for (i in 1:years){
    ls=1-(1-ploss[i])^(1/n_intrvl)
    dro=1-(1-pnoncmpl[i])^(1/n_intrvl)
    dri=1-(1-pdropin[i])^(1/n_intrvl)
    pc1=1-(1-pc[i])^(1/n_intrvl)
```

```
    pe1=1-(1-pe[i])^(1/n_intrvl)
   for (j in 1:n_intrvl){
    trans[,3]=c(ls,pe1, 1-(ls+pe1+dro), dro)
    trans[,4]=c(ls,pc1, dri, 1-(ls+pc1+dri))
    trans_a[1,3:4]=ad_cens[j+(i-1)*n_intrvl]
    trans_a[3,3]=trans_a[4,4]=1-ad_cens[j+(i-1)*n_intrvl]
    distr_e=(trans_a%*%trans)%*%distr_e
    distr_c=(trans_a%*%trans)%*%distr_c
    dstr_e=cbind(dstr_e, distr_e)
    dstr_c=cbind(dstr_c, distr_c)
    logr0=cbind(logr0,logr[i])}}}
 if (length(ratio)==1)
 {r1=1; r2=1}
 else {r1=ratio[1]; r2=ratio[2]}
 event_c = dstr_c[2,]-c(0, dstr_c[2,1:(ncol(dstr_c)-1)])
 event_e = dstr_e[2,]-c(0, dstr_e[2,1:(ncol(dstr_e)-1)])
 loss_c  = dstr_c[1,]-c(0, dstr_c[1,1:(ncol(dstr_c)-1)])
 loss_e  = dstr_e[1,]-c(0, dstr_e[1,1:(ncol(dstr_e)-1)])
 atrisk_c= apply(dstr_c[3:4,], 2, sum) + loss_c + event_c
 atrisk_e= apply(dstr_e[3:4,], 2, sum) + loss_e + event_e
 phi = atrisk_c*r1/(atrisk_e*r2)
 theta = log(1 - (event_c/atrisk_c))/log(1 - (event_e/atrisk_e))
 rho =  (event_c*r1 + event_e*r2)/sum(event_c*r1 + event_e*r2)
 gamma=(phi*theta)/(1+phi*theta)-phi/(1+phi)
 eta=phi/(1+phi)^2
 sig2=sum(logr0^2*rho*eta)
 sig=sum(logr0*rho*gamma)
 p_e = distr_e[2,]
 p_c = distr_c[2,]
 z_alpha=qnorm(1-alpha/2)
 z_beta=qnorm(1-beta)
 d_LR=sig2*(z_alpha+z_beta)^2/sig^2
 n_LR=(r1+r2)*d_LR/(p_c*r1+p_e*r2)
 ans=list(d_LR=d_LR, n_LR=n_LR, p_e=p_e, p_c=p_c)
 return(ans)}
```

D.4 R code for the sample size calculation under the Weibull mixture cure model by using formula (8.24)

```
############################# Input parameters ##############################
### kappa is shape parameter of the Weibull dist. S(t)=exp(-lambda t^kappa)###
### lambda0 is the hazard parameter of the Weibull dist. of control group; ###
### pi0 and pi1 are cure rates under the null and alternative hypothesis;  ###
### p is the sample size allocation ratio for the control group;           ###
### ta and tf are the accrual period and follow-up time;                   ###
### HR is hazard ratio of control to treatment; alpha is the type I error; ###
### Note: the code can be easily modified for other mixture cure model.    ###
#############################################################################
SizeMC=function(kappa, lambda0, pi0, pi1, p, ta, tf, HR, alpha, power)
{ z0=qnorm(1-alpha/2); z1=qnorm(power)
  tau=ta+tf; delta=1/HR
  gamma=log(pi1/(1-pi1))-log(pi0/(1-pi0))
  q=function(t){num=pi0*exp(gamma)+(1-pi0)*S0(t)^delta
   den=(pi0*exp(gamma)+(1-pi0))*(pi0+(1-pi0)*S0(t))
   ans=num/den; return(ans)}
```

```
S0=function(t){exp(-lambda0*t^kappa)}
h0=function(t){kappa*lambda0*t^(kappa-1)}
G=function(t){1-punif(t, tf, tau)}
q1=function(t){den=(p+(1-p)*q(t))^2
 num=q(t)*(p*(1-pi0+pi0*exp(gamma))+(1-p)*delta*S0(t)^(delta-1))
 ans=num/den; return(ans)}
q2=function(t){den=p+(1-p)*q(t)
 num=q(t)*(delta*S0(t)^(delta-1)/(q(t)*(1-pi0+pi0*exp(gamma)))-1)
 ans=num/den; return(ans)}
f1=function(t){q1(t)*G(t)*S0(t)*h0(t)}
f2=function(t){q2(t)*G(t)*S0(t)*h0(t)}
A=integrate(f1, 0, tau)$value
B=integrate(f2, 0, tau)$value
nXW=ceiling((z0+z1)^2*A/(p*(1-p)*(1-pi0)*(1-pi0+pi0*exp(gamma))*B^2))
ans=c(nXW=nXW); return(ans)}
SizeMC(kappa=1.018,lambda0=0.836,pi0=0.35,pi1=0.45,p=0.5,ta=4,tf=3,
    HR=1.5,alpha=0.05,power=0.90)
nXW
468
SizeMC(kappa=1.018,lambda0=0.836,pi0=0.35,pi1=0.35,p=0.5,ta=4,tf=3,
    HR=2.0,alpha=0.05,power=0.90)
nXW
762
SizeMC(kappa=1.018,lambda0=0.836,pi0=0.35,pi1=0.50,p=0.5,ta=4,tf=3,
    HR=1.0,alpha=0.05,power=0.90)
nXW
505
```

E

Derivation of the Asymptotic Distribution

Derivation of the Asymptotic Distribution of the Weighted Log-Rank Test under the Proportional Hazards Mixture Cure Model

The weighted log-rank score test is given by

$$U_w = \int_0^\infty W(t) \left\{ \frac{Y_2(t)}{Y(t)} dN_1(t) - \frac{Y_1(t)}{Y(t)} dN_2(t) \right\},$$

where $W(t)$ is a weight function that converges to $w(t)$, $N_j(t)$ is the number of observed failures by time t, $Y_j(t)$ is the number of subjects at risk just prior to t, in group $j = 1, 2$, and $Y(t) = Y_1(t) + Y_2(t)$. If we define martingale processes such that $M_j(t) = N_j(t) - \int_0^t \lambda_j^*(s) Y_j(s) ds, j = 1, 2$, then the weighted log-rank score test can be written as

$$
\begin{aligned}
U_w &= \int_0^\infty W(t) \left\{ \frac{Y_2(t)}{Y(t)} dM_1(t) - \frac{Y_1(t)}{Y(t)} dM_2(t) \right\} \\
&+ \int_0^\infty W(t) \frac{Y_1(t) Y_2(t)}{Y(t)} \{\lambda_1^*(t) - \lambda_2^*(t)\} dt.
\end{aligned}
$$

Under the null hypothesis $H_0 : \gamma = 0$ and $\eta = 0$, we have $\lambda_1^*(t) = \lambda_2^*(t) = \lambda_0^*(t)$, and $\pi_1 = \pi_2 = \pi_0$, where

$$\lambda_0^*(t) = \frac{(1 - \pi_0)\bar{S}(t)}{\pi_0 + (1 - \pi_0)\bar{S}(t)} \bar{\lambda}(t)$$

and $\bar{\lambda}(t) = \delta^{1/2} \lambda(t)$. Then, the weighted log-rank score reduces to

$$U_w = \int_0^\infty W(t) \left\{ \frac{Y_2(t)}{Y(t)} dM_1(t) - \frac{Y_1(t)}{Y(t)} dM_2(t) \right\}.$$

By the martingale property, the mean of U_w is 0 and the variance of U_w is given by

$$\mathrm{Var}(n^{-1/2} U_w) = n^{-1} E \int_0^\infty W^2(t) \frac{Y_1(t) Y_2(t)}{Y(t)} d\Lambda_0^*(t).$$

where $\Lambda_0^*(t) = \int_0^t \lambda_0^*(u) du$. As

$$n^{-1} \frac{Y_1(t) Y_2(t)}{Y(t)} = \frac{n_1 n_2}{n^2} \frac{\{Y_1(t)/n_1\}\{Y_2(t)/n_2\}}{Y(t)/n} \to \omega_1 \omega_2 \frac{\pi_1(t) \pi_2(t)}{\pi(t)},$$

where $\omega_1 = \lim_{n \to \infty} n_1/n$, $\omega_2 = 1 - \omega_1$, $\pi_j(t) = P(X_{ij} > t)$ and $\pi(t) = \omega_1 \pi_1(t) + \omega_2 \pi_2(t)$, then, by the martingale central limit theorem (Fleming and Harrington, 1991), $n^{-1/2} U_w \to N(0, \sigma_w^2)$, where

$$\sigma_w^2 = \omega_1 \omega_2 (1 - \pi_0) \int_0^\infty w^2(t) G(t) \bar{S}(t) \bar{\lambda}(t) dt, \qquad (E.1)$$

for which $G(t) = P(C_{ij} > t)$ is the common survival distribution of the censoring time. A consistent estimate of the variance σ_w^2 is given by

$$\hat{\sigma}_w^2 = n^{-1} \int_0^\infty W^2(t) \frac{Y_1(t) Y_2(t)}{Y(t)} d\hat{\Lambda}_0^*(t),$$

where $d\hat{\Lambda}_0^*(t) = dN(t)/Y(t)$ and $N(t) = N_1(t) + N_2(t)$. Therefore, the weighted log-rank test $L_w = n^{-1/2} U_w / \hat{\sigma}_w$ is asymptotically standard normal distributed under the null hypothesis.

To derive the asymptotic distribution of the weighted log-rank test under the alternative, consider a sequence of local alternatives $H_1^{(n)}$:

$$S_j^{*(n)}(t) = 1 - e^{(-1)^j \gamma_n} (1 - \pi_0) \{ 1 - \bar{S}(t)^{e^{(-1)^j \eta_n}} \}$$

or

$$\lambda_j^{*(n)}(t) = \frac{e^{(-1)^j \gamma_n} (1 - \pi_0) \bar{S}(t)^{e^{(-1)^j \eta_n}}}{1 - e^{(-1)^j \gamma_n} (1 - \pi_0) + e^{(-1)^j \gamma_n} (1 - \pi_0) \bar{S}(t)^{e^{(-1)^j \eta_n}}} \bar{\lambda}(t) e^{(-1)^j \eta_n},$$

where $n^{1/2} \eta_n = \eta_a < \infty$ and $n^{1/2} \gamma_n = \gamma_a < \infty$, and define martingale processes as $M_j^{(n)}(t) = N_j(t) - \int_0^t Y_j(u) \lambda_j^{*(n)}(u) du$. Then, $U_w = U_{1w} + U_{2w}$, where

$$U_{1w} = n^{-1/2} \int_0^\infty W(t) \left\{ \frac{Y_2(t)}{Y(t)} dM_1^{(n)}(t) - \frac{Y_1(t)}{Y(t)} dM_2^{(n)}(t) \right\}$$

and

$$U_{2w} = n^{-1/2} \int_0^\infty W(t) \frac{Y_1(t) Y_2(t)}{Y(t)} \{ \lambda_1^{*(n)}(t) - \lambda_2^{*(n)}(t) \} dt.$$

As $\gamma_n \to 0$, $\eta_n \to 0$, $H_1^{(n)} \to H_0$, and $\lambda_j^{*(n)}(t) \to \lambda_0^*(t)$, and by the martingale central limit theorem, U_{1w} converges to a normal variable with mean $EU_{1w} = 0$ and variance

$$\begin{aligned} EU_{1w}^2 &= n^{-1} E \int_0^\infty W^2(t) \left\{ \frac{Y_2^2(t)}{Y^2(t)} Y_1(t) \lambda_1^{*(n)}(t) + \frac{Y_1^2(t)}{Y^2(t)} Y_2(t) \lambda_2^{*(n)}(t) \right\} du \\ &\to \omega_1 \omega_2 \int_0^\infty w^2(t) \left\{ \omega_2 \frac{\pi_2^2(t) \pi_1(t)}{\pi^2(t)} \lambda_0^*(t) + \omega_1 \frac{\pi_1^2(t) \pi_2(t)}{\pi^2(t)} \lambda_0^*(t) \right\} dt \\ &= \omega_1 \omega_2 \int_0^\infty w^2(t) \frac{\pi_1(t) \pi_2(t)}{\pi(t)} \lambda_0^*(t) du \\ &= \omega_1 \omega_2 \int_0^\infty w^2(t) G(t) S_0^*(t) \lambda_0^*(t) dt = \sigma_w^2. \end{aligned}$$

By Taylor's expansion of $\lambda_j^{*(n)}(t)$ at $(\gamma_n, \eta_n) = (0,0)$, it follows that

$$
\begin{aligned}
\lambda_j^{*(n)}(t) &= \frac{(1-\pi_0)\bar{S}(t)}{\pi_0 + (1-\pi_0)\bar{S}(t)}\bar{\lambda}(t) + \frac{(-1)^j(1-\pi_0)\bar{S}(t)}{[\pi_0 + (1-\pi_0)\bar{S}(t)]^2}\gamma_n\bar{\lambda}(t) \\
&\quad + (-1)^j\left\{\frac{\pi_0(1-\pi_0)\bar{S}(t)\log\bar{S}(t)}{[\pi_0 + (1-\pi_0)\bar{S}(t)]^2} + \frac{(1-\pi_0)\bar{S}(t)}{[\pi_0 + (1-\pi_0)\bar{S}(t)]}\right\}\eta_n\bar{\lambda}(t) \\
&\quad + O_p(n^{-1})
\end{aligned}
$$

and

$$
\begin{aligned}
\lambda_1^{*(n)}(t) - \lambda_2^{*(n)}(t) &= \frac{2(\pi_0-1)\bar{S}(t)\bar{\lambda}(t)}{\pi_0 + (\pi_0-1)\bar{S}(t)}\left\{\eta_n + \frac{\gamma_n + \eta_n\pi_0\log\bar{S}(t)}{[\pi_0 + (1-\pi_0)\bar{S}(t)]}\right\} \\
&\quad + O_p(n^{-1}).
\end{aligned}
$$

As $n^{1/2}\gamma_n = \gamma$ and $n^{1/2}\eta_n = \eta$, we obtain

$$
\lim_{n\to\infty} n^{1/2}\{\lambda_1^{*(n)}(t) - \lambda_2^{*(n)}(t)\} = \frac{2(\pi_0-1)\bar{f}(t)}{\pi_0 + (1-\pi_0)\bar{S}(t)}\left\{\eta_a + \frac{\gamma_a + \eta_a\pi_0\log\bar{S}(t)}{\pi_0 + (1-\pi_0)\bar{S}(t)}\right\},
$$

where $\bar{f}(t) = \bar{\lambda}(t)\bar{S}(t)$. By substituting the above equation into U_{2w}, we can show that U_{2w} converges in probability to $\mu_w = \mu(w, \gamma_a, \eta_a)$, where

$$
\begin{aligned}
\mu_w &= 2\omega_1\omega_2(\pi_0-1) \\
&\quad \times \int_0^\infty w(t)\left\{\eta_a + \frac{\gamma_a + \eta_a\pi_0\log\bar{S}(t)}{\pi_0 + (1-\pi_0)\bar{S}(t)}\right\}G(t)\bar{S}(t)\bar{\lambda}(t)dt. \quad (\text{E.2})
\end{aligned}
$$

Thus, under the local alternatives $H_1^{(n)}$, the weighted log-rank test is asymptotically normal distributed with mean μ_w/σ_w and unit variance, that is,

$$
L_w = U_w/\hat{\sigma}_w \to N(\mu_w/\sigma_w, 1).
$$

As

$$
\lambda_j^{*(n)}(t) = \frac{e^{(-1)^j\gamma_n}(1-\pi_0)\bar{S}(t)^{e^{(-1)^j\eta_n}}}{1 - e^{(-1)^j\gamma_n}(1-\pi_0) + e^{(-1)^j\gamma_n}(1-\pi_0)\bar{S}(t)^{e^{(-1)^j\eta_n}}}\bar{\lambda}(t)e^{(-1)^j\eta_n},
$$

then by Taylor's expansion of $\lambda_j^{*(n)}(t)$ at $(\gamma_n, \eta_n) = (0,0)$, it follows that

$$
\begin{aligned}
\lambda_j^{*(n)}(t) &= \frac{(1-\pi_0)\bar{S}(t)}{\pi_0 + (1-\pi_0)\bar{S}(t)}\bar{\lambda}(t) + \frac{(-1)^j(1-\pi_0)\bar{S}(t)}{[\pi_0 + (1-\pi_0)\bar{S}(t)]^2}\gamma_n\bar{\lambda}(t) \\
&\quad + (-1)^j\left\{\frac{\pi_0(1-\pi_0)\bar{S}(t)\log\bar{S}(t)}{[\pi_0 + (1-\pi_0)\bar{S}(t)]^2} + \frac{(1-\pi_0)\bar{S}(t)}{[\pi_0 + (1-\pi_0)\bar{S}(t)]}\right\}\eta_n\bar{\lambda}(t) \\
&\quad + O_p(n^{-1})
\end{aligned}
$$

and

$$\lambda_1^{*(n)}(t) - \lambda_2^{*(n)}(t) = \frac{2(\pi_0 - 1)\bar{S}(t)\bar{\lambda}(t)}{\pi_0 + (\pi_0 - 1)\bar{S}(t)} \left\{ \eta_n + \frac{\gamma_n + \eta_n \pi_0 \log \bar{S}(t)}{[\pi_0 + (1 - \pi_0)\bar{S}(t)]} \right\}$$
$$+ O_p(n^{-1}).$$

As $n^{1/2}\gamma_n = \gamma$ and $n^{1/2}\eta_n = \eta$, we obtain

$$\lim_{n\to\infty} n^{1/2}\{\lambda_1^{*(n)}(t) - \lambda_2^{*(n)}(t)\} = \frac{2(\pi_0 - 1)\bar{f}(t)}{\pi_0 + (1 - \pi_0)\bar{S}(t)} \left\{ \eta_a + \frac{\gamma_a + \eta_a \pi_0 \log \bar{S}(t)}{\pi_0 + (1 - \pi_0)\bar{S}(t)} \right\}.$$

F

Derivation of Equations for Chapter 8

$$\pi(t)(1 - \pi(t))V(t)$$

$$= \frac{\omega_1\omega_2 S_1(t)S_2(t)}{[\omega_1 S_1(t) + \omega_2 S_2(t)]^2}\{\omega_1\lambda_1(t)S_1(t) + \omega_2\lambda_2(t)S_2(t)\}G(t)$$

$$= \frac{\omega_1\omega_2 S_1(t)S_1^\delta(t)}{[\omega_1 S_1(t) + \omega_2[S_1(t)]^\delta]^2}\{\omega_1\lambda_1(t)S_1(t) + \omega_2\delta\lambda_1(t)[S_1(t)]^\delta\}G(t)$$

$$= \frac{\omega_1\omega_2[S_1(t)]^\delta}{[\omega_1 + \omega_2[S_1(t)]^{\delta-1}]^2}\{\omega_1 + \omega_2\delta[S_1(t)]^{\delta-1}\}G(t)\lambda_1(t). \tag{F.1}$$

$$\frac{\pi(t)(1 - \pi(t))}{[\pi(t) + \{1 - \pi(t)\}\delta]}V(t)$$

$$= \frac{\omega_1\omega_2[S_1(t)]^\delta}{[\omega_1 + \omega_2[S_1(t)]^{\delta-1}]^2}\{\omega_1 + \omega_2\delta[S_1(t)]^{\delta-1}\}G(t)\lambda_1(t)$$

$$\times\frac{[\omega_1 + \omega_2[S_1(t)]^{\delta-1}]}{[\omega_1 + \omega_2\delta[S_1(t)]^{\delta-1}]}$$

$$= \frac{\omega_1\omega_2[S_1(t)]^\delta}{[\omega_1 + \omega_2[S_1(t)]^{\delta-1}]} \times \lambda_1(t)G(t). \tag{F.2}$$

$$\frac{\pi(t)(1 - \pi(t))}{[\pi(t) + \{1 - \pi(t)\}\delta]^2}V(t)$$

$$= \frac{\omega_1\omega_2[S_1(t)]^\delta}{[\omega_1 + \omega_2[S_1(t)]^{\delta-1}]^2}\{\omega_1 + \omega_2\delta[S_1(t)]^{\delta-1}\}G(t)\lambda_1(t)$$

$$\times\frac{[\omega_1 + \omega_2[S_1(t)]^{\delta-1}]^2}{[\omega_1 + \omega_2\delta[S_1(t)]^{\delta-1}]^2}$$

$$= \frac{\omega_1\omega_2[S_1(t)]^\delta}{[\omega_1 + \omega_2\delta[S_1(t)]^{\delta-1}]} \times \lambda_1(t)G(t). \tag{F.3}$$

Bibliography

Aalen OO, Borgan O, Gjessing HK. *Survival and Event History Analysis: A Process Point of View.* Springer-Verlag, New York, 2007.

Abe T, Kakemura T, Fujinuma S, Maetani I. Successful outcomes of EMR-L with 3D-EUS for rectal carcinoids compared with historical controls. *World Journal of Gastroenterology*, 2008; **14**: 4054-4058.

Ahnn S, Anderson SJ. Sample size determination for comparing more than two survival distributions. *Statistics in Medicine* 1995, **14**:2273-2282.

Ahnn S, Anderson SJ. Sample size determination in complex clinical trials comparing more than two groups for survival endpoints. *Statistics in Medicine*, 1998; **17**:2525-2534.

Andrews DF, Herzberg AM. *Data* Springer, New York, 1985.

Anderson TW. *An Introduction to Multivariate Statistical Analysis.* Wiley, New York, 1958.

Anderson PK, Borgan O, Gill RD, Keiding N. *Statistical Methods Based on Counting Processes* Springer, New York, 1993.

Ando R, Nakamura A, Nagatani M, Yamakawa S, Ohira T, Takagi M, Matsushima K, Aoki A, Fujita Y, Tamura K. Comparison of past and recent historical control data in relation to spontaneous tumors during carcinogenicity testing in Fischer 344 rats. *Journal of Toxicologic Pathology* 2008; **21**:53-60.

Babb J, Rogatko A, Zacks S. Cancer phase I clinical trials: efficient dose escalation with overdose control. *Statistics in Medicine*, 1998; **17**:1103-1120.

Barthel FMS, Babiker A, Royston P, Parmar MKB. Evaluation of sample size and power for multi-arm survival trials allowing for non-uniform accrual, non-proportional hazards, loss to follow-up and cross-over. *Statistics in Medicine*, 2006; **25**:2521-2542.

Bernardo PMV, Lipsitz SR, Harrington DP, Catalano PJ. Sample size calculations for failure time random variables in non-randomized studies. *Journal of the Royal Statistical Society. Series D (The Statistician)* 2000; **49**:31-40.

Borgan O. Maximum likelihood estimation in parametric counting process models, with applications to censored failure time data. *Scandinavian Journal of Statistics* 1984; **11**:1-16.

Cantor AB. Sample size calculations for the log rank test: a Gompertz model approach. *Journal of Clinical Epidemiology* 1992; **45**:1131-1136.

Cantor AB. *Extending SAS Survival Analysis Techniques for Medical Research*, SAS Institute Inc: Cary, NC, 1997, pp. 84-85.

Case LD and Morgan TM. Design of phase II cancer trials evaluating survival probabilities. *BMC Medical Research Methodology*, 2003; **3**:1-12.

Chang MN, Shuster JJ, Kepner JL. Group sequential designs for phase II trials with historical controls. *Controlled Clinical Trials*, 1999; **20**:353-364.

Cho SD, Krishnaswami S, Mckee JC, Zallen G, Silen ML, Bliss DW. Analysis of 29 consecutive thoracoscopic repairs of congenital diaphragmatic hernia in neonates compared to historical controls. *Journal of Pediatric Surgery*, 2009; **44**:80-86.

Chow SC, Shao J, Wang H. *Sample Size Calculations in Clinical Research*. 2nd Edition. CRC Press, Florida, 2007.

Collett D. *Modeling Survival Data in Medical Research*. 2nd Edition, Chapman and Hall, London, 2003.

Cook TD, DeMets D. *Introduction to Statistical Methods for Clinical Trials*. CRC Press, New York, 2007.

Corbière F, Joly P. A SAS macro for parametric and semiparametric mixture cure models. *Computer Methods and Programs in Biomedicine* 2007; **85**:173-180.

Cox DR. Regression models and life tables (with discussion). *Journal of the Royal Statistical Society B*, 1972; **74**:187-220.

Cox DR, Oakes DV. *Analysis of Survival Data*. Chapman and Hall, London, 1984.

Cytel Software Corporation. EAST version 5.4. Cytel, Cambridge MA, 2007.

DasGupta A. *Asymptotic Theory of Statistics and Probability*. Springer, New York, 2008.

Dixon DO, Simon R. Sample size considerations for studies comparing survival curves using historical controls. *Journal of Clinical Epidemiology* 1988; **41**:1209-1213.

Efron B. The two sample problem with censored data. *Proceedings of the Fifth Berkeley Symposium on Mathematical Statistics and Probability*, Volume 4: Biology and Problems of Heath. University of California Press, Berkeley, CA, 1967. pp.831-853.

Emrich LJ. Required duration and power duration determinations for historically controlled studies of survival times. *Statistics in Medicine* 1989; **8**:153-160.

Ewell M, Ibrahim JG. The large sample distribution of the weighted log rank statistic under general local alternatives. *Lifetime Data Analysis* 1997; **3**:5-12.

Farewell VT. The use of mixture models for the analysis of survival data with long-term survivors. *Biometrics* 1982; **38**:1041-1046.

Farewell VT, D'Angio GJ. A simulated study of historical controls using real data. *Biometrics* 1981; **37**:169-176.

Fleming TR. Historical controls, data banks, and randomized trials in clinical research: a review. *Cancer Treatment Reports*, 1982; **66**:1101-1105.

Fleming TR, Harrington DP. *Counting Processes and Survival Analysis*. Wiley, New York, 1991.

Freedman LS. Tables of the number of patients required in clinical trials using the logrank test. *Statistics in Medicine* 1982; **1**:121-129.

Freireich EJ et al. The effect of 6-mercaptopurine on the duration of steroid-induced remissions in acute leukemia. *Blood* 1963; **21**:699-716.

Gangnon RE, Kosorok MR. Sample-size formula for clustered survival data using weighted log-rank statistics. *Biometrika* 2004; **91**:263-275.

Gehan EA. Design of controlled clinical trials: use of historical controls. *Cancer Treatment Reports* 1982; **66**:1089-1093.

Gehan EA, Freireich EJ. Cancer clinical trials: a rational basis for use of historical controls. *Seminars in Oncology* 1981; **8**:430-436.

George SL, Desu MM. Planning the size and duration of a trial studying the time to some critical event. *Journal of Chronic Disease* 1973; **27**:15-24.

Grambsch PM, Therneau TM. Proportional hazards tests and diagnostics based on weighted residuals. *Biometrika* 1994; **81**:515-526.

Gray RJ, Tsiatis AA. A linear rank test for use when the main interest is in differences in cure rates. *Biometrics* 1989; **45**:899-904.

Green SG, Byar DP. Using observational data from registries to compare treatments: the fallacy of omnimetrics. *Statistics in Medicine* 1984; **3**:361-370.

Greenwood M. The natural duration of cancer. *Reports on Public Health and Medical Subjects* 1926; **33**:1-26.

Guyot P, Ades AE, Ouwens M, Welton NJ. Enhanced secondary analysis of survival data: reconstructing the data from published Kaplan-Meier survival curves. *BMC Medical Research Methodology* 2012; **12**:9.

Halabi S, Singh B. Sample size determination for comparing several survival curves with unequal allocations. *Statistics in Medicine* 2004; **23**:1793-1815.

Halpern J, Brown BW. Designing clinical trials with arbitrary specification of survival functions and for the log rank or generalized Wilcoxon test. *Controlled Clinical Trials* 1987; **8**:177-189.

Harrington DP, Fleming TR. A class of rank test procedures for censored survival data. *Biometrika* 1982; **69**:553-566.

Haybittle JL. Repeated assessment of results in clinical trials of cancer treatment. *British Journal of Radiology* 1971; **44**:793-797.

Hasegawa T. Sample size determination for the weighted log-rank test with the Fleming-Harrington class of weights in cancer vaccine studies. *Pharmaceutical Statistics* 2014; **13**:128-135.

Heo M, Faith MS, Allison DB. Power and sample size for survival analysis under the Weibull distribution when the whole lifespan is of interest. *Mechanisms of Ageing and Development* 1998; **102**:45-53.

Hsieh FY. Comparing sample size formulae for trials with unbalanced allocation using the logrank test. *Statistics in Medicine* 1992; **11**:1091-1098.

Hsieh FY, Lavori PW. Sample-size calculations for the Cox proportional hazards regression model with nonbinary covariates. *Controlled Clinical Trials* 2000; **21**:552-560.

Jennison C, Turnbull BW. Group-sequential analysis incorporating covariate information *Journal of the American Statistical Association*, 1997; **92**:1330-1341.

Jennison C, Turnbull BW. *Group Sequential Methods with Applications to Clinical Trials*. Chapman and Hall, New York, 2000.

Julious SA. *Sample Sizes for Clinical Trials*. CRC Press, Florida, 2010.

Jung SH, Chow SC. On sample size calculation for comparing survival curves under general hypothesis testing. *Journal of Biopharmaceutical Statistics* 2012; **22**:485-495.

Jung SH, Kim C, Chow SC. Sample size calculation for the log-rank tests for multi-arm trials with a control. *Journal of the Korean Statistical Society* 2008; **37**:11-22.

Kalbfleisch JD, Prentice RL. *The Statistical Analysis of Failure Time Data.* 2nd Edition. Wiley, New York. 2002.

Kalish LA, Harrington DP. Efficiency of balanced treatment allocation for survival analysis. *Biometrics*, 1988; **44**:815-821.

Kantoff PW, Higano CS, Shore ND, Berger ER, Small EJ, et al. Sipuleucel-T immunotherapy for castration-resistant prostate cancer. *The New England Journal of Medicine*, 2010; 363:411-422.

Kaplan EL, Meier P. Nonparametric estimation from incomplete observations. *Journal of the American Statistical Association* 1958; **53**:457-481.

Kelly WK, Halabi S. *Oncology Clinical Trials* New York: Demos Medical Publishing, LLC. 2010.

Kirkwood JM, Straderman MH, Ernstoff MS, Smith TJ, Borden EC, Blum RH. Interferon alfa-2b adjuvant therapy of high-risk resected cutaneous melanoma: the Eastern Cooperative Oncology Group Trial EST 1684. *Journal of Clinical Oncology*, 1996; **14**:7-17.

Kooperberg C, Stone CJ. Logspline density estimation for censored data. *Journal of Computational and Graphical Statistics* 1992; **1**:301-328.

Korn EL, Freidlin B. Conditional power calculations for clinical trials with historical controls. *Statistics in Medicine* 2006; **25**:2922-2931.

Kosorok M. Two-sample quantile tests under general conditions. *Biometrika* 1999; **86**:909-921.

Krall JM, Uthoff VA, Harley JB. A step-up procedure for selecting variables associated with survival. *Biometrics* 1975; **31**:49-57.

Kuk AYC, Chen CH. A mixture model combining logistic regression with proportional hazards regression. *Biometrika*, 1992; **79**:531-541.

Lachin JM. Introduction to sample size determination and power analysis for clinical trials, *Controlled Clinical Trials*, 1981; **2**:93-114.

Lachin JM, Foulkes MA. Evaluation of sample size and power for analyses of survival with allowance for nonuniform patient entry, losses to follow-up, noncompliance, and stratification. *Biometrics* 1986; **42**:507-519.

Lakatos E. Sample sizes based on the log-rank statistic in complex clinical trials. *Biometrics* 1988; **44**:229-241.

Lakatos E. Designing complex group sequential survival trials. *Statistics in Medicine* 2002; **21**:1969-1989.

Lakatos E, Lan KKG. A comparison of sample size methods for the log-rank statistic. *Statistics in Medicine* 1992; **11**:179-191.

Lan KKG, DeMets DL. Discrete sequential boundaries for clinical trials. *Biometrika* 1983; **70**:659-663.

Lan KKG, Lachin JM. Implementation of group sequential logrank tests in a maximum duration trial. *Biometrics* 1990; **46**:759-770.

Lan KKG, Wittes J. The B-value: a tool for monitoring data. *Biometrics* 1988; **44**:579585.

Lan KKG, Zucker DM. Sequential monitoring of clinical trials: the role of information and Brownian motion. *Statistics in Medicine* 1993; **12**:753-765.

Lee JW, Sather HN. Group sequential methods for comparison of cure rates in clinical trials. *Biometrics* 1995; **51**:756-763.

Lee FT, Wang JW. *Statistical Methods for Survival Data Analysis*. 3rd Edition. Wiley, New York.

Lin DY, Yao Q, Ying Z. A general theory on stochastic curtailment for censored survival data. *Journal of the American Statistics Association* 1999; **94**:510-521.

Loudon I. The use of historical controls and concurrent controls to assess the effects of sulphonamides, 1936-1945. *Journal of the Royal Society of Medicine* 2008; **101**:148-155.

Maki E. Power and sample size considerations in clinical trials with competing risk endpoints. *Pharmaceutical Statistics* 2006; **5**:159-171.

Makuch RW, Simon RM. Sample size considerations for non-randomized comparative studies. *Journal of Clinical Epidemiology* 1980; **33**:175-181.

Mantel N. Evaluation of survival data and two new rank order statistics arising in its consideration. *Cancer Chemotherapy Reports* 1966; **50**:163-170.

O'Brien PC, Fleming TR. A multiple testing procedure for clinical trials. *Biometrics* 1979; **35**:549-556.

O'Quigley J, Pepe M, and Fisher L. Continual reassessment method: a practical design for phase I clinical trials in cancer, *Biometrics* 1990; **46**:33-48.

Peng Y, Dear KBG. A nonparametric mixture model for cure rate estimation. *Biometrics* 2000; **56**:237-243.

Peng Y, Dear KBG, Denham JW. A generalized F mixture model for cure rate estimation. *Statistics in Medicine* 1998; **17**:813-830.

Piantadosi S. *Clinical Trials: A Methodologic Perspective.* Wiley, New York, 1997.

Pintilie M. Dealing with competing risks: testing covariates and calculating sample size. *Statistics in Medicine* 2002; **21**:3317-3324.

Pintilie M. *Competing Risks: A Practical Perspective.* Wiley, New York, 2007.

Pocock SJ. Randomized versus historical controls: a compromise solution. *Proceedings of the 9th International Biometric Conference*, Volume 1, 2nd Edition, 1976. pp.245-260.

Pocock SJ. Group sequential methods in the design and analysis of clinical trials. *Biometrika* 1977; **64**:191-199.

Proschan MA, Lan KKG, Wittes JT. *Statistical Monitoring of Clinical Trials: A Unified Approach.* Springer, New York, 2006.

Rahbar MH, Chen Z, Jeon S, Gardinerd JC, Ning J. A nonparametric test for equality of survival medians. *Statistics in Medicine* 2012; **31**:844-854.

Randales RH, Wolfe DA. *Introduction to the Theory of Nonparametric Statistics.* Wiley, New York, 1979.

Reid N. Estimating the median survival time. *Biometrika* 1981; **68**:601-608.

Rosenbaum PR, Rubin DB. The central role of the propensity score in observational studies for causal effects. *Biometrika* 1983; **70**:41-55.

Rubinstein LV, Gail MH, Santner TJ. Planning the duration of a comparative clinical trial with loss to follow-up and a period of continued observation, *Journal of Chronic Diseases* 1981; **34**:469-479.

Schoenfeld DA. The asymptotic properties of nonparametric tests for comparing survival distributions. *Biometrika* 1981; **68**:316-319.

Schoenfeld DA. Sample-size formula for the proportional-hazards regression model, *Biometrics* 1983; **39**:499-503.

Schoenfeld DA, Ritcher JR. Nomograms for calculating the number of patients needed for a clinical trial with survival as an endpoint. *Biometrics* 1982; **38**:163-170.

Sellke T, Siegmund D. Sequential analysis of the proportional hazards model. *Biometrika* 1983; **79**:315-326.

Skolnik JM, Barrett JS, Jayaraman B, et al. Shortening the timeline of pediatric phase I trials: the rolling six design. *Journal of Clinical Oncology* 2008; **26**:190-195.

Slud EV. Sequential linear rank tests for two-sample censored survival data. *Annals of Statistics* 1984; **12**:551-571.

Sprott DA. Normal likelihoods and relation to a large sample theory of estimation. *Biometrika* 1973; **60**:457-465.

Song JY, Chung BS, Choi KC, Shin BS. A 5-year period clinical observation on herpes zoster and the incidence of postherpetic neuralgia (2002-2006); a comparative analysis with the historical control group of a previous study (1995-1999). *Korean Journal of Dermatology* 2008; **46**:431-436.

Storm C, Steffen I, Schefold JC, Krueger A, Oppert M, Jorres A, Hasper D. Mild therapeutic hypothermia shortens intensive care unit stay of survivors after out-of-hospital cardiac arrest compared to historical controls. *Critical Care* 2008; **12**:R78.

Sy JP, Taylor JMG. Estimation in a Cox proportional hazards cure model. *Biometrics* 2000; **56**:227-236.

Tarone RE, Ware J. On distribution-free tests for equality of survival distributions. *Biometrika*, 1977; **64**:156-160.

Tsiatis AA. Repeated significance testing for a general class of statistics used in censored survival analysis. *Journal of the American Statistical Association* 1982; **77**:855-861.

Tsiatis AA, Rosner GL, Tritchler DL. Group sequential tests with censored survival data adjusting for covariates. *Biometrika* 1985; **72**:365-373.

Van Rooij WJ, de Gast AN, Sluzewski M. Results of 101 aneurysms treated with polyglycolic/polylactic acid microfilament nexus coils compared with historical controls treated with standard coils. *American Journal of Neuroradiology* 2008; **29**:991-996.

Wang S, Zhang J, Lu W. Sample size calculation for the proportional hazards cure model. *Statistics in Medicine* 2012; **31**:3959-3971.

Wang Y. *Sample Size Calculation Based on the Semiparametric Analysis of Short-Term and Long-Term Hazard Ratios*. PhD thesis, Columbia University, New York, 2013.

Whitehead J, Stratton I. Group sequential clinical trial with triangular continuation regions. *Biometrics* 1983; **39**:227-236.

Wu J. Confidence intervals for the difference of median failure times applied to censored tumor growth delay data, *Statistics in Biopharmaceutical Research* 2001; **3**:488-496.

Wu J. Comments on "Sample size calculation for the proportional hazards cure model" by Songfeng Wang, Jianjian Zhang and Wenbin Lu. *Statistics in Medicine* 2015; **34**:2576-2577.

Wu J. Power and sample size for randomized phase III survival trials under the Weibull model, *Journal of Biopharmaceutical Statistics* 2015; **25**:16-28.

Wu J. Sample size calculation for testing differences between cure rates with the optimal log-rank test, *Journal of Biopharmaceutical Statistics* 2017; **27**:124-134.

Wu J, Xiong X. Group sequential trial design against historical controls under the Weibull model, *Journal of Biometrics and Biostatistics* 2014; **5**:209.

Wu J, Xiong X. Group sequential design for randomized phase III trials under the Weibull model, *Journal of Biopharmaceutical Statistics* 2015; **25**:1190-1205.

Wu J, Xiong X. Survival trial design and monitoring using historical controls. *Pharmaceutical Statistics* 2016; **15**:405-411.

Wu J, Xiong X. Group sequential survival trial design and monitoring using the log-rank test, *Statistics in Biopharmaceutical Research* 2017; **9**:35-43.

Wu L, Gilbert PB. Flexible weighted log-rank tests optimal for detecting early and/or late survival differences. *Biometrics* 2002; **58**:997-1004.

Xie J, Liu C. Adjusted Kaplan-Meier estimator and log-rank test with inverse probability of treatment weighting for survival data. *Statistics in Medicine* 2005; **24**:3089-3110.

Xiong X. A class of sequential conditional probability ratio tests. *Journal of the American Statistical Association* 1995; **15**:1463-1473.

Xiong X. SCPRT on information time, 2017. http://www.stjuderesearch.org/depts/biostats/scprt.

Xiong X, Tan M, Boyett J. Sequential conditional probability ratio tests for normalized test statistic on information time. *Biometrics* 2003; **59**:624631.

Xiong X, Tan M, Boyett J. A sequential procedure for monitoring clinical trials against historical controls. *Statistics in Medicine* 2007; **26**:1497-1511.

Xiong X, Tan M, Kunter MH. Computation methods for evaluating sequential tests and post-estimations via sufficiency principle. *Statistica Sinica* 2002; **12**:1027-1041.

Xiong X and Wu J. A novel sample size formula for the weighted log-rank test under the proportional hazards cure model. *Pharmaceutical Statistics* 2017; 16:87-94.

Xu Z, Zhen B, Park Y, Zhu B. Designing therapeutic cancer vaccine trials with delayed treatment effect. *Statistics in Medicine* 2016; **36**:592-605.

Yateman NA, Skene AM. Sample sizes for proportional hazards survival studies with arbitrary patient entry and loss to follow-up distributions. *Statistics in Medicine* 1992; **11**:1103-1113.

Young WR, Chen DG. *Clinical Trial Biostatistics and Biopharmaceutical Applications.* CRC Press, Florida, 2015.

Zhang D, Quan H. Power and sample size calculation for log-rank test with a time lag in treatment effect. *Statistics in Medicine* 2009; **28**:864-879.

Zhang S, Gao J, Ahn C. Calculating sample size in trials using historical controls. *Clinical Trials* 2010; **7**:343-353.

Index